Get Fit with Technology: How to Lose Weight Using Your PC

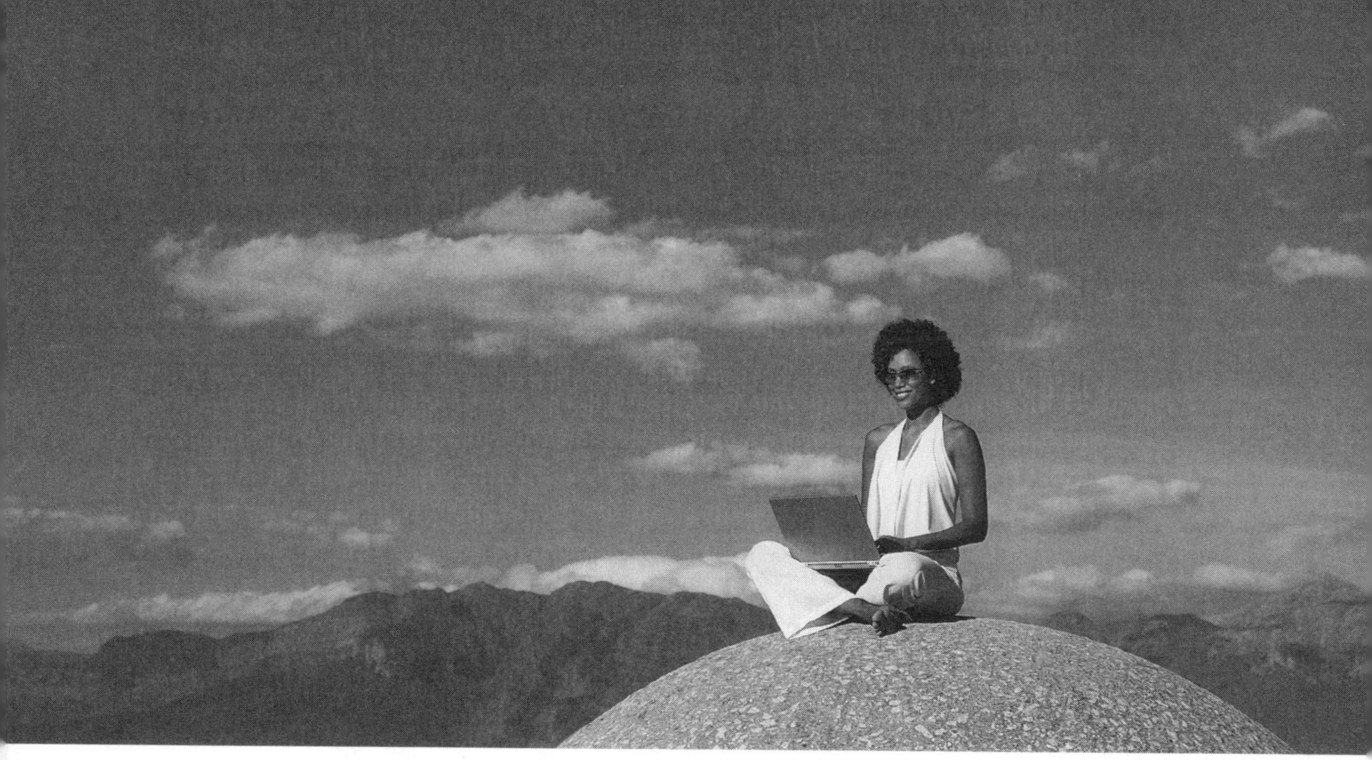

Jordan Gold

THOMSON
COURSE TECHNOLOGY
Professional ■ Trade ■ Reference

ISBN: 1-59200-615-9

Library of Congress Catalog Card Number: 2004114413

Printed in the United States of America

04 05 06 07 08 BH 10 9 8 7 6 5 4 3 2 1

THOMSON
COURSE TECHNOLOGY
Professional ■ Trade ■ Reference

Thomson Course Technology PTR,
a division of Thomson Course Technology
25 Thomson Place
Boston, MA 02210
http://www.courseptr.com

SVP, Thomson Course Technology PTR:
Andy Shafran

Publisher:
Stacy L. Hiquet

Senior Marketing Manager:
Sarah O'Donnell

Marketing Manager:
Heather Hurley

Manager of Editorial Services:
Heather Talbot

Senior Editor and Acquisitions Editor:
Mark Garvey

Associate Marketing Manager:
Kristin Eisenzopf

Marketing Coordinator:
Jordan Casey

Project Editor/Copy Editor:
Cathleen D. Snyder

PTR Editorial Services Coordinator:
Elizabeth Furbish

Interior Layout Tech:
Shawn Morningstar

Cover Designer:
Abby Scholz

Indexer:
Katherine Stimson

Proofreader:
Sandy Doell

Dedication

For Karen and Adam

Acknowledgments

Writing any book takes a lot of effort, and there are always a lot of people to thank for helping to make a book informative and interesting. This one is no exception.

First, thanks to my fiancée, Karen, and my son, Adam, for putting up with my late nights and weekends while writing this book, and for continuing to put up with my calorie counting, label reading, gadget wearing, and workout tracking ways. And for tolerating the fact that I think all of this is great fun!

Second, thanks to the wonderful folks at Thomson and Course Technology, including Andy Shafran, who came up with the idea for this book; Stacy Hiquet, one of my favorite people in publishing, who published it; Mark Garvey, who provided great support and encouragement along the way; Cathleen Snyder, the best copy editor any author could hope to work with; plus Heather Hurley and Sarah O'Donnell in marketing, who make sure that people like you know that this book exists.

Thanks also to the many people at many different companies who provided help, information, and encouragement along the way, including Grace Ann Arnold (Weight Watchers), Eddy Chavey (Mr. Breakfast), John Collins (Fitness Expert), Sara Delekta (Prevention.com), Terry Dunkle (DietPower), Eric Goldman (eDiets), Maclean Guthrie (WebMD), Julie Helmstetter (OMRON), Lisa Hulme (SportBrain), Thom Kirby (bearykirby.com), GinaMarie MangiaRacina (Atkins), Ed Prestwood (NutriBase), Allison Tanner (eDiets), and Mark Wistrow (Pam).

I'd also like to thank the people who were kind enough to share their success stories with me (and you): Kathy Anderson, Michelle B., Paula Johnson, Lynn Key, Sharon Ranch, Pete Riley, and Denise and Matt Tausig.

About the Author

Jordan Gold is the author of nine books and hundreds of magazine and online articles about a wide variety of topics, including computing, health, finance, fitness, sports, and movies. He is also a fitness and gadget freak, and he used many of the products mentioned in this book to help him lose 26 pounds in 2000. He has kept that weight off, thanks to technology.

Contents at a Glance

Contents

Introduction

I've been using PCs since 1981, when I bought one of the first IBM PCs on the market. I've been losing weight since before that, when I gained too much weight in college after falling off the vegetarian diet wagon. This book is the result of my experience when I realized that weight loss and PCs could work well together.

I'm not the only one who has discovered this. Researchers at Brown University found that people using their PCs in conjunction with a weight loss program lost three times more weight on average than people who didn't use their PCs to aid in weight loss. The researchers wrote up their findings in the *Journal of the American Medical Association*, so chances are, your doctor knows this too.

My real weight loss experience began with weight gain. From 1992 to 1998 I lived in Indiana and gained 26 pounds thanks to too many business dinners and not enough exercise (although I thought I was exercising enough).

Determined to fix this and lose that weight when I moved back to California in 1998, I started a weight loss program at Weight Watchers. I used software, WW Points (a product that is no longer available), which worked on my Palm PDA to track what I ate, and I found that tracking my dietary intake on my PDA kept me in line. When I hit my ***POINTS*** limit for the day, I stopped eating. I also kept an exercise diary on my PC using Excel.

The weight came off, albeit fairly slowly—it took me nearly 18 months to lose those 26 pounds. But I did it, and they've stayed off for the last four years thanks to perseverance, hard work, the Internet, and gadgets. I've also found that it's much better to lose weight slowly because you're more likely to keep that weight off if you lose it over a longer period of time.

In February, 2001, I got a SportBrain Web-enabled pedometer as a gift from my fiancée, Karen. I wasn't too excited about it until I started using it. I was amazed at how much fun it was once I realized that I could compete with other SportBrain users, get rewards for my efforts, and join a community of other fitness enthusiasts like myself. We kept each other motivated in much the same way that my friends at Weight Watchers had worked together in person. This helped the weight stay off.

In July, 2001, SportBrain went out of business for a time as part of the dot-com bust. (They came back to life in December, 2002, and are still in business in a much less ambitious form.) In that 16-month period, I bought several pedometers and a heart rate monitor, and I experimented with other devices in an attempt to keep my fitness going. I was successful in doing this, but I was delighted when SportBrain came back in business.

Over the years, I've discovered the usefulness of food diaries as well. Tracking what you eat is very important in a weight loss program because most people don't know how much they eat in a day. Plus, you're less likely to eat that cookie if you know you have to "tell" on yourself when you write it down. Also, a food diary provides you with a better picture of your eating habits because it can tell you exactly how many fats, proteins, carbs, calories, and vitamins you're getting on a daily, weekly, monthly, or even yearly basis. There are many food diaries available, and we cover them in depth in Chapter 2, "Diet and Exercise Diaries."

This book teaches you how to use the Internet and fitness-related gadgets effectively to manage your weight and to become more fit. We cover the best sites for cooking, eating, exercising, and getting health information and support. There's lots of advice, stories of others who've succeeded in losing weight, and tips and tricks from experts for navigating the tricky highway that is weight loss and fitness.

You've made the right decision in picking up this book. I'll help you get the rest of the way by giving you some useful advice.

We have a companion Web site for this book that contains links and other information. The address is http://www.GetFitWithTechnology.com. I invite you to visit often and to provide me with any feedback you have for suggested improvements for later editions. I'll post the best advice and the best recommendations on the Web site. You also can contact me via e-mail at jordango@gmail.com. I welcome your feedback.

The most important advice I can give you about losing weight is to have fun doing it. If you approach it as fun and challenging instead of boring and dreadful, you'll be much more successful. That's why I recommend that you get a gadget or two to make your efforts more fun!

Jordan Gold
Arcadia, California

Chapter 1

Health and Fitness with Help from Your PC

"I've been on a diet for two weeks and all I've lost is two weeks."

—Totie Fields

So, you got on the scale and you weren't happy with the results. You'd like to lose a few pounds, or more than a few. And you want to have fun doing it. You've picked up the right book! This is not a book that will teach you how to lose 20 pounds in a month, only to gain it back. And it's not a book that's going to advise you to eat only blue foods on Mondays, orange foods on Tuesdays, green foods on Wednesdays, and purple foods on Thursdays.No, this book is going to help you lose weight and get in shape and have fun doing it. It will give you the tools you need to harness the power of your PC and make the experience enjoyable, fun, and permanent.

Congratulations on buying this book. According to the *Journal of the American Medical Association*, you've made the right choice. They found that using a personal computer in conjunction with weight loss makes you much more likely to lose weight. In fact, people who used computers to help them lose weight lost three times more than people who didn't use computers to aid in weight loss. A few other facts about weight loss in America (supplied by SparkPeople.com):

- 65% of U.S. adults are overweight or obese. 15% of children under 19 are overweight. (Data supplied by the Centers for Disease Control and Prevention.)
- The rate of obesity in the U.S. has grown nearly 150% since 1960. (Data supplied by the Centers for Disease Control and Prevention.)
- Excess weight can be attributed to approximately 70% of the risk of diabetes in the U.S. (Data supplied by the National Institute of Diabetes and Digestive and Kidney Diseases.)
- If you are even moderately obese, your life expectancy is likely shortened by two to five years. (Data supplied by the *Journal of the American Medical Association.*)
- Obesity costs corporations in the U.S. approximately $12 billion annually in medical costs and claims, lost productivity, and higher insurance premiums. (Data supplied by the National Business Group on Health.)
- Three-hundred thousand deaths per year are related to obesity and inactivity. (Data supplied by the U.S. Surgeon General.)
- Weight loss and exercise reduce your risk of cancer by 30%. (Data supplied by the *Journal of the American Medical Association.*)

Steps to Success

It's not hard to lose weight; it's hard to keep it off. Many of us lose lots of weight and then gain it (and more) back when we change our eating habits back to how they were before we started dieting. Follow the steps in this chapter, and you'll get off the boomerang lose-and-gain cycle once and for all.

Step One: Get a Plan!

There's an old saying: "If you don't know where you're going, who does?" What's your goal? How much do you want to lose, by when, and how are you going to get there? You have to figure this out before you or anyone else can help you get there.

Before you decide how much you want to weigh, you should find out how much you should weigh. A popular measurement for this is the Body Mass Index, or BMI. The BMI, which is good for both men and women, measures your body fat based on your weight. BMI is calculated by measuring your weight in pounds divided by your height in inches squared, and then multiplying the result by 703. In the metric system, BMI is calculated by measuring your weight in kilograms divided by your height in meters squared, or by measuring your weight in kilograms divided by your height in centimeters squared, and multiplying the result by 10,000. In any case, once you determine your BMI, this is what it means:

- 18.5 or less: Underweight
- 18.5 to 24.9: Normal Weight
- 25.0 to 29.9: Overweight
- 30.0 or greater: Obese

There are lots of BMI calculators on the Web. A good one is at the National Institutes of Health at http://nhlbisupport.com/bmi/bmicalc.htm. It's shown in Figure 1.1.

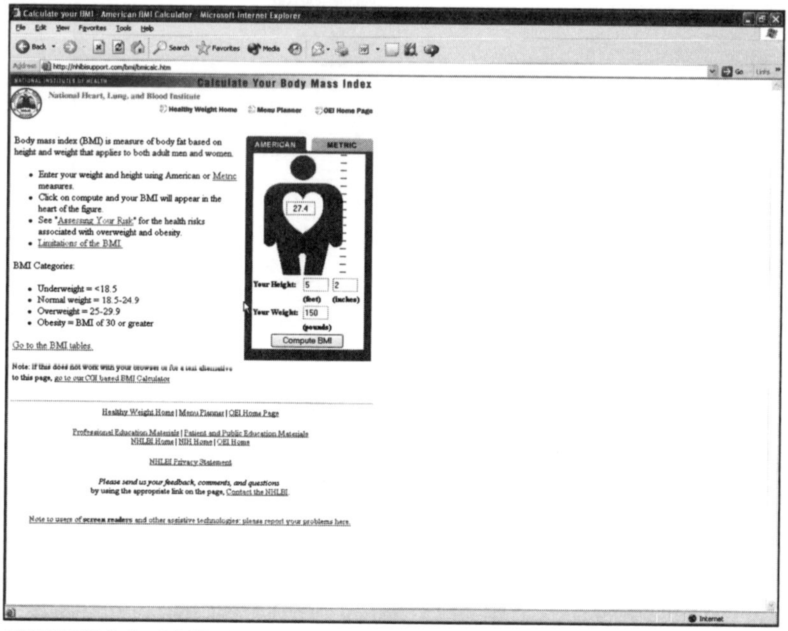

FIGURE 1.1 *BMI calculator at the National Institutes of Health*

For example, suppose you are 5'2" and you weigh 150 pounds. Your BMI is 27.9, which puts you in the overweight category. You'd like to weigh 125 and get your BMI down to 22.9, which puts you in the normal weight category. It's reasonable to make a plan where you'll lose a pound or so per week, so let's say that you decide to give yourself six months to lose 25 pounds.

You know that you can do this by eating right and exercising often. You also need to know a few facts:

- Your activity level: How often do you exercise now?
- The number of calories you eat per day to maintain your current weight.
- Your desired activity level: How often do you want to exercise?
- The number of calories you need to eat each day to reach your goal weight.

You can find out most of this information using a calorie calculator. You can find a nice one on the Web at About.com. (I told you this would be fun!) Specifically, you can find this calculator at http://walking.about.com/cs/calories/l/blcalcalc.htm. It's also shown in Figure 1.2.

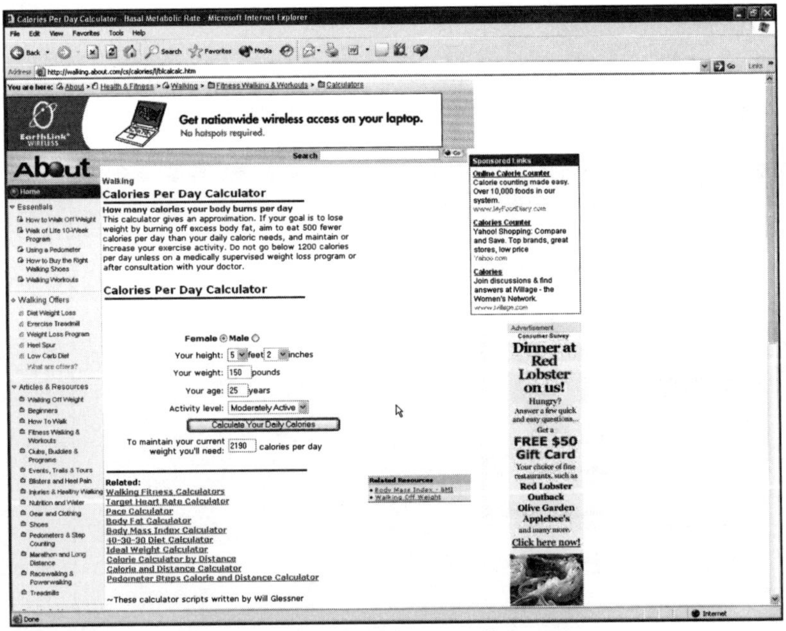

FIGURE 1.2 *Calories Per Day Calculator on About.com*

Suppose you are a moderately active 25-year-old female who is 5'2" and weighs 150 pounds. According to the calculator, you need to eat 2,190 calories per day to maintain your weight. However, note that *moderately active* is the key phrase. Suppose you are sedentary, and you sit at a desk all day and rarely work out. You need only 1,825 calories per day to maintain your weight. However, if you're a workout monster, always working out and extremely physically active, you need 2,920 calories per day to maintain your weight.

Realize also that you might think you are more active than you really are. Walking a mile a day is admirable, but to be really active (and to lose weight), you should be working out at least 45 minutes five times a week, at a much more ambitious pace than walking. Running for a mile per day would burn many more calories than walking.

It's easy to see that you need many more calories per day to maintain your weight if you are physically active. Put another way, if you want to lose weight, you can get more active, eat the same number of calories, and still lose weight. One pound of body weight is equal to roughly 3,500 calories. So, to lose a pound per week, you need to eat 500 less calories per day while keeping the same level of physical activity, or you can get more active, burn more calories, and eat only a few hundred fewer calories per day.

Using the example above, if you become very active, you'd have to eat 2,482 calories per day to maintain your body weight. So, suppose you resolve to get more physically active, working out for a minimum of 45 minutes per day, and you set your calorie intake at 1,982 per day. You're burning 292 more calories per day (2,482 minus 2,190) and you're eating 208 less calories than the 2,190 you were eating before, for a total of 500 calories.

In practice, to lose a pound a week, if you fit into this category, you need to eat *no more* than 1,982 calories per day, and you need to work out *at least* 45 minutes per day.

Write your goal on a piece of paper (or on your PC). For example:

> April 10, 2005
>
> I'm going to lose 25 pounds by October 10th. I'm going to eat no more than 1,982 calories per day, and I'm going to work out for at least 45 minutes per day.

Step Two: Use Your PC and/or PDA

We've been kicking PCs around for decades. They cause physical ailments: People gain weight using them, and they get eyestrain, carpal tunnel syndrome, and many other maladies. You're going to turn that around and use your PC and/or your PDA to help you reach and maintain a healthier lifestyle. Your computer and/or PDA offer you a world of flexibility that you wouldn't have otherwise. You have health and fitness information at your fingertips, and you can track all of your activities, including where you've been, how far you've traveled, how many calories you ate, and so on. And, you get the support of thousands of people who have been through the same challenges and struggles as you. You can analyze what you eat, see how much you've exercised, and travel the globe, all from the comfort of your chair in front of your computer. But you need a little more than a computer to get started. In addition to your PC, you'll need a few more items:

- A food diary
- An exercise log
- A gadget (I use the term "need" lightly.)
- A food scale (There aren't any that are PC-enabled, but I'm sure they're coming.)
- Support, both online and offline

- Determination
- Perseverance
- A sense of humor
- Patience

I will discuss food diaries in much more detail in Chapter 2, "Diet and Exercise Diaries." They are essential to winning the battle of the bulge. There are many food diaries available for your computer or PDA. You can buy software products, such as DietPower, use Weight Watchers' eTools online, or try a variety of other products that I'll talk about in much more detail in Chapter 2.

I've found that exercise logs work hand-in-hand with food diaries. Writing down my activities makes me do more. I use an Excel spreadsheet to log my activities. Figure 1.3 shows a sample spreadsheet.

Exercise Diary

Date	Activity	Minutes	Distance	Calories	Calories per minute
Monday	Treadmill	45	3 miles	475	10.56
Tuesday	Elliptical Trainer	42	4.3 miles	575	13.69
Wednesday	Biking	75	15 miles	450	6.00
Thursday	Walking	90	4 miles	500	5.56
Friday	Swimming	45	20 laps	300	6.67
Saturday	Treadmill	50	3.2 miles	525	10.50
Sunday	Biking	45	10 miles	300	6.67
total for week		392		3125	7.97

FIGURE 1.3 *Sample Excel workout spreadsheet*

Gadgets are the most fun, and I will talk about them in detail in Chapter 6, "Fun Fitness Gadgets." My favorite gadget for weight loss is the SportBrain Web-enabled pedometer. This little device (see Figure 1.4) tracks how many steps you've taken, how fast you've gone, how many calories you've burned, and a number of other measurements, and then logs it all on your own personal SportBrain Web site. You'll find yourself parking a little farther from the office, taking the long way to the store, and walking a lot more if you have a device that motivates you to do more. There are many other devices out there, and I will cover them extensively in Chapter 6.

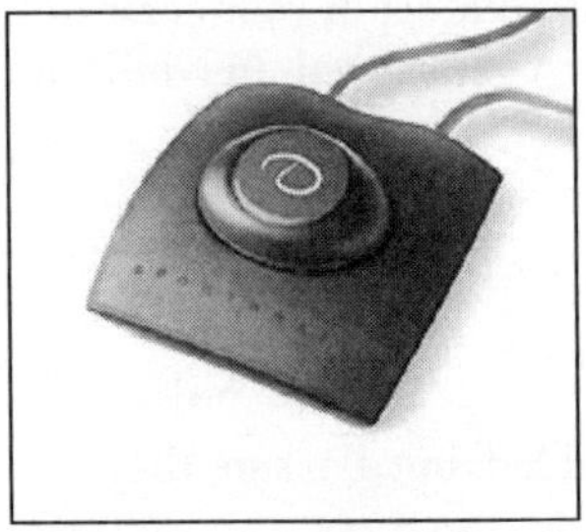

FIGURE 1.4 *SportBrain Web-enabled pedometer*

Step Three: Eat Right

The world is a minefield for dieters. Pick up any women's, fitness, or health magazine, and you'll see a major discord. On the one hand, there are articles about eating right and getting into shape. On the other hand, there are ads for foods that aren't healthy.

To be successful at dieting, you have to be vigilant. You have to work hard to eat the right foods in the right quantities. But you can't totally deprive yourself or you'll set yourself up for failure.

Measure Up!

You can't really tell how much you're eating if you don't measure it. In order to measure it, you need to weigh it in some cases, or just use old-fashioned measuring cups and spoons.

THE IMPORTANCE OF FOOD SCALES AND MEASURING CUPS AND SPOONS

Okay, so there are no PC-enabled food scales (but there are remote-controlled thermometers, a fun invention!), but I wouldn't have lost the weight I lost if I didn't have a food scale. I suggest spending about $30 and getting a very good one, such as the Weight Watchers Digital Food Scale. Figure 1.5 shows a picture of a digital food scale. Use it to weigh everything you eat (at least for a few months), and you'll be shocked at how quickly the pounds come off. Go ahead and have those potato chips; just don't have more than one ounce. When you buy something at the grocery store, get some Ziploc bags and measure out individual servings using your food scale. Then put those plastic bags in a large bag in your house. Food lasts longer and your waistline will stay smaller. And, you won't feel deprived.

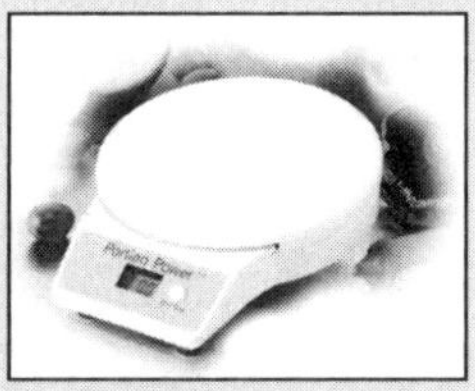

FIGURE 1.5 *Digital food scale*

Also, don't forget about measuring cups and spoons. Weight Watchers and other vendors offer complete sets of measuring devices that let you portion out items from one-quarter teaspoon up to two cups. An entire set should cost less than $10.

Shopping for Groceries

Remember the scene in *Moscow on the Hudson* in which Robin Williams, playing a Russian, walks into an American grocery store for the first time? When he gets to the coffee aisle, he faints straightaway. There are so many choices that he's overwhelmed.

Many of us feel overwhelmed when we shop for groceries (although I haven't seen anyone faint in a grocery store recently). There are too many food choices and too many temptations. It's very hard to eat the right things without a tremendous amount of willpower. Walk into the grocery store, and you'll often see aisles of prepared foods, many of which have no nutritional information on them. End caps, those little displays at the end or front of each aisle, are usually stacked high with tempting, unhealthy food that's on sale. Plus there's the bakery, which has cakes, muffins, cupcakes, donuts, and other terrible foods for you. Most of these items are loaded with trans-fatty acids, which are proven to increase your risk of heart disease.

AVOID TRANS-FATS

In recent years, there have been many studies that point out the dangers of so-called trans-fats, or trans-fatty acids. These artificial fats were created to increase the shelf life of foods. You can tell that a food has trans-fats in it if one or more of the ingredients has something that is partially hydrogenated. Avoid these foods! They are often found in heavily processed foods, including cookies, crackers, baked goods, margarine, and microwave popcorn.

Trans-fats are bad for you because they increase your risk of heart disease. They raise total cholesterol levels, just like saturated fats, while decreasing good cholesterol (HDL).

Look for foods that don't have trans-fats in them. Many manufacturers are making versions of their products that don't include trans-fats. Although these won't last as long on the shelf or in your cupboard, they are better for you, so buy them instead.

I like grocery shopping, but I know that the store is there to make a profit. They often put items that they want me to buy on end caps or on shelves at eye level. And they often offer foods that aren't so healthy at blowout sale prices, while healthier choices are offered at higher prices.

One example is cheese. I love cheese, but I try to eat low-fat cheeses, which don't taste quite as good as high-fat alternatives but are a lot healthier. Often, stores will put the full-fat versions on sale while the low-fat products are at full price. Those of us who buy the alternative are somewhat of a captive audience, so they take advantage of us.

SMART GROCERY SHOPPING

Want to buy healthy foods in the grocery store? Concentrate on the perimeter of the store, where all the fresh foods are, such as fruits, vegetables, meat, and seafood. Enter those inner aisles with caution! And try to ignore those end caps!

Eating in Restaurants

In the 1950s and 1960s, going to restaurants was a treat. A family might eat in a restaurant once a week or even less often. Everyone ate meals at home or brought their lunch to work. And portions were much smaller!

Today, most of us eat in restaurants several times per week. It's no longer a treat; it's more of a necessity because our lives are too busy for us to cook dinner every night. But eating out is a problem because portions are too big. Plus there are no nutritional guidelines provided in a typical restaurant. Restaurant owners know that if you knew the nutritional information for many of your favorite dishes, you wouldn't order them! And soon, you wouldn't eat in their restaurants. The dirty secret of restaurants is the way they get that food to taste so good: They douse it in butter and other fats. Fatty food might not be good for you, but it sure tastes good!

If you are serious about losing weight, you should cut down on your visits to your favorite restaurants. That doesn't mean you should avoid them altogether. Many restaurants have healthy choices on the menu. If you stick to those, you'll be okay. However, I've found that the times I lose the most weight are the times when I go to restaurants the least.

Some notable restaurant stars in the weight loss business are Subway and Applebee's. Subway has devoted much of its advertising budget to promoting healthy eating, and their ads even feature someone who lost hundreds of pounds eating their food. Applebee's has a whole line of foods geared toward healthy eating that even includes Weight Watchers ***POINTS*** values.

SMART EATING AT RESTAURANTS

We have several rules in our family for eating at restaurants. While we don't always make the healthiest choices, we try to limit our portions by splitting meals, drinking lots of water, avoiding the bread basket, and taking some food and putting it into a to-go box even before we start eating.

For the most part, if you insist on eating at restaurants, avoid fast food. You'll be hard-pressed to make a healthy choice. And those french fries are just too tempting! Table 1.1 shows some typical fast food "meals" and the resulting calorie counts. For those chains that offered salads, I chose one as well.

Table 1.1 Fast Food Minefields

Chain	Meal	Nutritional Data
McDonald's	Big Mac, Medium Fries, Diet Soda	950 calories, 50 grams of fat, 1,270 mg of sodium
McDonald's	Grilled Chicken Cobb Salad, Dressing, Diet Soda	390 calories, 20 grams of fat, 1,500 mg of sodium
Burger King	Angus Steak Burger with Bacon and Cheese, Medium Fries, Diet Soda	1,150 calories, 62 grams of fat, 2,530 mg of sodium
Burger King	Fire-Grilled Shrimp Caesar Salad with Creamy Garlic Caesar Dressing, Diet Soda	450 calories, 32 grams of fat, 2,300 mg of sodium
Jack in the Box	Sourdough Grilled Chicken Club, Onion Rings, Diet Soda	1,005 calories, 57 grams of fat, 1,640 mg of sodium
Jack in the Box	Asian Chicken Salad, Low-Fat Balsamic Dressing, Diet Soda	635 calories, 34.5 grams of fat, 1,915 mg of sodium
KFC	Three Crispy Strips, Potato Wedges, Diet Soda	640 calories, 36 grams of fat, 2,080 mg of sodium
Taco Bell	Fresco Style Chicken Gordita Supreme, Rice, Beans, Mild Sauce, Diet Soda	520 calories, 14.5 grams of fat, 1,990 mg of sodium
Carl's Jr.	Six Dollar Burger, CrissCut Fries, Diet Soda	1,363 calories, 86 grams of fat, 2,640 mg of sodium
Carl's Jr.	Buffalo Ranch Chicken Salad, Buffalo Ranch Dressing, Diet Soda	714 calories, 51 grams of fat, 1,902 mg of sodium
Wendy's	Classic Double with Cheese, Biggie Fries, Diet Soda	1,110 calories, 56 grams of fat, 1,900 mg of sodium
Wendy's	Homestyle Chicken Strips Salad, Creamy Ranch Dressing, Diet Soda	670 calories, 45 grams of fat, 1,770 mg of sodium

The recommended daily allowance for sodium is 2,400 mg. One visit to the fast food outlet per day ensures that you'll eat way more sodium than you need, and more than likely you'll eat too many calories as well.

Pyramids to Live By: Check with Your Doctor

Every diet that you go on tells you to ask your doctor before beginning any new plan. While this is largely a disclaimer to avoid getting sued, it's also common sense. Have a checkup and ask your doctor his or her opinion of the best way to lose weight. Although most doctors are not dieticians, they have lots of experience and can give you some good advice. They can also tell you if you're ready to go on a different diet and if the diet you are contemplating is a healthy choice for you.

They might tell you to use the USDA Food Guide Pyramid as a guide for eating right. The Food Guide Pyramid is actually pretty easy to understand: Eat a low-fat diet heavy in grains, fruits, and vegetables and light in meats, cheese, sugar, and fat.

This Pyramid, which is due for an update, is shown in Figure 1.6. It provides strong guidelines for eating right.

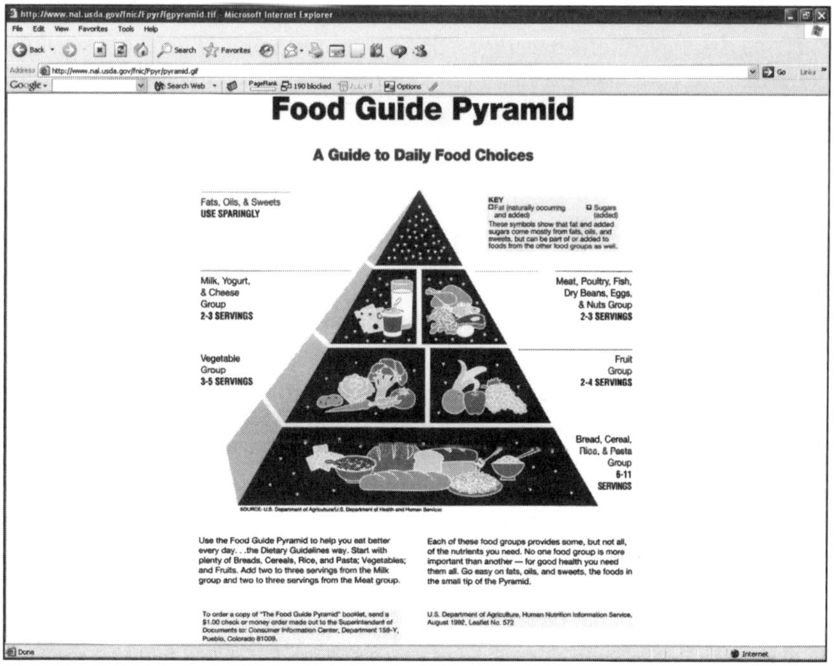

FIGURE 1.6 *USDA Food Guide Pyramid*

- **Eat a variety of foods.** The USDA recommends this so that you get all the vitamins, fiber, energy, and protein that you need. A good way to do this is to make sure that you have a wide variety of colors on your plate. For example, carrots, green beans, corn, a single serving of meat, and whole-wheat bread provides a colorful plate and a healthy and tasty meal.

- **Balance the food you eat with physical activity to maintain or improve your weight.** Basically, you need to exercise.
- **Choose a diet with plenty of grain products, vegetables, and fruits.** This is really the same idea as the first bullet.
- **Choose a diet low in fat, saturated fat, and cholesterol.** Eat a low-fat diet to reduce your risk of heart disease and cancer.
- **Choose a diet moderate in sugars.** Sugar is 14 calories per teaspoon. It's very difficult to lose weight if you eat too much of it. The easiest way to lose weight is to drastically reduce the amount of sugar you eat. It's amazing how many calories are in a donut or a breakfast muffin.
- **Choose a diet moderate in salt and sodium.** This one is very difficult because it requires you to read labels and be vigilant. The recommended daily allowance of sodium is 2,400 milligrams. You can get that much in a single meal at a fast food restaurant.
- **If you drink alcoholic beverages, do so in moderation.** There are many studies that outline the benefits of drinking one or two glasses of wine per day, particularly red wine. However, a glass of wine has approximately 140 calories in it. There are no recommendations that say you should drink wine if you don't already drink it. And, because alcohol is addictive, you need to be careful not to overindulge.

Dietary Changes: As the Pyramid Turns

The Food Guide Pyramid was last updated in 1996. The USDA is updating the Pyramid and might have a new one available by the time you read this. One of the reasons they are changing the Pyramid is because studies have shown that a low-fat diet by itself is not necessarily healthy. You should also avoid trans-fats and cut down on simple carbohydrates found in sugar, potatoes, white flour, and white rice. This emphasis on cutting carbs has been popularized by the wildly successful Atkins and South Beach diets.

Simple versus Complex Carbs

A *simple carbohydrate* is one that goes almost directly into your bloodstream, similar to sugar. Simple carbohydrates are more processed than complex carbohydrates, so your body doesn't have to work as hard to absorb them. This is not good, because although simple carbs make you feel satisfied, once you eat some, your body wants more of them. This becomes a vicious cycle that leaves many people overweight and craving carbs. Because white flour is a simple carbohydrate, you should try to avoid anything with white flour. Other simple carbs are sugar, white rice, and potatoes.

By contrast, *complex carbohydrates* are not processed, and your body must work much harder to absorb them. Complex carbs are higher in dietary fiber and don't cause the cravings that simple carbs do. So, instead of eating white bread, eat a whole-grain bread, such as whole wheat or rye. Instead of eating white rice, eat brown rice. Sweet potatoes are an option for potatoes, and the Potato Board is working on a low-carb potato that might be out by the time you read this.

Simple carbs have a high glycemic index. This means that they turn to sugar very quickly in your bloodstream, they raise your blood sugar abnormally, they make you feel lethargic, and they make you crave more of them.

If you limit your intake of simple carbs, you will lose weight because you will eat fewer calories. A baked potato or white rice isn't bad for you; it's the cravings they cause that are the problem. You'll crave sugar and other simple carbs if you eat potatoes and white rice.

Phase One of the South Beach diet eliminates most carbs completely. This phase lasts two weeks for most people. Author Arthur Agatson claims you'll lose 10 to 14 pounds in that first two weeks. He also claims that you'll lose your cravings for sugar and other simple carbs if you follow his plan. Well, I've tried the South Beach diet on two occasions. On the first occasion, I lost seven pounds in seven days, but I felt terrible. The book says you'll feel bad if you don't eat three meals a day plus frequent snacks. I did that, to no avail. However, my cravings for sugar and other simple carbs disappeared within a day or two. It was amazing! To feel better, I switched to Phase Two and kept the weight off. In Phase Two, you are allowed to eat complex carbohydrates.

Unlike South Beach, Atkins espouses a high-fat, low-carb diet; almost 60% of its calories come from fat. It espouses eating no simple carbs or trans-fats. In all other ways, it turns the USDA Pyramid upside down, as shown in Figure 1.7.

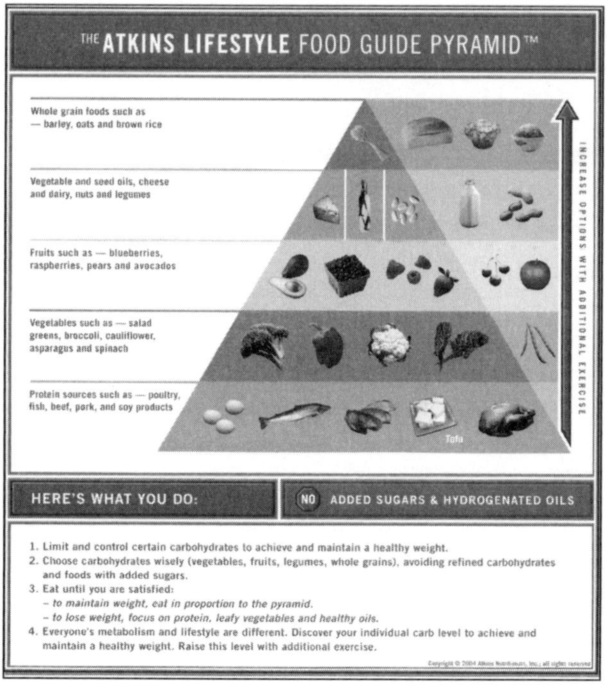

FIGURE 1.7 *The Atkins Lifestyle Food Guide Pyramid*

Atkins breaks the process into four stages: Induction, Ongoing Weight Loss, Pre-Maintenance, and Lifetime Maintenance. Like South Beach, it concentrates on limiting simple carbohydrates. Unlike South Beach, it limits complex carbohydrates significantly as well. In Stage One, which lasts two weeks, you can eat up to 20 grams of net carbs per day (net carbs are total carbs minus fiber), drink eight to 10 glasses of water per day, and eat liberal amounts of fats, oils, and proteins. Stage One allows no starchy vegetables, fruit, legumes, grains, nuts, or seeds.

In Stage Two, you can add up to five grams daily of net carbs per week as your weight loss allows. Then, as you reach Stage Three, you can add another 10 grams daily of net carbs per week. In Stage Four, you can eat whatever your daily net carb threshold is, typically 40 to 100 net carbs per day.

The people that I've known who have tried Atkins have lost lots of weight in a very short period of time. However, they've generally gained it back as soon as they started eating carbs again. But the Atkins folks argue that their diet is healthy and does help people maintain a healthy lifestyle if followed correctly. Perhaps the people I've known didn't follow it correctly. Investigate Atkins if you're interested. If it works for you, great.

Instead of low-carb, it's wiser to adopt a low *simple* carb diet and eat whole grains, fruits, and vegetables. In fact, many diets that claim to be low-carb are actually low *net* carb. You get net carbs by subtracting fiber from total carbs. Whole-grain foods have more dietary fiber in them, so they result in lower net carbs.

To that end, the Harvard School of Public Health has released its own food pyramid, shown in Figure 1.8. This pyramid espouses the diet that the South Beach diet advocates in Phase Two—a high fiber, low-fat diet.

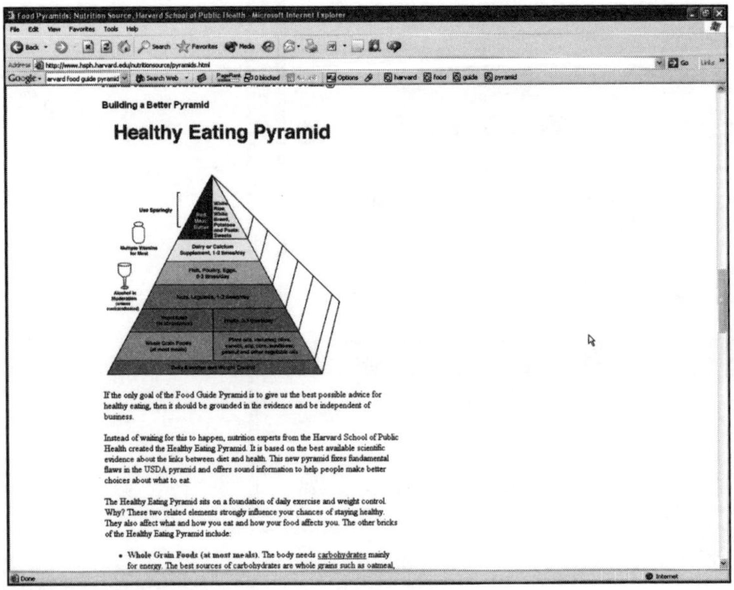

FIGURE 1.8 *Harvard Food Guide Pyramid*

Like South Beach, the Harvard pyramid argues for low consumption of red meat, butter, and simple carbohydrates (white rice, white bread, potatoes, pasta, and sweets), with a diet low in dairy products plus a moderate intake of fish, poultry, eggs, nuts, legumes, vegetables, fruits, whole grains, and plant oils. A healthy diet is then balanced by weight control and daily exercise.

Low-Fat versus Low-Carb

In the early 1990s, low-fat diets were the craze. Everything in the grocery store was light, low-fat, or fat-free. Nabisco couldn't keep up with the demand for SnackWell's. (Ever the company to jump on a trend, Nabisco now offers low-carb SnackWell's, called CarbWell.) The problem with low-fat is that people were concentrating solely on how much fat they had in their diet. If their diet was too low-fat, such as Dr. Dean Ornish's plan for heart patients (which has less than 10% of calories coming from fat), people couldn't stick to it.

In other cases, people would stay on low-fat diets for years and never lose weight. In fact, they gained weight. I was one of those people. On my typical day, I'd have a bagel with low-fat cream cheese for breakfast (or a low-fat blueberry muffin), a sandwich with low-fat potato chips for lunch, low-fat SnackWell's in the afternoon, a baked potato with low-fat margarine, vegetables, and soy sauce for dinner, and then low-fat ice cream for dessert. I didn't lose weight; in fact, I gained weight—about four pounds per year. Why was I gaining weight? Simple—I was eating too many calories! My overindulgence in simple carbohydrates from bread, potatoes, and sugar was resulting in a feeding frenzy because I continued to want those things in my diet. To make matters worse, many of the foods I was eating had trans-fatty acids, which kept my bad cholesterol high and my good cholesterol low. When I stopped eating those foods, I stopped craving them and was able to lose weight. And, my cholesterol went down.

DRINK WATER, AND LOTS OF IT

I know that it's counterintuitive, but it's true. If you want to lose weight faster, drink lots of water—at least eight glasses per day, more if you exercise a lot. This will keep your body hydrated and flush out fat cells. I always keep a water bottle with me and make sure that I get my eight glasses per day. Those 24-ounce bottled-water containers are great. Drink three of those in a day and you've got nine glasses of water. And it's easy to do this. One in the morning, one in the afternoon, and one in the evening.

Common Sense

Perhaps it all just comes down to common sense. Do you really think that you'll lose weight and keep it off and be healthier if you eat a steak with butter and high-fat ice cream for dessert? Or do you think that if you eat a diet rich in vitamins and minerals and exercise sensibly that you'll be better off?

WHAT AMERICANS EAT (OR ATE) ACCORDING TO THE FDA

It takes a while to compile survey data, so the USDA recently released a study that showed what Americans were eating from 1994 to 1996. The study is called "Continuing Survey of Food Intakes by Individuals." I like the popular title much better: "What We Eat in America."

The study showed that Americans were eating less fat, an average of 33% of total calories compared to 40% in the late 1970s. Unfortunately, they weren't eating more fruits and vegetables. In fact, only a little more than one-half of the population ate fruit on any given day.

What were Americans eating more of? Grains, of course. Consumption of grains had increased by 110% since the late 1970s. Consumption of snack foods and ready-to-eat cereals also increased.

Children were drinking less milk, down by 16% from the late 1970s. They had replaced that with carbonated soft drinks, up by 16%, and non-citrus juices, which increased by a whopping 280%. No wonder kids were becoming overweight!

Also up was the percentage of people who ate away from home on any given day. It had increased by one-third, as 57% of Americans ate away from home.

What this showed is that Americans were eating less fat, but not quite getting to the less than 30% recommended by the USDA, and eating more grains and sugars. What the study didn't show is that they were gaining weight. And this weight gain led to Atkins and other low-carb diets in the early part of this century.

I strongly suggest the Harvard food pyramid as a good starting point for determining what to eat. Of course, check with your doctor first before beginning any diet plan. However, whatever you eat, if you reduce your caloric intake, exercise more, and follow the instructions in this book, you'll lose weight. Now, let's talk about exercise.

Get Motivated

Motivation comes from within. If you are not ready to lose weight, you won't. You'll just come up with a lot of excuses for why you're not being successful. If you don't want to get in shape, you won't. You'll come up with lots of reasons not to exercise. Here are some of my favorite excuses, along with my rejoinders:

- **We don't have any healthy food in the house.** Go shopping! And throw out the bad stuff!

- **I don't have any willpower.** Is there an invisible force opening your mouth and forcing the food in? Seriously, make sure that the foods that cause you the most difficulty are not in your house. These are called *trigger foods* because they trigger eating binges in you. Get rid of them!
- **It's too cold outside to exercise (or too hot, or raining, etc.).** Exercise inside, or exercise at a different time of the day.
- **My bicycle is broken.** Walk, run, swim, or do something else. Just get active!
- **I'm bored with using the treadmill.** Join an exercise class and do something different.
- **Nobody wants to exercise with me.** Sometimes you have to do things by yourself.
- **It's okay; it's a special occasion.** This is okay, but only if you don't have a special occasion every day or week. Same thing for making exceptions. Try to limit these to one per month.
- **It's hot outside; I'm going to get some ice cream.** That's okay too, as long as you work those calories into the rest of the day.
- **I can't afford a gym membership.** Go outside, walk in the park, on a walking trail, or in an arboretum or a mall, or run on the track at your local high school.

You have to want to lose weight or it just won't work. If you find yourself making excuses, maybe you just aren't ready. You need something to inspire you. The fact that you've picked up this book is a good sign, but it's not necessarily going to mean that you are ready to go on a life-changing diet program that results in you being more fit than you've ever been before. You need perseverance and determination for this. You also need support. You need someone to tell you that it's okay that you overate yesterday. Everyone falls off the wagon once in a while. You need someone to motivate you because they are losing weight and you're not. You need someone who has done it and can tell you which pitfalls to watch out for. Dieting and losing weight is hard work. You simply cannot do it all alone.

You can get support offline at Weight Watchers meetings or from your friends, family, and coworkers. You can also get support online through a number of sources, including Weight Watchers, SportBrain, SparkPeople, and many other sites. I will cover support sites and the different types of support you can get online in Chapter 3.

To diet with the help of your computer, you can join Weight Watchers online for support and their eTools food diary software, keep a careful diary of what you eat, and work out judiciously, tracking your progress with a SportBrain Web-enabled pedometer. I will discuss food diaries in Chapters 2 and 3.

Exercising Right

You should exercise at least 20 minutes per day. If you're like me, you'll exercise more than that because you'll do something you really like to do and you'll do it well. Or you'll use an "extra-credit gadget" to help you with exercise.

In my case, that's a TiVo digital video recorder in the same room as my elliptical trainer. Let me digress for a second and wax poetic on the joys of TiVo, particularly as a weight-loss tool.

TiVo is an amazing invention. As you probably know, most people who have one absolutely love it. And most people who don't have one can't understand the fuss. That's because its benefits are hard to understand until you have one. It's a big challenge for TiVo. Realize, however, that having a TiVo can help you exercise more. Here are the biggest benefits of TiVo along with reasons why it helps you exercise more.

- **You can watch the beginning of a program while you're recording the end.** TiVo is essentially a computer with a hard disk, so the fact that TiVo is recording a program doesn't mean that you can't watch what it has already recorded. No tape is involved and you don't have to rewind anything, so you can watch what's been recorded while it's recording the same program. If there's a particular program that you want to watch while you are exercising, there's no need to wait for the program to be completely recorded.
- **Wish lists are amazingly powerful.** One time I wanted to watch all the movies that Alfred Hitchcock made, so I set up a wish list that had TiVo automatically record every Alfred Hitchcock movie, no matter what channel it was on or at what time. This gives you a wider variety of programs to choose from when you're starting your exercise.
- **You can watch a program in a fraction of the time it takes to watch it in real time.** I can watch a baseball game in about 40 to 45 minutes instead of three hours. This is a nice benefit for my family and me. They get to spend more time with me, and I get to spend less time in front of the TV while still getting to watch my favorite teams play. (Since I'm from Chicago I'm a glutton for punishment, suffering with the Bears and the Cubs.) I also can plan my workout around watching a game, something I probably wouldn't do if I was watching the game for several hours.

With TiVo in the same room as my elliptical trainer, I can watch a game or something else on TV while I'm working out. It's a great way to make the time pass while burning calories. I notice that if it's a particularly close game (I always make sure I don't know the score in advance), I work out harder. Of course, I'm disappointed if my team loses, but at least I burned some calories in the process.

I keep an exercise diary on my computer so I know when I've worked out, how many miles I've gone, and how many calories I've burned for each workout. I work out at least 20 minutes per day, but more often, I spend 45 to 60 minutes each day working out. I try not to just use the elliptical trainer; instead, I do a variety of exercises, including walking, biking, swimming, and playing tennis.

Remember, the more you exercise, the more calories you'll burn. A pedometer, such as a SportBrain, will calculate how many calories you've burned, but there are also exercise calculators on the Web that will help. One nice one is at http://www.caloriecontrol.org/exercalc.html. It's shown in Figure 1.9.

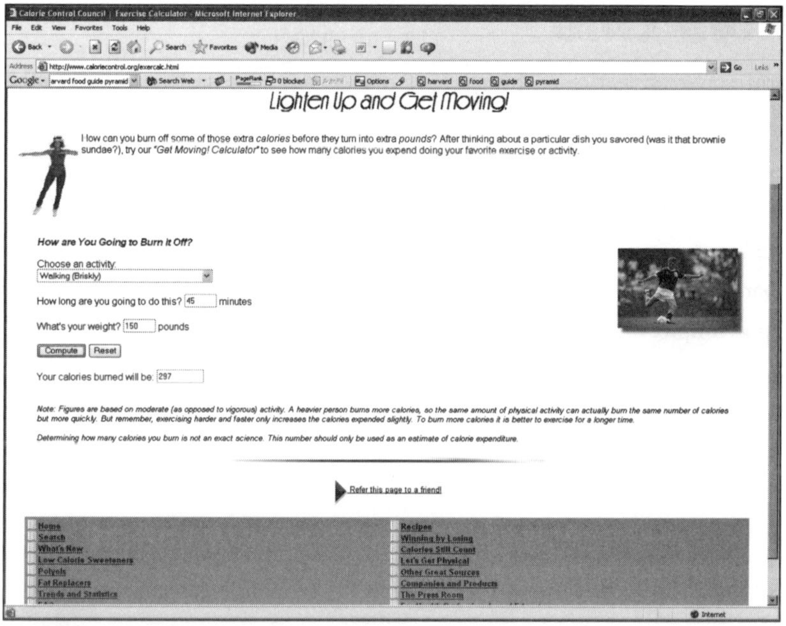

FIGURE 1.9 *Web-based exercise calculator*

Even before you calculate your exercise on the Web, Table 1.2 will give you a good idea of how many calories you'll burn in an hour of doing the following activities. (These values are based on a 150-pound person.)

Table 1.2 Exercise Chart

Activity	Calories Burned
Basketball	450
Biking (12 mph)	410
Golf (Carrying clubs)	324
Jogging (10-minute mile)	654
Racquetball	588
Swimming	500
Tennis (Doubles)	312
Tennis (Singles)	450
Walking (3 mph)	320

Source: About.com

The Bottom Line

To lose weight you need to do six things:

- Eat right.
- Drink lots of water.
- Exercise at least 20 minutes each day.
- Have fun.
- Be patient.
- Keep it simple.

Keep reading. We'll get you there.

Chapter 2

Diet and Exercise Diaries

"You have to stay in shape. My grandmother, she started walking five miles a day when she was 60. She's 97 today and we don't know where the hell she is."

—Ellen DeGeneres

When I was in my most active period of weight loss a few years ago, I would write down whatever food and portion I ate immediately and put it into my Palm. I used a software program called WW Journal (no longer available due to legal issues with Weight Watchers), which allowed me to write down the foods I ate and their portions. Then, using calorie, fat, and other nutritional information, the program helped me calculate the Weight Watchers points. When I got to my allotted points portion for the day, I stopped eating. No exceptions. On the weeks that I diligently kept a food diary in this manner, I lost weight. On the weeks when I didn't do this, either by estimating food portions or by not writing things down when I ate them and then guessing later, I didn't know whether I stayed in my points total, and I was much less successful on those weeks.

Over time, I wanted more power, something that analyzed the foods I ate and told me the number of calories I ingested, the percentage of calories from fat, the vitamin intake, and more. I also wanted something that told me how I was doing over time, not just one day or one week at a time. So I started looking for a better diary that worked with my PC.

Why Keep a Food Diary?

It's been proven in many studies that you eat less when you write down what you eat. A recent study by the USDA Human Nutrition Research Center showed that women on average underreported their calories by 500 per day. Men were better, and heavier people were the worst guessers. For whatever reason, if you write down what you've eaten or what you're about to eat, you'll eat less. Part of the reason for this is because once you see how many calories something contains, you'll automatically eat less. It's also because you don't want to disappoint yourself by eating too much.

Also, you learn by analyzing. A food diary shows you what you eat and when you eat it. That's informative in itself. If you know that you tend to have a mid-afternoon snack each day, perhaps you can change from M&Ms to some peanuts or fruit. If you know that you're eating 3,000 calories per day when you thought you were eating 2,000, you'll make the changes necessary to get those calories down.

However, the difference between a handwritten food diary and an electronic one is like the difference between a paper check register and Quicken. It's one thing to balance your checkbook each month; it's quite another to analyze your spending and get reports that show you where the money went and when. Think of an electronic food diary as a very powerful version of Quicken for your health and fitness.

The most powerful part of an electronic food diary is its nutritional analysis and reporting capabilities. As long as the food that you're eating is in its database, a good food diary program will tell you how many calories you ate, what percentage came from fat, what vitamins you got, and so on. And like Quicken, a good reporting capability will show you, graphically, how you're doing over time.

Also, although we call these products *food diaries*, they also help you track your fitness levels as you enter in the exercise you do each day. Some of the programs give you extra credit for this, allowing you to eat more calories if you exercise more.

FitDay, a software- and Web-based food diary product discussed later in this chapter, offers seven reasons for keeping a food diary:

- You are more likely to lose weight if you keep a food diary.
- If you keep a food diary, you are more likely to make healthy choices and eliminate unhealthy ones.
- You no longer have to guess whether you're on track for the day; you'll know it.
- You'll improve your nutrition because you'll eat healthier foods.
- Keeping a food diary helps you stay motivated. It also keeps you focused.
- By recording what you eat, you eliminate unconscious eating. You'll know what you ate at all times.
- A food diary helps you overcome the barriers to weight loss by identifying the things that are making it more difficult for you to lose weight.

Electronic food diaries come in several forms. You can use a Web site, a software program on your computer, or a program on your PDA. Some programs are a combination of two or all of these options. In addition to FitDay, a number of other very good food diary software products are available. I'll cover many of them in this chapter; Appendix B, "More Food and Exercise Diaries," contains a more extensive product listing.

Choosing the Right Diary for You

A number of factors go into choosing the right food diary. These include price, compatibility with your computer or PDA's operating system, database size, ease of adding foods into the database, reports, and a number of other factors. This chapter includes an overview of some of the most popular food and exercise diaries. Again, Appendix B contains a more complete list of available products.

CHOOSE CAREFULLY

Almost all of the food diaries in this chapter and in Appendix B offer a "try before you buy" option. Take advantage of this. No program is perfect for everyone, and once you start using a food diary, you'll find idiosyncrasies in the program that might bother you. No program is likely going to be perfect for you, but if you look around enough, you'll find the software that suits you best.

The following sections detail some factors that you should consider when choosing the right product for you.

Price and Operating System

You can spend as much as $100 for the diaries mentioned in this chapter. You can also spend as much as $40 per month to use those diaries online. You can get a perfectly good online diary for free using Web-based software such as FitDay. A higher price might indicate more power and flexibility than a lower price. On the other hand, it might not. Do not make your decision based solely on price.

Operating system is a much more important choice. If you are among the more than 90% of the market that uses Windows, you're in luck. All of the software programs discussed in this chapter will work on your computer. Linux and Mac users have fewer options because most vendors do not offer Linux or Mac versions of their software. One exception for Mac users is CalorieKing, which offers a Macintosh version of its software that is designed to work in conjunction with the Web version of the software.

Database Size and Expandability

The bigger the database that comes with your food diary, the less time you'll have to spend entering nutritional data into the computer when you're adding foods into the database. One program, CalorieKing, claims to include more than 30,000 entries. Most of the programs discussed here have around 20,000 foods in their database, but the content of those 20,000 often varies wildly. Perhaps the way that one of your favorite foods is listed in a particular program bothers you—for example, peaches might be shown as 4" round in one program and small, medium, and large in another. Weight Watchers Online offers a great feature that has pictures of various portion sizes to help you estimate how much you ate. And of course, food scales and measuring cups and spoons are very helpful for enabling you to accurately input the amount of calories you've eaten in a day.

To evaluate a program, think about the foods you eat the most, and then search for them in the program's database. The ease of adding foods and entering them in your food log is also critical, because if it's difficult, you won't do it. And, of course, if a program is not easily expandable, don't use it.

To add foods into the database of any food diary, you need Nutrition Facts information, which is on all packages of food sold in grocery stores (per the USDA). Also called the *food label*, Nutrition Facts information has changed over the years, getting progressively more detailed over time. Figure 2.1 shows a sample food label for a macaroni-and-cheese product.

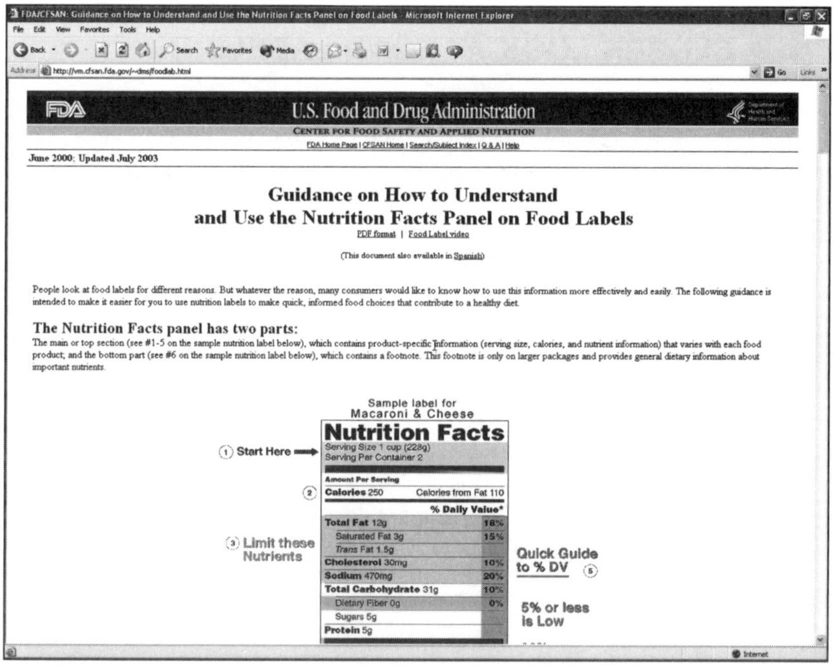

FIGURE 2.1 *Nutrition Facts label*

EASILY ENTERING FOODS INTO A DATABASE

No food diary has all of the foods you want in its database. You'll invariably eat a food that isn't there. Often, it's better to simply add the food anyway because generic versions of the food might not be accurate. For example, DietPower lists one ounce of low-fat cheddar cheese at 49 calories, quite a bit less than the typical low-fat cheddars that I've seen, which have 80 calories per ounce.

To easily enter a food, get the Nutrition Facts label from the package, or if you ate at a restaurant, go to the company's Web site and get the data there.

Sometimes, you'll have a hard time finding the Nutrition Facts information. For example, in many of the food databases I've used, ethnic foods, such as California rolls or pad thai, are very hard to find. When I get into that situation, I break the foods down into ingredients (nori, rice, avocado, and crab, in the case of California rolls) and make a rough estimate. Of course, it's better to know the amount of calories you're eating *before* you do it, so try to input this information in advance.

A CLOSER LOOK AT FOOD LABELS

The Nutrition Facts label (refer to Figure 2.1) provides at-a-glance information about the foods that you might be considering purchasing in the grocery store. The values are based on a 2,000-calorie-per-day diet. Of course, the label isn't worth anything unless you understand what you're reading. Here's a quick look at each individual component:

- **Serving size.** This is the size of what the manufacturer considers a serving. Always view this dubiously and read the label carefully. A can of soda, for example, usually has two servings in it.
- **Servings per container.** This is a key measure. A bag of tortilla chips that you think is single serving can have five or six servings in it. Eating the whole bag can set you back 700 or more calories for the day. Note that the rest of the label is based on one serving. So if you eat two servings, double the data (calories, fat, vitamins, and so on) so you get a clear picture of what you've actually consumed.
- **Calories and calories from fat.** Calories are roughly calculated by multiplying the grams of protein and carbohydrates by four and the grams of fat by nine. That's because there are nine calories per gram of fat, but only four calories per gram of carbohydrate and protein. The USDA recommends that you get only 30% of your calories from fat, so a product like the one shown in Figure 2.1 is not necessarily a good choice because 44% of its calories are from fat. As part of a meal, however, it might be a good choice, if you balance it with lots of vegetables and other low-fat foods.
- **Total fat, saturated fat, and trans-fat.** In this example, total fat is 12 grams, with three of those coming from saturated fat and 1.5 coming from the dreaded trans-fats. Note that the 12 grams of fat is 18% of the total value recommended by the USDA for someone on a 2,000-calorie-per-day diet.
- **Other values.** The label breaks down the amount of cholesterol, sodium, carbohydrate, fiber, sugars, and protein in the food, along with a reading of what percentage each is of the daily value.
- **Vitamins and minerals.** The label shows the percentage of the daily value for four important vitamins and minerals—vitamins A and C, calcium, and iron. Some labels show information for other vitamins and minerals as well.
- **Footnote.** If there is room on the package, the label includes a footnote section that explains that the percentage of daily value is based on a 2,000-calorie-per-day diet. It also includes recommendations for a 2,500-calorie-per-day diet. The USDA says that any percent of daily value less than 5% is low and anything greater than 20% is high. This is why serving size is so important. If you eat three servings of a food that has 400 mg of sodium per serving, the product is not 16.67% of your daily value, as it would be for one serving—it is 50%. Note also that no matter the calories, the recommended intake of cholesterol and sodium remain constant.

Entering Data

Many of the programs discussed in this chapter allow you to use more than one device to enter food information. That's good, because you don't eat all your meals in one place. Being able to use a PDA or the Web to enter data is very important. Many programs also let you enter data on your PC at work, copy the files to a disk, and then copy them on your computer at home, so that you have all food information in one place. NutriBase and Diet & Exercise Assistant let you enter data into your PDA, and then copy that data to your PC. If you have a PDA that is Web-enabled, programs such as eDiets, FitDay, CalorieKing, and others will work for you.

Nutrients and Water

A good food diary should track at least the number of nutrients that are on the Nutrition Facts label. All of the programs mentioned in this chapter do that. However, if you are on a cholesterol-, carbohydrate-, or sodium-reduced diet, make sure the program you're considering allows you to change the thresholds for these items accordingly. Or you might care about a particular mineral, such as zinc. Make sure the program you're considering tracks this for you.

There is also a potential for overkill in this area. Do you really need to know how much you are getting of more than 100 nutrients?

Exercise Database

In losing weight, exercise is just as important as diet. In general, the more you exercise, the easier it is to lose weight. However, if your software program doesn't know running from walking or swimming from sailing, you're not going to know how many calories you've expended. Most food diaries don't do a good job in this category. Because they were designed by dieticians, they concentrate on food, and exercise is almost an afterthought.

Programs are getting better, but they aren't there yet. For example, they might allow you to say that you've walked at a moderate pace for a certain period of time, but they don't let you enter the exact amount of time you exercised and how fast you went. Also, most food diaries don't have a category for use of an elliptical trainer, which is one of the most popular pieces of exercise equipment, but which is relatively new.

Reports and Graphs

Reports and graphs are very important to any diet plan because they provide feedback about how well you're doing in your quest to lose weight. Most programs have a large number of reports, many of which you'll never use. However, there are a few key reports and graphs that you'll want to look at when you're using a food diary.

- **Weight lost over time.** You'll love this one, particularly as you lose weight in the beginning.

- **Percentage of calories from fat, carbs, and protein.** A pie chart does nicely for this, and it's an eye-opening experience when you think that you're eating a low-fat diet and you discover that 45% of your calories come from fat. (Remember, fat is nine calories per gram, while carbs and protein are four.)
- **Calories eaten per day.** This is a nice chart that shows you your calories per day over a set amount of days.
- **Exercise log.** This provides feedback about how much and what kinds of exercises you do.
- **Goals achieved.** Many programs have a goal-setting feature, and then give you reports to show the goals that you have achieved. This is important because reaching goals helps you stay motivated.

Although these reports are the basics, many food diaries provide a wide variety of additional reports that add power and flexibility to your analysis. DietPower lets you graph your intake of any one of 35 nutrients so, for example, you can see how much calcium you ate over the last few weeks. NutriBase lets you analyze your meals or snacks one at a time so you can analyze whether what you've eaten for breakfast over the past month has been healthy, for example.

Number of People per Copy

When you start a diet, you become the Pied Piper of your household. Once you start losing weight, others in the family will follow your motivational lead and will want to lose weight also. Or, you could just make your diet a family affair and get everyone to join in from the start. In any case, make sure the software you buy can accommodate as many people as there are in your family who want to lose weight.

Support

I will cover support in more detail in Chapter 3, "Support Sites," but it's important to know how good the support is for the software you use. Is there a well-traveled online forum for your software? Chat rooms? A resource library? A store? Online experts? Events? Mentors? Many of these programs have all that and more, allowing you to share your experiences and work with others in your weight loss journey. Weight Watchers, of course, has a great community of users; support has been the key ingredient in Weight Watchers for decades, both online and off. eDiets makes support a key part of its process as well. And other programs, such as SparkPeople, offer excellent online support.

Is There a Professional Version Available?

This might be a negative or positive, depending on your viewpoint. However, many of the programs do offer professional versions so that dieticians and other health care professionals can help multiple patients with weight loss issues. Using these programs as an individual gives you more data than you would get with some other programs, but they are often less personal and not as user friendly. This is even the case for the versions of these programs that are designed for end users. For example, the personal version of NutriBase still feels clinical to me, and it includes "patient" data in many places.

A Closer Look at Some Popular Food Diaries

There are a number of excellent food diaries available. They come in several forms—Web-based, software-based, PDA-based, and a combination of these. Using a Web-based food diary is convenient because no matter what computer you use, all you have to do is log in and enter the foods you've eaten. In the end, the type of food diary you choose should be based on what works best for you. There are no real advantages in performance when you are considering a Web- or software-based diary. The following sections give you a look at some of the most popular choices; Appendix B provides a more complete list.

CalorieKing.com

$19.95/year, Web site

Database software and diet diary (PC, Mac, Palm, and Pocket PC), $19.95 each (Mac or PC version is free with annual membership.)

http://www.calorieking.com

Pros: Best food database with most foods, good information site, easy to enter foods into a diary, good reports, low price.

Cons: Not as flexible as some other products, shopping list feature is a little clumsy.

Family Health Network, the owner of CalorieKing.com, has been around for a long time, since long before the Internet. The Web site is built around a 30,000-food database that serves as the basis for the best-selling *The Doctor's Pocket Calorie, Fat & Carbohydrate Counter: Plus 170 Fast-Food Chains & Restaurants* by Dr. Allan Borushek. CalorieKing features a food and exercise diary, an online university with 13-week courses on health-related issues, a community site with bulletin boards and other support, articles about weight loss and motivation, and much more (see Figure 2.2).

After taking your profile information, including your current weight and goal weight, CalorieKing designs meal plans for you to follow. If you opt to go with a meal plan, CalorieKing also develops a shopping list for you. If you decide to make your meal plan convenience-food–oriented, you might have a shopping list that includes a large number of frozen dinners.

The shopping list can be disconcerting, however. My shopping list showed the following for fruit:

- Three small servings of fruit
- Five medium servings of fruit
- One large serving of fruit
- One extra-large serving of fruit

In other words, don't take this shopping list to the grocery store without looking at it first!

Alternatively, you can forego meal plans and simply input the calories you are eating. Figure 2.3 shows the CalorieKing Diet Diary.

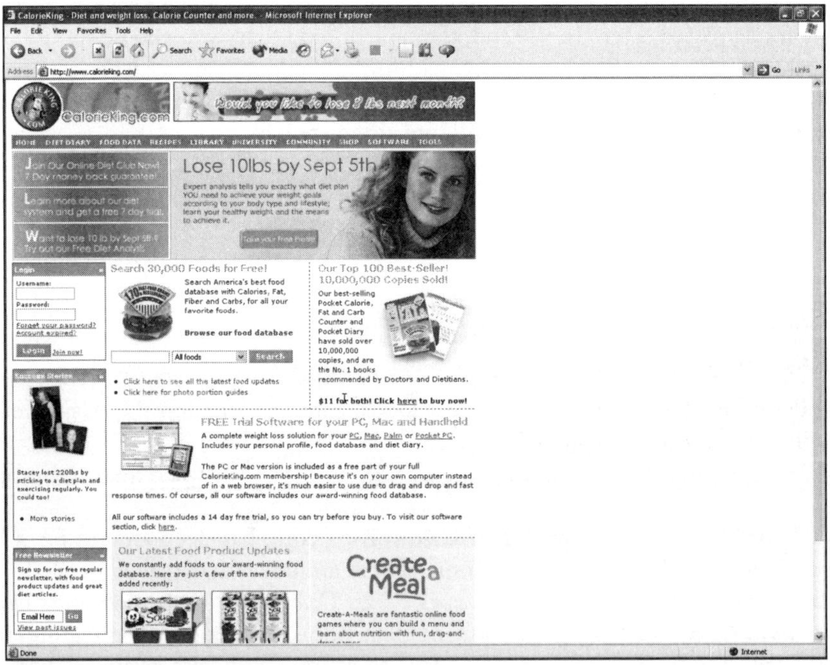

FIGURE 2.2 *CalorieKing home page*

The heart of CalorieKing, and the feature that no other database has, is its extensive food database. At more than 30,000 foods, including information for 230 fast-food chains and restaurants, CalorieKing features the menus of many restaurants, well beyond the normal fast-food fare included in other databases. Foods included in the database are from such national restaurant chains as Applebee's, The Cheesecake Factory, Chevy's, Denny's, The Olive Garden, Papa John's, Pizza Hut, Red Lobster, and others. Plus, the database is updated on a daily basis, so you are always up to date with food and nutritional information. All updates are summarized on a monthly basis on the CalorieKing Web site.

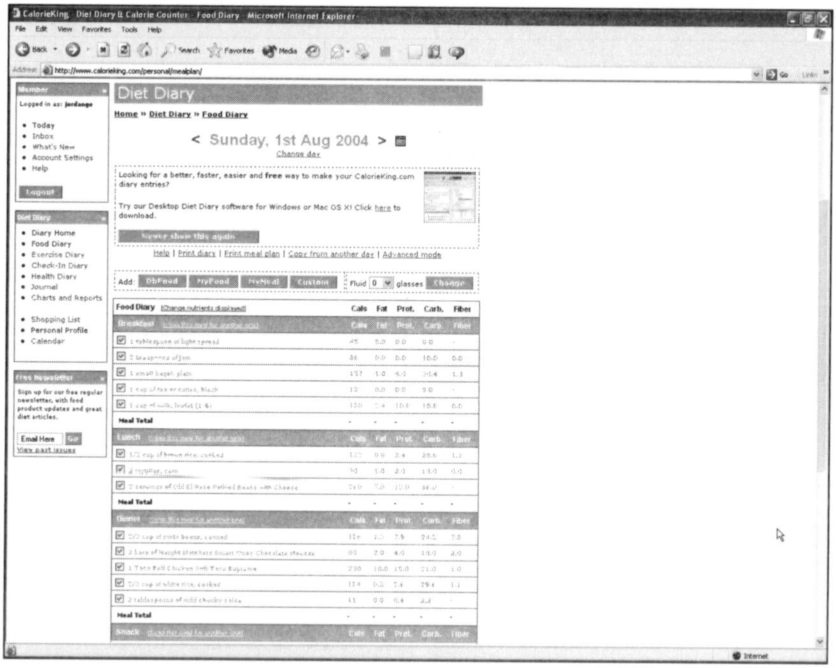

FIGURE 2.3 *CalorieKing Diet Diary*

CalorieKing's Portion Watch feature helps you visually see how big portion sizes really are. Figure 2.4 shows portion sizes for rice and pasta, for example.

CalorieKing also features an exercise diary that lets you choose from a variety of different exercises to plan your weight loss activities for the day.

Diet & Exercise Assistant

$9.95 (Windows)

$19.95 (Pocket PC and Palm OS)

http://www.keyoe.com

Pros: Low price, easy to use, reasonable power, and convenient format on PDA.

Cons: Not as powerful as other programs, smallest food database.

It's very convenient to keep a food diary using a PDA. After all, it's cumbersome to enter foods on your computer while you're eating; it's much easier to use a PDA. Diet & Exercise Assistant lets you do just that. It features most of the bells and whistles of competing products, sans the support group. It features a food diary, an exercise diary, a weight tracker, and the flexibility of adding foods to the database, although you do this on your PC, not your PDA (see Figure 2.5). Diet & Exercise Assistant works on both Pocket PC and Palm devices.

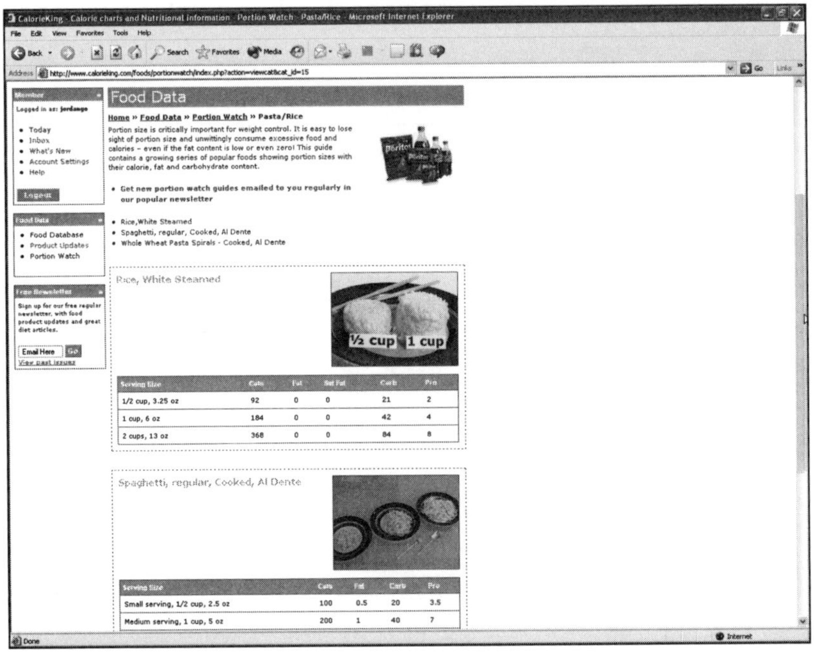

FIGURE 2.4 *CalorieKing Portion Watch*

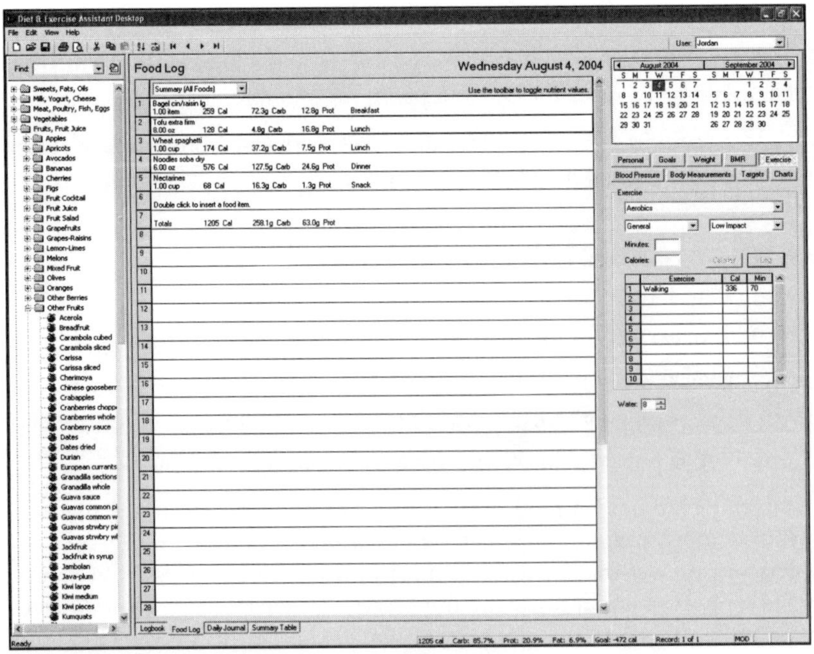

FIGURE 2.5 *Diet & Exercise Assistant Food Log*

The Diet & Exercise Assistant provides you with the ability to calculate the calories you burn from exercise each day by analyzing your personal information (height, weight, age, gender, and activities). After you set a weight loss goal and target date, the calorie calculator will set how many calories you can consume each day to reach your goals. The program monitors your progress with charts and graphs. Diet plans are available to ensure that you are eating the right nutrients each day. You log diet and exercise activities in the Logbook, which summarizes your daily activities and tells you how you are doing (see Figure 2.6).

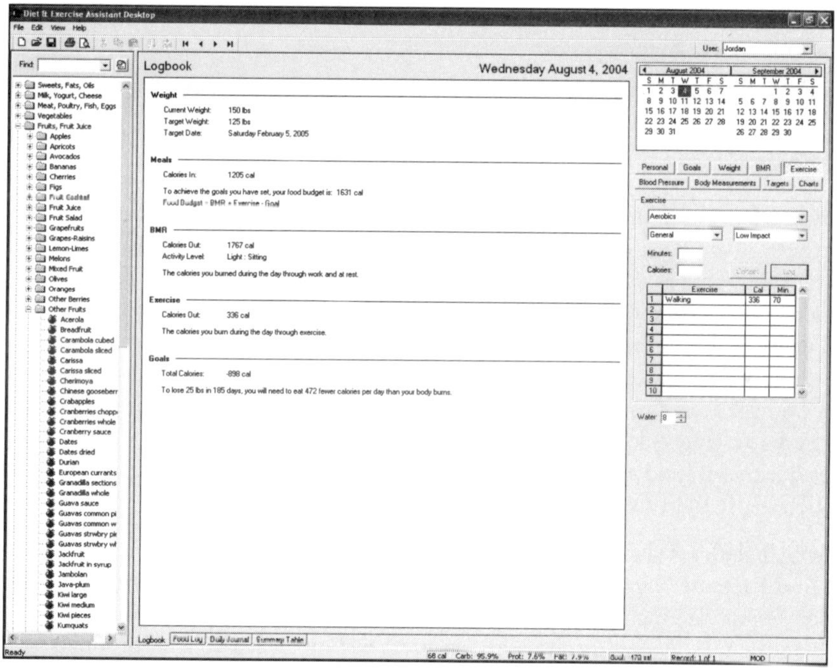

FIGURE 2.6 *Diet & Exercise Assistant Logbook*

The database includes 8,000 foods and tracks calories, carbs, protein, fiber, fat, and saturated fat. Finding foods in the Food Log is not easy. Because everything is categorized according to a group (fats, sweets, and so on), I had a hard time finding foods such as pizza, and there is no search function in the program to help you find them. Plus, for fruits, instead of listing one large, small, or medium-sized piece of fruit (nectarine, for instance), the program only shows cups, ounces, and other measurements that are difficult to gauge when you're eating a piece of fruit.

The exercise database calculates calories burned by taking the amount of time you spent exercising and the type of exercise. Users can log their own exercises as well, and the program also tracks blood pressure. Food items are summarized based on the USDA Food Guide Pyramid.

The Windows product is designed to be used in conjunction with the PDA software. It features HotSync conduits that synchronize your user data and the food database. It supports multiple users as well. The company is continually updating their food database, so users can increase the size of their database by linking to the company's Internet site and downloading database updates.

DietPower

$49.99 download, $54.99 CD-ROM (Windows only)

http://www.dietpower.com

Pros: Excellent interface, great help site, unique metabolism feature, easy to use.

Cons: Much less community support than competing products, some features are not intuitive.

DietPower takes a unique approach to weight loss (see Figure 2.7). Most software packages assume that you are burning calories at an average level—in other words, that your basal metabolic rate is the same as everyone else's. This is most likely not true. Some of us have slower or faster metabolisms than other people. Therefore, while one person can eat 2,000 calories per day and exercise for 30 minutes a day and lose weight, another person at the same weight eating the same foods and exercising at the same rate will not. Assuming you've entered your calories, exercise activities, and weight correctly, DietPower will determine your true metabolic rate and adjusts your calorie needs accordingly. Of course, you need to enter your foods and activities accurately, and the software takes some time (at least a week) to get a feel for your metabolic rate. It then constantly adjusts your caloric need based on your input.

DietPower includes a database of more than 21,000 foods and tracks up to 33 nutrients. Its WaterMinder feature bugs you to drink enough water, and its Exercise Log tracks your exercises. Plus, user forums are included on the DietPower Web site to provide support and encouragement along the way. An online store allows users to buy health-related products at a discount.

DietPower also comes with a great help system (100,000 words) that provides lots of nutrition information and tips to help you lose weight. It includes context-sensitive help and animated tutorials to make learning more fun. It also answers many more questions than a typical software help system, including questions such as:

- If you're a moderate drinker, how many beers can you have each day?
- Which fats protect you against heart disease?
- Why does eating sardines help you adapt to cold weather?
- How does peanut butter fight depression?
- What vitamins do you need if you smoke?

It's easy to find foods in DietPower's database. Type a few letters of the food's name, and the program will go directly to the correct food. Then you can view nutrients in either pie or bar chart form. You can also easily enter foods into the database by entering the nutrition facts from the food's label.

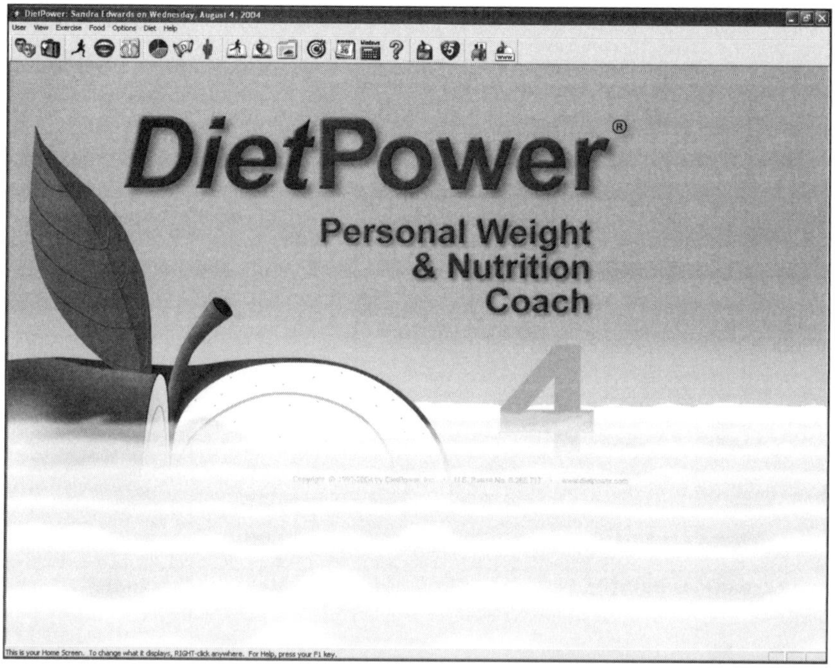

FIGURE 2.7 *DietPower*

Logging foods is very easy. DietPower claims that you can easily enter a meal in less than two minutes. Its database is very accessible and easy to use, and entering foods is a snap. Simply copy the information on the Nutrition Facts label on the box, or go on the restaurant's Web site and get the nutritional information. Figure 2.8 shows a sample DietPower Food Log.

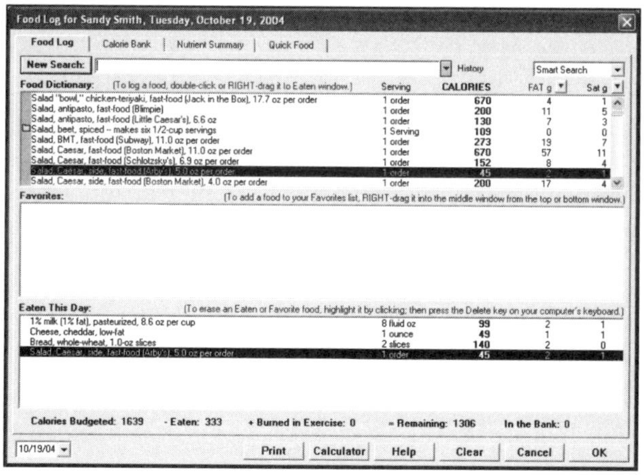

FIGURE 2.8 *DietPower Food Log*

Exercises are logged as well, with more than 1,000 activities in the database. The burn rates for these activities are adjusted based on your current weight. If exercises increase your metabolic rate, DietPower adjusts your calorie budget accordingly.

DietPower also gives you a nutrient summary for the day, which shows at a glance all of the nutrients that you've consumed that day. The program also grades you with a Nutrient Quotient based on your food choices. This is shown in Figure 2.9.

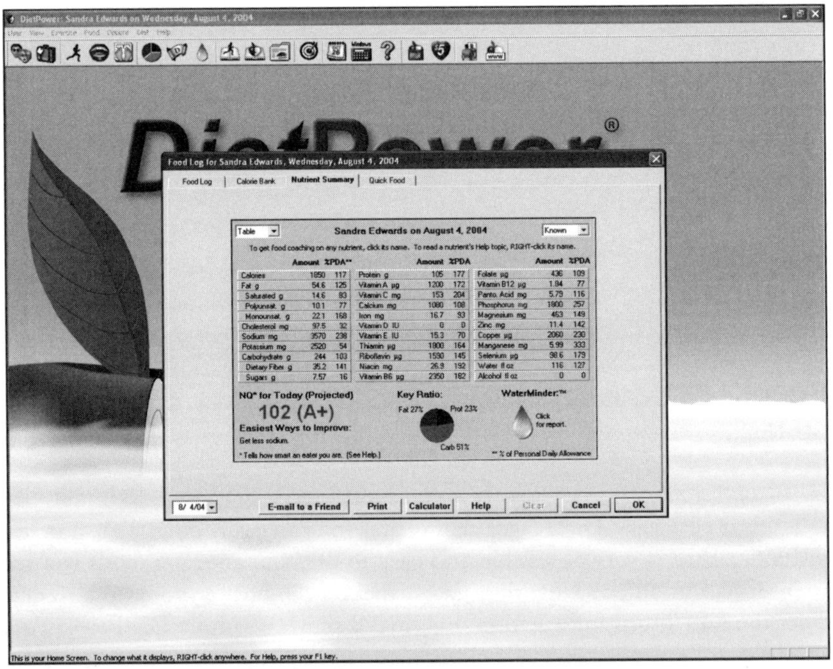

FIGURE 2.9 *DietPower Nutrient Summary*

DietPower includes a number of reports, including your intake of any single nutrient over time, as shown in Figure 2.9, and a daily progress graph, which includes your goal weight, the target date you set for reaching that weight, the weights you've entered, and a date for reaching your goal weight based on your diet and exercise. You can print a diet plan, a nutrient profile, or any other report.

You can also create custom goals, such as not eating more than 1500 mg of sodium per day, or drinking 15 glasses of water per day.

DietPower's Web site includes a store where you can get bargains on health products, lots of information about the software, a newsletter providing tips and health news, and a great feature called Diet Killers, which lists 29 foods that are almost guaranteed to sabotage your diet, along with tips on avoiding those foods. My favorite diet killers and their comments include the following:

- **Alcohol.** Alcohol is a major diet killer. At 199 calories per fluid ounce, it provides ten times as many calories as whole milk and 16 times as many as carbonated soft drinks. DietPower also shows how much weight you'll gain in a week if you drink one of these per day. A 4-ounce martini each day will make you gain a half pound per week. DietPower recommends that if you must drink, drink light beer. It has lots of water in it and it fills you up so you don't overeat.
- **Bologna.** Bologna is one of DietPower's ten worst foods. Eighty percent of its calories come from fat, it's loaded with sodium, and it includes nitrites, which possibly cause cancer. DietPower recommends avoiding bologna entirely.
- **Brownies.** Brownies are 132 calories per ounce. This is thirty percent more than chocolate cake! They call brownies a great food if you're trying to gain weight.
- **Cookies.** DietPower says "cookies are to dieting as land mines are to a picnic." Funny but true. At more than 100 calories per ounce, you'll find yourself eating 300 or more calories at a sitting. Avoid them. DietPower recommends low-fat oatmeal cookies if you must eat them.
- **Cream.** If you drink two cups of coffee per day and use one tablespoon of cream per cup, you can lose seven pounds in a year by switching to half-and-half. You can lose another three pounds by switching to skim milk.
- **Donuts.** DietPower reminds you that donuts are just lumps of dough boiled in oil. (Sounds great, huh?)
- **French fries.** Big fat fries usually have fewer calories and sodium than thin fries. (Oh, that's why they don't taste as good!) Of course, most dieters today are on low-carb diets, so french fries are pretty unpopular these days.
- **Potato chips.** High in sodium, fat, and calories, potato chips are a horrible food. Switching to pretzels is a good idea.
- **Slim Jim.** Slim Jim is DietPower's candidate for the world's worst food, at 50 percent fat and 500 milligrams of sodium per ounce. Also, it's a mystery as far as what part of the cow it comes from.

You can try a fully functional version of DietPower on your PC for free for 15 days. You can get a copy at http://www.dietpower.com.

LOSING WEIGHT THROUGH SCIENCE

Pete Riley had always been overweight. By the time he was 27, the 6'1" Riley had reached 250 pounds. However, once his weight gain got out of control, he decided to change his ways. He quit smoking, started running and cycling, and tried to stay away from buffets. That led him to lose 40 pounds over the first three years of his quest and get his weight down to 210 pounds. But he couldn't get any lower than that. With a goal of 190, he looked for help.

Riley, a space physicist, had been thinking about how energy conservation works in weight loss. He decided that losing weight was as simple as tracking your energy minus how much energy you burned. He wrote some computer programs to help him do this, but couldn't create what he wanted.

Then he found DietPower. "It's a scientist's dream program," Riley says. "It doesn't matter what type of foods you eat, just the calories." Riley's favorite feature of the program is the bank account, which tracks your calories in and out and adjusts your basal metabolic rate accordingly. "This works really well because if I eat something every day that I think is 200 calories, but it's really 500, then this mistake is accounted for by a change in the allowed calories."

He also found that his weight loss goal was too modest. Riley had become a competitive cyclist during his weight loss quest and he decided that to become successful at it, he had to get his weight down to 170. DietPower helped him do this; he lost 30 pounds using the software over a 15-month period. Riley now races in a bicycle league in Southern California with a team called Viejas.

Riley, an avid Macintosh user, wishes that DietPower would release a Mac version. He's tried Macintosh versions of food diaries and has found them lacking.

He uses the Garmin Forerunner 201 GPS for fun while he's training, and he also uses the S-Polar 720i heart rate monitor. Those products help him monitor his workouts. (Both products are discussed in detail in Chapter 6, "Fun Fitness Gadgets.") He considers exercise to be the essential ingredient in any weight loss plan because if you exercise long enough, you can eat whatever you want and still lose weight.

Riley, now 37, has reached a healthy point in his weight loss. His before-and-after pictures are shown in Figures 2.10 and 2.11. After years of being overweight, Riley is now underweight. His doctor has even told him not to lose any more weight. "I've got a handle on my calories now. I can keep my weight where it is." When he needs to, Riley uses DietPower to keep his weight stable; he's been able to do so for several years.

Riley realizes that his gadgets and software aren't the real key to his losing weight—he is. "For any program to work, you have to want to make the change," he says. "DietPower provided a framework for me to be disciplined. I had to do the rest."

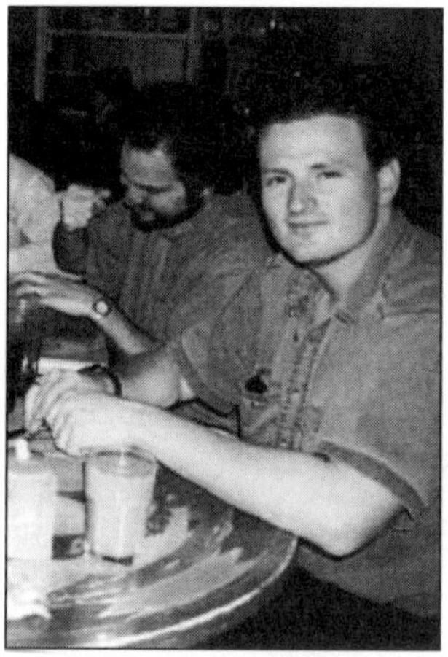

FIGURE 2.10 *Pete Riley before weight loss*

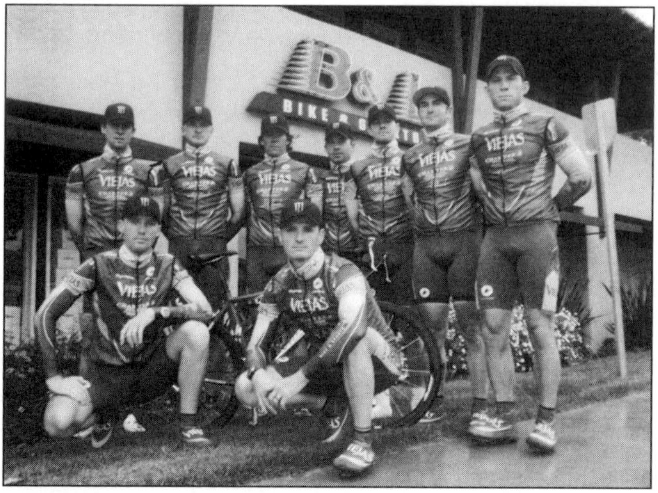

FIGURE 2.11 *Pete Riley and his bicycle team. Riley is crouching in the center.*

LOSING WEIGHT AND GETTING TALLER!

When Kathy Anderson moved from Washington state to Massachusetts in early 2001, she made an appointment to see the doctor to discuss some medications she was taking. Her new doctor treated her badly. "He treated me like I was subhuman because of my weight," she says. Now 35, Anderson, who is 5'4", reached 236 pounds in 2001. She decided to lose weight. "I decided that if I wasn't treating myself with respect by being overweight, I couldn't expect anyone else to, either."

LOSING WEIGHT AND GETTING TALLER! *(CONTINUED)*

Anderson had been overweight since she was a child. Due to problems at home, Anderson had turned to food for comfort and weighed 207 pounds by her senior year in high school.

In June, 2001, Anderson decided to change all that. She started with a few rules—she ate only when she was truly hungry, she didn't need to clean her plate, and she cut down dramatically the number of meals she ate in restaurants. She also started a walking program with her husband, reaching an average of 3.5 miles per day.

These efforts got her weight down to 190 within nine months, where she plateaued. She then found out about DietPower from an online support group for the show Cooking Thin, broadcast on the Food TV network. Host Kathleen Daelemans, who was a spa chef at a resort in Hawaii, lost a great deal of weight herself, started a show, and wrote a cookbook to help others lose weight.

Anderson loves online groups for support. She belonged to others on Yahoo! Groups and MSN. "When I was having bad days, I could post and get support, and when I was having good days, I could support other people," she says.

Anderson wanted to get to 145 pounds, and she used DietPower to help her get there. "DietPower helped me track my calories and get control over binge eating," Anderson says. "It was like balancing the checkbook. I could see exactly what I had left to spend, and could store calories ahead for a rainy day."

Using DietPower plus eating at home and exercising, Anderson got her weight down to 145 by October, 2002. While she has backslid a bit, she is now starting to use DietPower again to get her weight down to 135.

Anderson's favorite DietPower feature is the ability to enter recipes into the database. Her favorites are BBQ and turkey burgers. She also likes that she can log a whole day in just a few minutes.

As a learning experience, Anderson also logs recipes that she used to prepare into the database to see how bad they were. "It's a very dangerous experience," she laughs.

Although Anderson likes DietPower, she warns that it isn't a magic bullet. "It's only as useful as the person using it," she says. "Someone who is looking for an easy solution is going to be sadly disappointed. The only way to lose weight is to grit your teeth and get prepared to do some tough work, both mentally and physically."

Anderson says that deciding to lose weight is the best gift that she could have given herself. She's happier and more self-confident than she has ever been. She has gone back to school to get a medical degree, and she hopes to pursue a career in Bariatrics, which is a medical field that helps people reduce their weight. "I won't practice weight loss surgery, though," she says. "Surgeries don't address the root causes of obesity—just the symptoms."

LOSING WEIGHT AND GETTING TALLER! *(CONTINUED)*

She also has enjoyed a remarkable side effect—she has grown by one and a half inches due to her weight loss. Anderson's doctor says that occasionally people who lose large amounts of weight grow in height. Their spine uncompresses due to the weight loss. Figures 2.12 and 2.13 show Anderson before and after her weight loss.

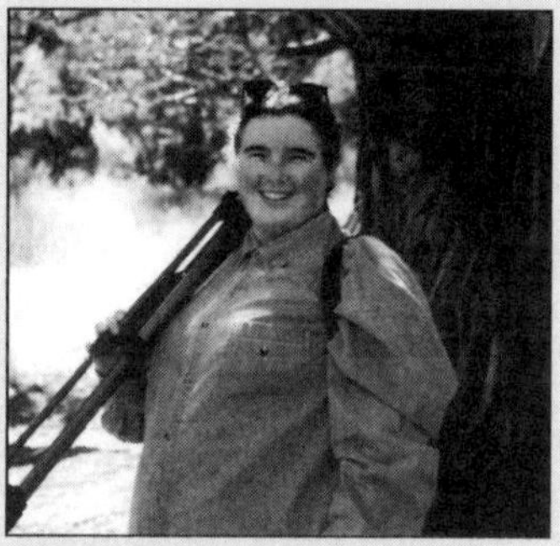

FIGURE 2.12 *Kathy Anderson at her highest weight*

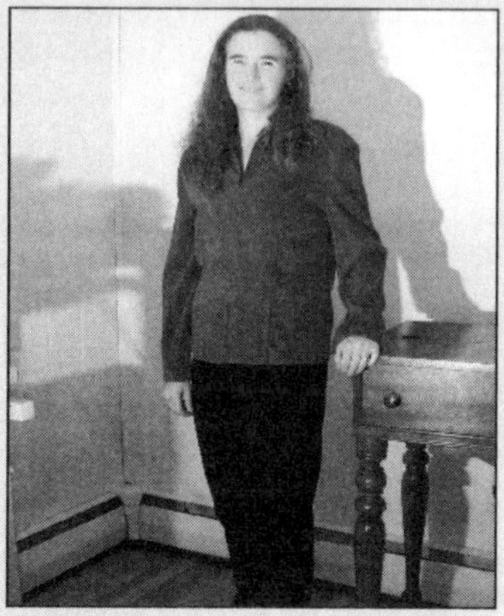

FIGURE 2.13 *Kathy Anderson at 160 pounds*

eDiets

$1.99 per week to $6.99 per week, depending on how many options you choose

http://www.eDiets.com

Pros: Most comprehensive site available, with classes, information, many different meal plans, and professional support on a 24/7 basis.

Cons: Expensive, food diary is not as flexible as other products.

Like Weight Watchers, eDiets is a complete weight loss program, more than a food and exercise diary (see Figure 2.14). In fact, it really doesn't allow much in the way of entering your own foods into a database. Instead, it features a wide variety of meal plans based on 19 different diet choices, as well as fitness programs based on two different fitness solutions.

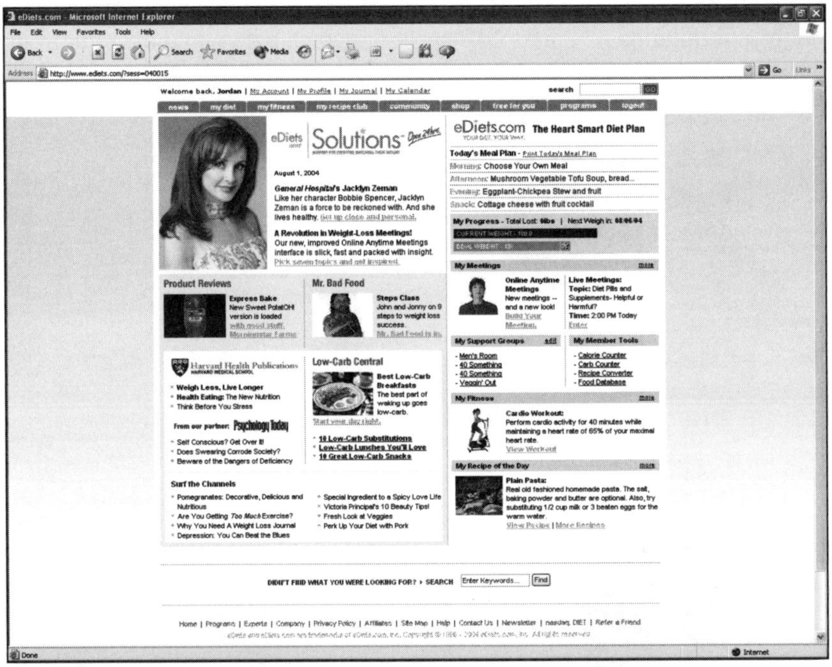

FIGURE 2.14 *eDiets.com*

eDiets also includes message boards, an online e-zine with the latest health and fitness news, and a wide variety of other health-related information.

Because everyone is different, eDiets offers more than 20 different diet options, including:

- Atkins
- The Zone
- Slim-Fast
- Shape Up! (With Dr. Phil McGraw)
- The Perricone Nutritional Face-Lift
- Bob Greene's Get with the Program!
- Bill Phillips' Eating for Life
- Special needs healthy living diets
- An eDiets.com alternative to Jenny Craig
- Trim Kids diet for children

Because 20 different options might be intimidating to some of us, eDiets recommends a program for you based on the results of their Diet Needs Analysis questionnaire. Once you select a diet, eDiets creates a meal plan for you based on your food preferences and needs. The meal plans come complete with recipes and shopping lists so you can take your shopping list to the grocery store and get all the foods you need for a week. Figure 2.15 shows a sample meal plan.

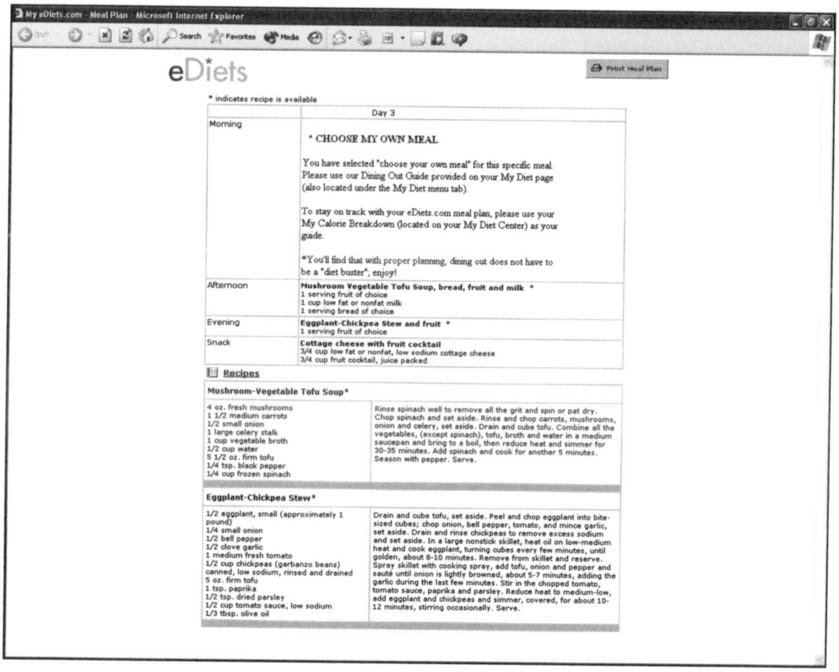

FIGURE 2.15 *eDiets.com sample meal plan*

The rest of the eDiets home page shows all of the features of eDiets.com, which include reviews of health-related products, articles from a variety of publications, including Harvard Medical School's *Harvard Health* publications and *Psychology Today* magazine, columns from a variety of experts, recipes, meetings, support groups, a fitness log, and member tools for counting calories and carbs. There's also an always-available live online help desk and a mentor program to help people lose weight. It's like an online health and fitness club. I'll focus on the support aspects of eDiets.com in Chapter 3.

eDiets has been recognized by a variety of publications as one of the best sites on the Web. More than 225,000 people are members of eDiets, which costs between $1.99 and $6.99 per week to belong. Another 13 million people regularly receive one of eDiet's electronic newsletters, which offer a variety of health-related information to end users for free. Table 2.1 shows eDiets' pricing.

Table 2.1 eDiets.com Pricing

Item	Cost per Week
Newsletters	Free
eDiets Solutions	$1.99
Meals and Support (includes Solutions)	$2.99
eDiets Fitness	$2.00
Recipe Club	$2.00

For those who only want support and who want to do their meal planning elsewhere, eDiets offers eDiets Solutions, which provides all of eDiets' support services for $1.99 per week. Also, a sister site of eDiets.com is eFitness.com, which is geared more toward men.

A new feature of the site tackles the problem of childhood obesity. eDiets worked with Melinda Southern, an expert on childhood obesity who developed the Trim Kids program. Although the program is for parents, it can help children develop healthier eating and exercise habits, which is very important in this day of PlayStations, fast food, and scheduled play dates instead of going outside and playing every day.

FitDay

Web version: Free

PC version: $19.95 download, $24.95 CD-ROM (Windows only)

http://www.FitDay.com

Pros: Nice product, low price, has everything that most people need in a nutrition software product.

Cons: Has no standout feature.

Although NutriBase boasts a plethora of features and DietPower offers basal metabolic tracking, FitDay is more plain vanilla. It does what you need, but it doesn't offer nearly the power of NutriBase or DietPower. However, it represents an excellent value as a diet diary. For one thing, the online version is free! It's very easy to use, it provides enough reports for most people, and it has a nice-sized database that is easy to add to. FitDay is a nice, easy-to-use software product that makes it easy to keep a food diary and that tracks all of the important activities and intakes. A free version of the software is available on the Web (see Figure 2.16), but you can purchase a more powerful version from the company (see Figure 2.17).

Like other software products, FitDay provides a diet and exercise diary. It also helps you get on the right track by starting you off with your own goals (see Figure 2.18). What's your BMI? How much weight do you want to lose and by when? Using that information, FitDay helps you design a meal plan that will get you to your goals.

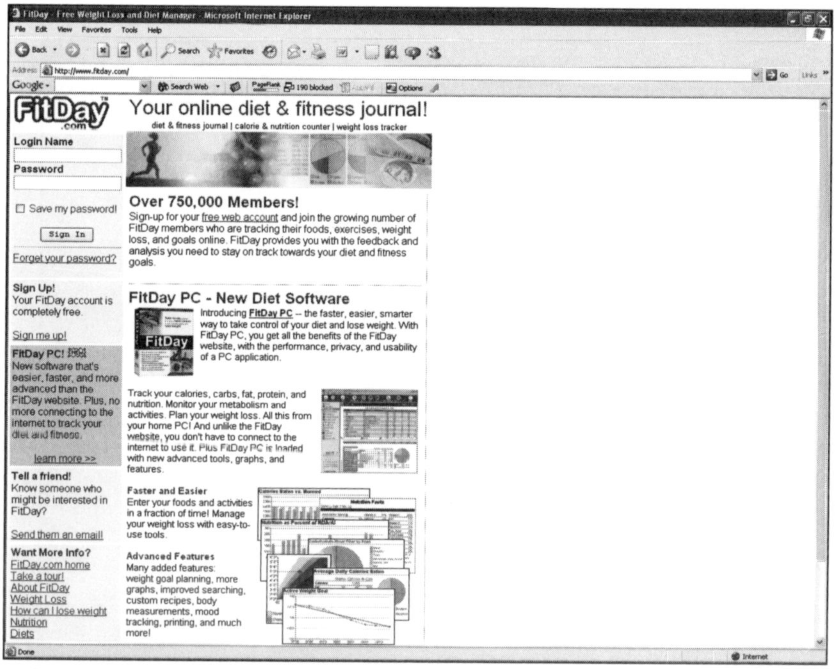

FIGURE 2.16 *FitDay Web home page*

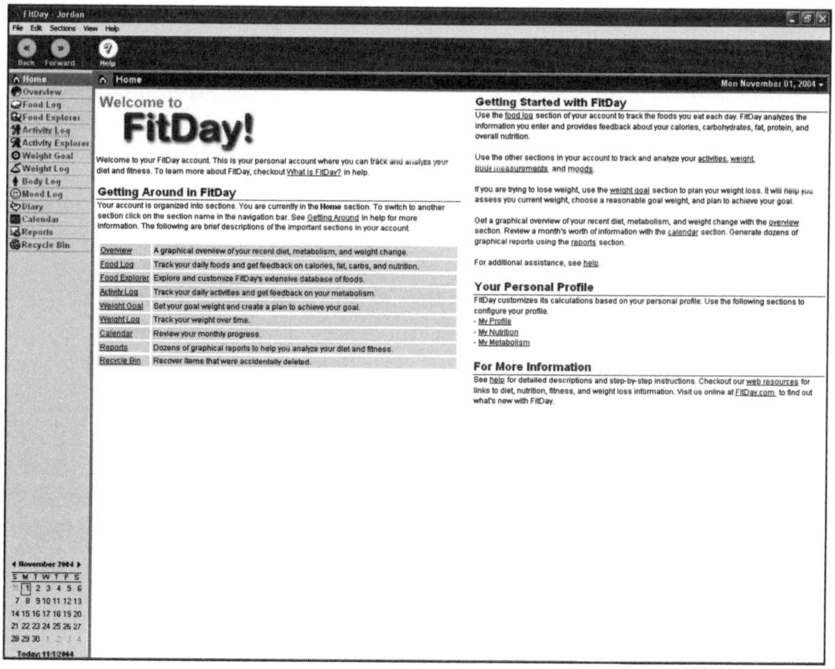

FIGURE 2.17 *FitDay PC home page*

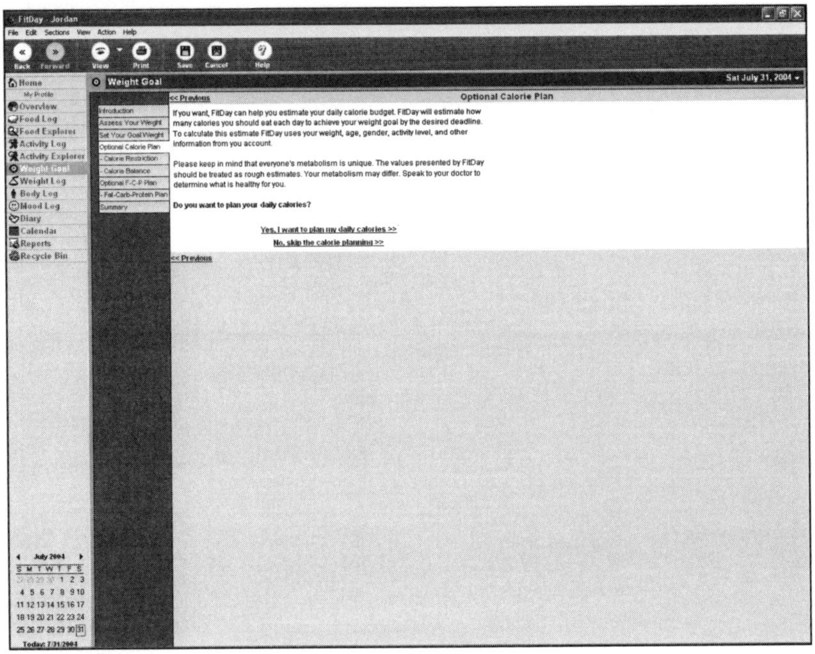

FIGURE 2.18 *Goal planning with FitDay*

FitDay also includes a number of reporting capabilities that let you analyze how well you're doing. Are you exercising enough? Eating properly? Getting the right vitamins and minerals? The reports monitor and track your weight over time. You can also monitor various body measurements, such as neck, bicep, forearm, chest, waist, hip, thigh, and calf size. You can then track and graph these measurements over time.

For many overweight people, there is a definite relationship between eating and emotions. FitDay's diary feature lets you write about your moods, including happiness, stress, anger, hunger, health, and mental clarity. You can then analyze the relationships between your mood and your diet. FitDay's PC software adds more power and functionality than the Web version of the software. It includes a number of additional niceties, including at-a-glance real-time reporting on your foods for a day. So, at breakfast, you can tell whether you're eating too much carbs, fat, or calories, with a pie chart added for good measure.

NutriBase

$29.95 to $69.95 to download

$39.95 to $89.95 on CD

Windows and Palm OS

http://www.dietsoftware.com

Pros: Many features, tons of flexibility and power.

Cons: Somewhat expensive; some versions are not as user friendly as competing products; originally designed for professionals, which leads to some confusion on the part of end users.

NutriBase is nutrition software on steroids. The personal version, which comes in four flavors, is downsized from the much more extensive professional versions intended for dieticians and other health professionals (see Figure 2.19). In fact, if you go to http://www.nutribase.com, you'll get the information about the professional version of the software. The personal editions are featured at http://www.dietsoftware.com.

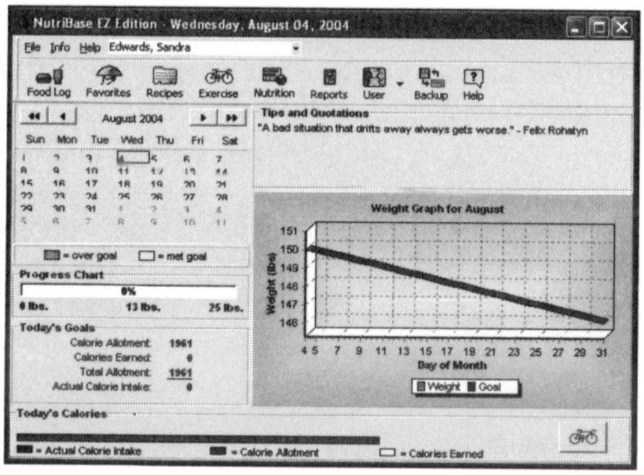

FIGURE 2.19 *NutriBase EZ*

As a result, NutriBase is much more powerful than competing programs, with more reports, options, and bells and whistles than the competition. However, because it is based on professional software, it sometimes seems too clinical for the consumer market. In fact, much of the online marketing material about NutriBase refers to clients, suggesting that the software's bias toward health professionals might make it inappropriate for end users. It isn't, but it does take some getting used to.

NutriBase works on both the Palm and Windows operating systems. The Palm version enables you to enter foods that you've eaten throughout the day on your PDA and then sync with your PC in the evening. Its database, which is based on the USDA's extensive nutrient database, tracks up to 88 nutrients. Plus, the database includes brand-name foods and restaurant menu items.

There are four different versions of NutriBase:

- **EZ Edition.** Single user version, tracks up to 30 nutrients. Includes up to 64 built-in meal plans. $39.99 as a download, $49.99 on CD.
- **Junior Edition.** Also tracks 30 nutrients. Does not track saturated fat. It handles up to two users. $29.95.
- **Personal Edition.** Same as the Junior Edition, but handles five users and 52 nutrients, including saturated fat and caffeine. $49.95.
- **Personal Plus Edition.** Same as the Personal Edition, but handles up to ten users and 88 nutrients. $69.95.

NutriBase automatically selects the appropriate recommended daily allowances (RDA) for foods based on your age and gender. It also boasts extensive reporting capabilities, including actual versus target weight and body fat. Entering meals into its database is easy because NutriBase lets you auto-record frequently eaten foods and enter them into a food diary for a day. However, NutriBase is not as easy to use as many products. When you search for a food, for example, the search results bring up food groups, which you then click on to find the appropriate food. For example, if you search for turkey breast, five categories come up—entrees; poultry; restaurant, fast food; restaurant, sit down; and sausages and lunch meats. You click on the appropriate section and select your food choice from there. This is one extra step that I would be happy not to have.

Among its more unique features, NutriBase provides a nutrient density view that compares equal caloric values of foods—for example, 100 calories of chocolate chip cookies versus 100 calories of lettuce. Guess which one wins? An alarm can alert you when you've eaten or you plan to eat a food that exceeds a particular calorie or nutrient limit—for example, too much fat or salt. Figure 2.20 shows a sample food log.

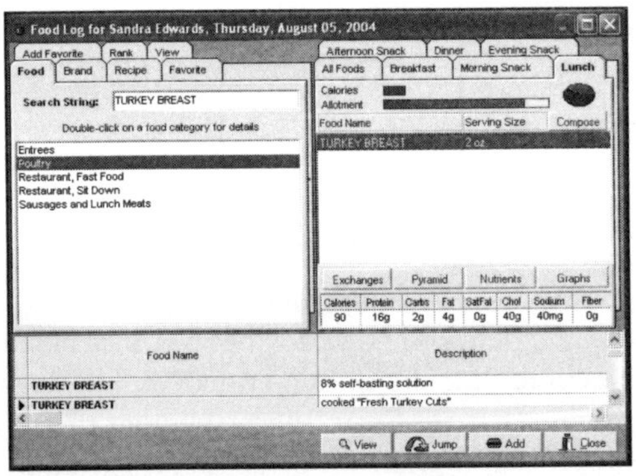

FIGURE 2.20 *NutriBase EZ Food Log*

A Fitness Manager tracks a variety of exercises, automatically calculating calorie expenditures for each based on gender, age, and body weight. It also provides you with an exercise history report, which shows how many calories you've burned on a daily basis through exercise activities (see Figure 2.21). You can also get a report that shows you the exercises you've done most often and the ones you've done least often.

NutriBase also features a meal plan capability that lets you determine your food choices for the next four weeks. There are eight different meal plans available, including diabetic, low-carb, low-fat, vegetarian, and others. This feature is a holdover from the professional version, in which dieticians can prepare meal plans for clients. This is an extremely powerful feature because you can check off the foods you've eaten, prepare a deviation report that shows what you've eaten that is different from the plan, and analyze the meal plans in many different ways. Figure 2.22 shows meal plans.

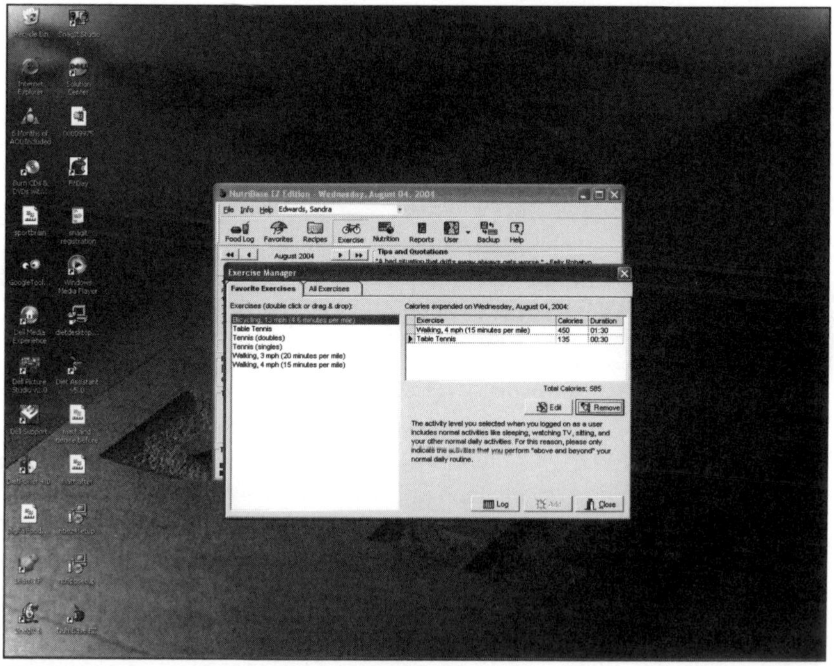

FIGURE 2.21 *NutriBase Exercise Manager*

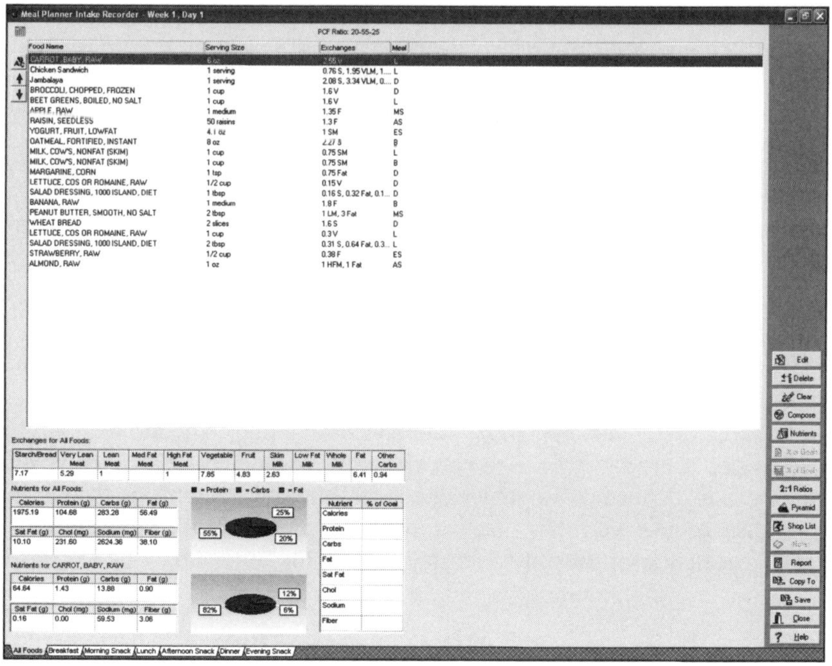

FIGURE 2.22 *NutriBase meal plans*

NutriBase has extensive reporting capabilities that let users create custom reports that could be hundreds of pages long. This can include eating analyses, recipe analyses, and meal plan analyses. It might be more than you want to know about what you eat, but it's hard to imagine wanting more data after you use NutriBase.

You can download a sample copy of NutriBase that works for 14 days before you have to purchase it.

LOSING WEIGHT WITH NUTRIBASE

At first, Paula Johnson's (not her real name) goal was to simply stop gaining weight. So, in the summer of 2002, Johnson, a professor, bought NutriBase EZ Edition and started analyzing her meals and calories. The first thing she found out was that she was eating a lot more calories than she thought. "I was eating about 2,500 to 3,000 calories per day," she says. Johnson decided to limit her calories to no more than 2,000 per day and set a goal of losing 25 pounds over the next year, or a half-pound per week.

The 5'8" Johnson easily maintained a weight of about 145 without dieting in her 20s and 30s, and even easily lost the weight she gained when pregnant without consciously dieting. But from age 40 on, she started to gain weight slowly. By age 52, she weighed about 225, 80 pounds more than she weighed in her 30s.

Her cholesterol and blood pressure were normal despite her elevated weight, but she grew concerned about the difficulties of being overweight as she aged. She also noted that she didn't want to go on a diet; she wanted a lifestyle change. "I was very aware that I had gained weight through eating more and exercising less," she says. "I knew that the way to lose weight was to eat less and exercise more."

After analyzing her diet habits for two months, Johnson started in earnest in late July, 2002. She would eat no more than 2,000 calories per day. With modest goals, she knew she was taking a long-term approach to weight loss.

However, Johnson was much more successful than she thought she'd be. She got her weight down to 200 pounds from 225 in 90 days, losing 1.5 pounds per week, or triple the rate she was expecting! She realized that her metabolism was much higher than NutriBase estimated. With her calories set at 1,859 per day, she set a new goal of 170 pounds. By late July, 2003, or one year after beginning the program, Johnson's weight was in the low 160s. She had lost more than 60 pounds in one year! Nine months later, Johnson's weight was back to 145, where it remains today. "I knew that eventually I'd lose weight at a slower rate," she says. "My goal at this point was to teach myself how to eat so I could stay in the 140s."

LOSING WEIGHT WITH NUTRIBASE *(CONTINUED)*

In the first year, Johnson purposely ate an extra 500 calories per day for a few days when she started to feel too hungry. "I wanted to avoid that starving feeling that leads you to eat everything in sight," she says.

Johnson likes using NutriBase and keeping track of her diet and exercise. She's also trying to train herself to have a more accurate feeling in her body of how much she should be eating. She considers using a program like NutriBase to be essential to a weight loss program. "It helps to have an automated system for recording food consumption," she says. "I also like having the long-term records to look back at to see what I was doing in the past."

Johnson is not the least bit strict in her program. "I go over my calorie allotment about 20 percent of the time," she says. "If I really want something, I will eat it. The only commitment I'm making is to be honest with myself and keep truthful records of what I am eating. Of course, this intentionally makes me think about whether I really want it."

She also finds that she exercises a lot more then she used to. "I find that simply recording the exercise motivates me to do more," she says. "When I exercise more, I eat more, and when I exercise less, I eat less," she says. Johnson shoots for 500 calories each day for breakfast, another 500 for lunch, and 700 to 800 for dinner. If she exercises more, she allows herself to have more calories. "If I exercise more, I can have a bigger dinner, a glass of wine, or a bedtime snack. This becomes a motivation to exercise, which has other health benefits."

It's not easy to lose weight. It's a long-term process, and Johnson knows that. She credits her positive mental attitude with helping her lose the weight she's lost, and she is certain that she'll be able to keep it off.

SparkPeople.com

$9.95 per year

http://www.sparkpeople.com

Pros: Low price, comprehensive product with lots of features.

Cons: Not quite as powerful as some competing products.

SparkPeople represents the "such a deal" part of the online diet and fitness world—a Web site with lots of support, a good food diary, and some excellent features for only $9.95 per year (see Figure 2.23). Given the smart design of the Web site and the support features offered, SparkPeople is a great value. A lot of other people think so, too; the company claims that a significant percentage of its users are people who have switched from Weight Watchers or eDiets, two much more expensive alternatives.

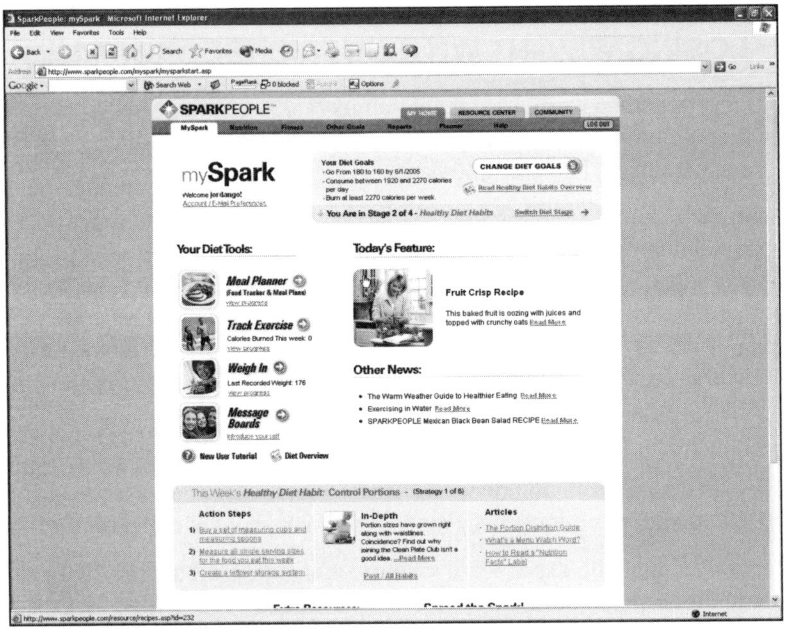

FIGURE 2.23 *SparkPeople.com*

Like Weight Watchers and eDiets, SparkPeople focuses on more than food for losing weight. The company's philosophy is to concentrate on the whole person. "Many companies think that dieting is all about what happens in the kitchen or on a treadmill," says company founder Chris Downey. "In reality, dieting is all about what's in the mind and the heart more than the kitchen."

The site features a meal planner, an exercise tracker, a message board, and health related articles. The articles are always interesting and feature very good information to help people lose weight. In the section shown in Figure 2.24, SparkPeople focuses on portion control, and articles support the notion that portion control is a key to losing weight. Products to help you control portions are available for purchase.

SparkPeople is goal-oriented. You set the goals and it provides you with feedback. Taking the approach that short-term goals should be easy to achieve so that you can reach your long-term goals, SparkPeople is built on a program of providing positive feedback. For example, suppose you set a goal of eating fruit one time per day every day for a week, and another goal of exercising every day for a week. SparkPeople helps you monitor your progress and provides you with positive feedback once you've achieved these goals.

SparkPeople is built on a philosophy that diets work in four stages:

- **Stage 1: Fast Break.** This stage generally lasts for the first two weeks of a diet, and it is the hardest stage. SparkPeople's philosophy is that you start with small goals, learn to use the Web site, and gain momentum on your diet.

- **Stage 2: Healthy Diet Habits.** During this six-week period, you do daily meal planning and tracking and develop the healthy habits that will help you stay on your plan.
- **Stage 3: Lifestyle Change.** During this 10-week period, you transition from being on a diet to making permanent changes to your diet and exercise program so that you continue to be on a healthy lifestyle path long after you've lost your weight. The goal, after all, is to keep the weight off.
- **Stage 4: Spread the Spark.** During this stage, which is ongoing, you move the habits you've learned into other areas of your life, which ultimately makes you not just physically healthy, but also mentally healthy. SparkPeople hopes that you like the program so much that you'll do a little evangelizing for them.

SparkPeople offers optional meal planning as well as food tracking capabilities, plus an exercise assistant that makes it easier to track and plan your exercises and meals. Figure 2.25 shows a sample meal plan.

SparkPeople also has some good reports that measure your progress for health and fitness goals (see Figure 2.26). Plus, it features a 12-week online weight loss class and some unique features, including a printable tape measure that can be downloaded in PDF and used by folks who want to measure their progress—literally.

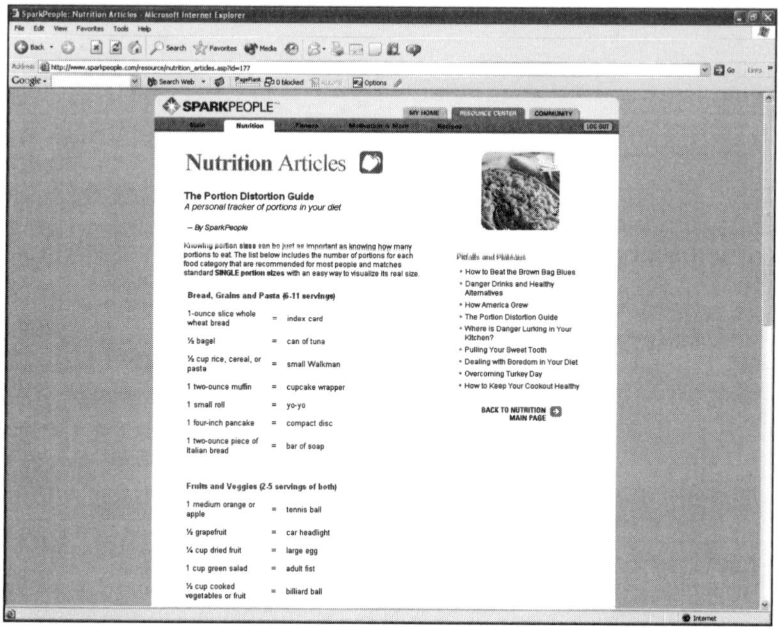

FIGURE 2.24 *Breaking the big-portion habit on SparkPeople.com*

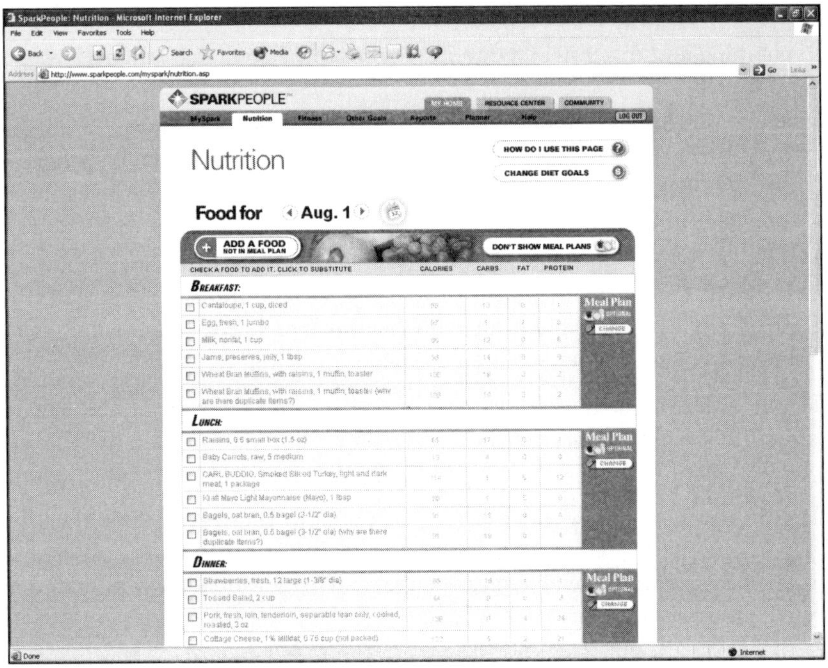

FIGURE 2.25 *SparkPeople.com's meal planner*

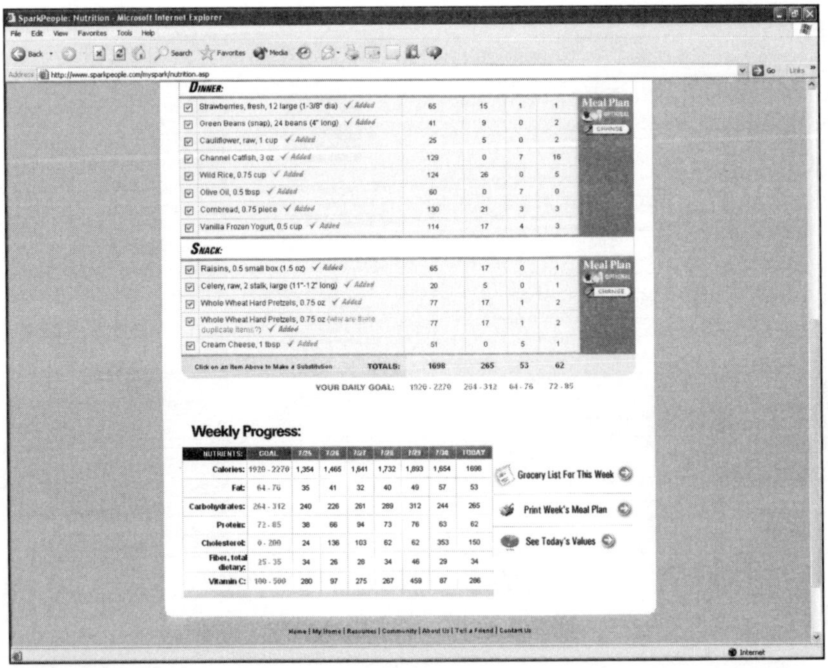

FIGURE 2.26 *SparkPeople.com's diet report*

SparkPeople is not as comprehensive as some of the other sites and products available. For example, there are only 10,000 foods in their database, and their fitness program isn't as extensive as others. However, it's a tremendous value, providing good food and exercise tracking and excellent support services. For $9.95 a year, it's hard to go wrong.

A HUSBAND AND WIFE SPARK TOGETHER

Denise and Matthew Tausig were tired of the grind. Both were overweight and both wanted to lose weight. Denise, a 26-year-old escrow assistant in Capitola, California, had 171 pounds on her 5'5" frame. Matthew, 28, a golf pro in Santa Cruz, had 265 pounds on his 5'8" body.

"We would start to eat better, but then we'd go back to our old routines and put whatever weight we lost back on again," she says.

Denise was afraid that she'd develop diabetes as her mother did. "I don't want to have to go through what she has gone through," she says. "So I figured it was time for a change in my eating habits."

Matt took a look at his family and decided that he had to do something. His parents were both overweight and had numerous health issues. Plus, his father, brother, and mother had all had back problems. "I had to do something about my weight to have a chance at a healthy life as I got older," Matt says. "But I had to do more than lose weight; I had to make a lifestyle change."

As a New Year's resolution, the Tausigs started their program on January 1, 2004. After evaluating several different programs, the Tausigs chose SparkPeople. "I like the way that the program stresses making lifestyle changes," Matt says. "That and the price are what made me choose them."

Denise set a goal of reaching 140 pounds by the end of 2004. Fortunately for her, she obliterated that goal and reached 132 pounds by the end of July.

Matt set a goal of 200 pounds by the end of the year. Both reached their goals in less than five months—on May 23, 2004. Matt also continues to lose weight; he reached 183 pounds by the end of July, 2004.

Denise credits SparkPeople with helping her and Matt reach their weights so quickly. "We followed the plan very closely. Also, having your partner doing it with you was very helpful. We really supported each other a lot and still do."

"I never cheated on any day," Matt adds. "I followed the program, exercised as much as possible, and lost weight very quickly."

Denise likes many SparkPeople features, particularly the food tracker. "It's easy to use and helps me know that I'm still on track with my calories," she says.

A HUSBAND AND WIFE SPARK TOGETHER *(CONTINUED)*

They also like the message boards. "There is so much support there, and I am able to help out others who are trying to meet their goals," Denise says. Matt also spends a lot of time on message boards, both getting support and helping others.

Denise did a variety of exercises along the way to help her reach her goal weight. "I use an elliptical trainer at home, and [I] have a small collection of workout videos that I do at home. These are enough to let me change my routine quite a bit," she says. Denise also uses free weights at home for strength training.

Denise credits Matt as well for helping her reach her goals. "Many people on the message boards complain about their significant others," she says. "Sometimes, significant others who aren't on a plan will hurt them because they bring foods home that sabotage diets." Denise stresses that this often is not intentional; it's just that most people who aren't on diets aren't as empathetic as they could be.

The Tausigs didn't have that. "I could always get the support that I needed from Matt," she says. Matt agrees. "I felt that I would be letting her down if I cheated on the program," he says.

Denise says that the most important part of weight loss is planning. "Plan your meals ahead of time so there aren't any surprises at the end of the day of how much you actually ate," she says.

Matt says the key is approaching a program as a lifestyle change, not a diet. "Diets don't work," he says. "I approached this as a lifestyle change so that I could become a healthier person."

Matt also believes that it's important to communicate to everyone that you are trying to change your lifestyle. "When people know what I am doing and see the progress that I'm making, they don't try to sabotage me. They are happy to see my progress," he says. Figures 2.27 through 2.29 show Matt and Denise before and after their weight loss.

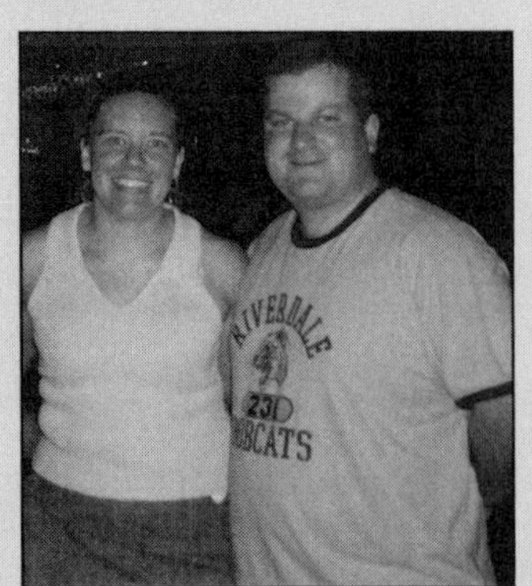

FIGURE 2.27 *Denise and Matt Tausig before their weight loss*

A HUSBAND AND WIFE SPARK TOGETHER *(CONTINUED)*

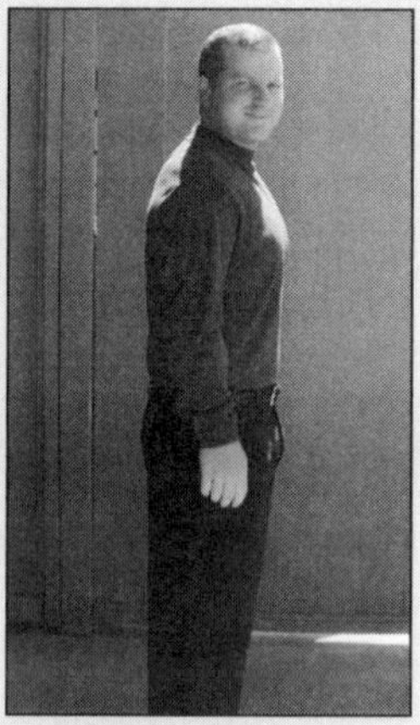

FIGURE 2.28
Matt Tausig with his new look

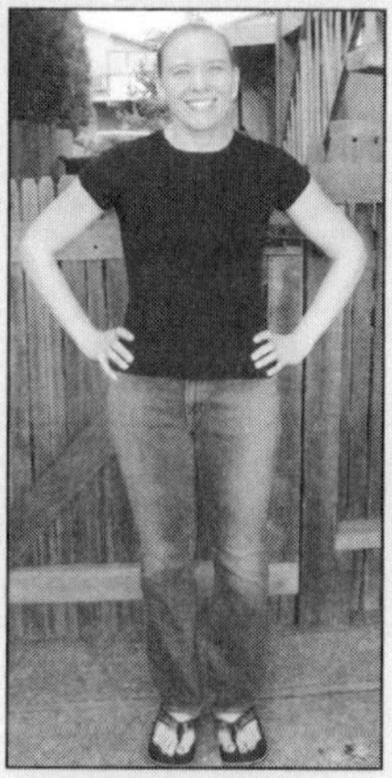

FIGURE 2.29
Denise showing off her new waistline

Weight Watchers Online/eTools

eTools (the online companion for Weight Watchers meetings members): $29.95 for prepaid three-month subscription or $12.95 per month

Weight Watchers Online (for people who don't attend meetings): $65 for prepaid three-month subscription and $16.95 per additional month, or $46.95 for the first month and $16.95 for each additional month

http://www.weightwatchers.com

Pros: Combines Weight Watchers' powerful offline support with an online product, great way to count *POINTS*, helpful features abound.

Cons: High price. If you aren't on Weight Watchers the *POINTS* system might not work for you because counting points is different than counting calories.

Weight Watchers Online (see Figure 2.30) and eTools are similar products, but offered at different prices. There are a few meeting-related items that eTools members don't get because it's expected that they go to meetings so they don't need the same materials that Weight Watchers Online members receive. Weight Watchers meetings members get eTools for a lower price than non-Weight Watchers members get Weight Watchers Online for. For the purposes of brevity, I'll call this product Weight Watchers Online for the rest of this section, but realize that I'm referring to both products.

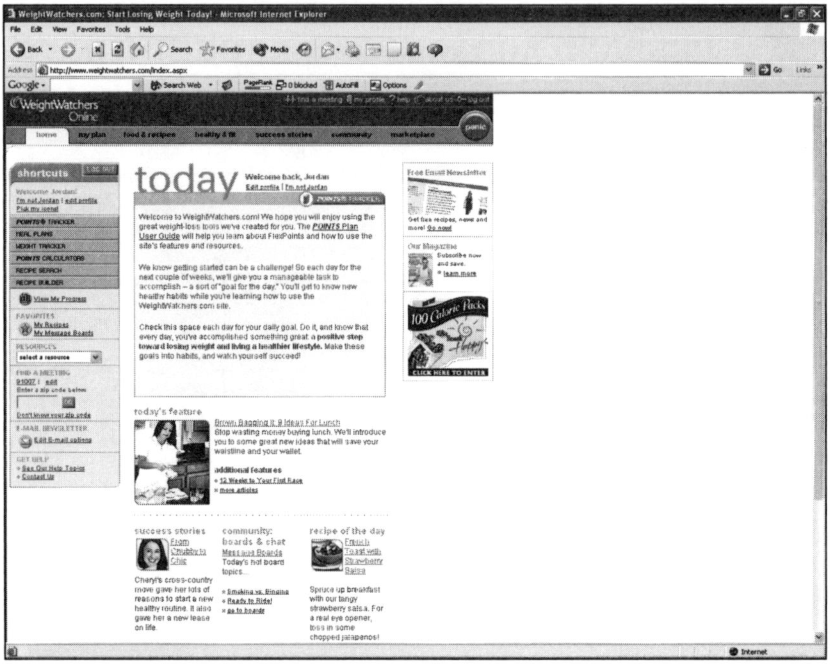

FIGURE 2.30 *Weight Watchers Online*

More expensive than other food diaries, these products have the support of Weight Watchers built in, so they are really much more than food diaries. (I'll discuss support sites, including the rest of the Weight Watchers site, in much more detail in Chapter 3.) However, Weight Watchers has been helping people lose weight for more than 40 years, and it's one of the best programs out there. And if it works for you, it's worth the money.

I used to have a neighbor who was a tailor. Because they often adjust people's clothes, tailors can be authorities on weight loss. He told me that the only program he found that would result in people keeping weight off is Weight Watchers. People on other programs often gained the weight back and came back to him to get their clothes let out again. But with Weight Watchers, they generally didn't come back once their clothes were taken in.

On Weight Watchers, both online and off, members can follow one of two plans—the Flex plan and the Core plan. In the Flex plan, each member is given a certain number of ***POINTS*** that he or she can eat in a day. If you exercise, you can eat additional ***POINTS***. ***POINTS*** are determined by a user's weight. One of the great things about ***POINTS*** is that many vegetables are zero ***POINTS*** because they are so nutrient-dense and calorie-free. Plus, for many people, ***POINTS*** are easier to follow than calories, fat grams, and carbs.

On the Core plan, you focus on eating a core group of foods, and you don't count ***POINTS*** much at all. As long as you eat foods in the core areas, which include fruits and vegetables, lean meats, whole grains, and fat-free dairy products and certain other types of foods, you don't count *POINTS*. (However, there are limits to how much of these foods you can eat in a day.) If you choose to eat foods outside of the Core plan, you have 35 *POINTS* per week that you can use.

Weight Watchers Online includes a food database with more than 20,000 foods, an activity database with more than 100 activities, a recipe database with more than 1,000 recipes, eating out guides, and a personal weight tracker. There are separate food guides for the Core plan and the Flex plan. The food diary is a *POINTS* Tracker; it calculates the number of *POINTS* that you've consumed in a day and continually tells you how many you have left (see Figure 2.31). Any activities result in additional *POINTS* that you can consume. The *POINTS* Tracker is one of the simplest and most user-friendly food diaries, although tracking *POINTS* instead of calories can be disconcerting for non-Weight Watchers users.

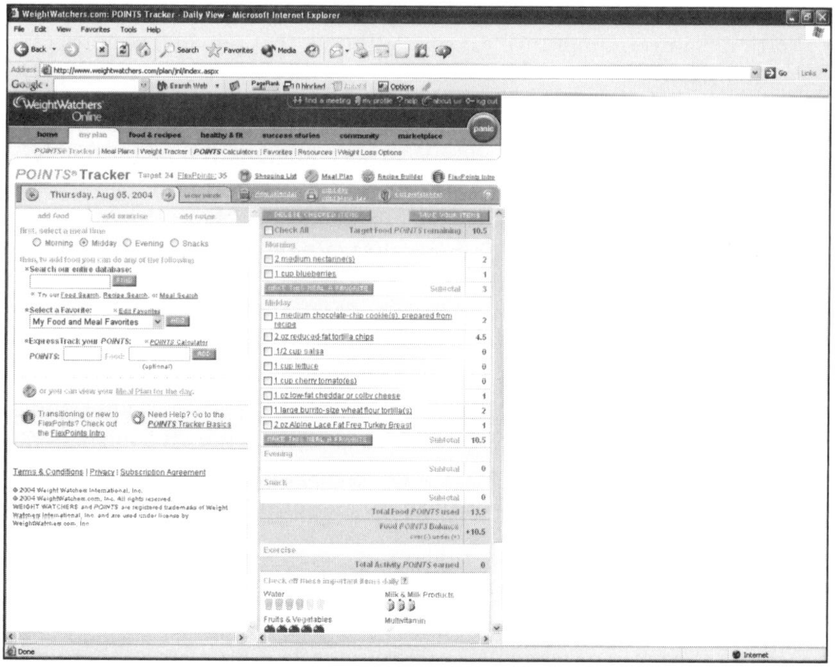

FIGURE 2.31 *Entering meals in the* ***POINTS*** *Tracker*

In true Weight Watchers fashion, Weight Watchers Online features many very helpful features:

- **Recipe Renovation.** Lets users take fattening recipes and "thin them up," removing high-fat, high-*POINTS* ingredients and substituting other ingredients.
- **Recipe Builder.** Users add the ingredients, and the software calculates the ***POINTS*** for the recipe.

- **Online *POINTS* Calculator.** Determines *POINTS* values for foods based on information from Nutrition Facts food labels. Also calculates activity *POINTS* burned by measuring your body weight against the type, intensity, and duration of the activity.
- **Community.** Message boards, recipe swaps, newsletters, and chat rooms highlight a very active community.
- **Weight Tracker.** Users weigh in just as they would when going to a weekly Weight Watchers meeting. The software tracks their progress over time.
- **Meal Plans.** Users select the type of meals they'd like to eat—regular, low-carb, or vegetarian—and Weight Watchers creates the meal plan for them.
- **Eating Out Guide.** Includes *POINTS* values for a variety of international cuisine, plus most fast food restaurants. There are separate guides for the Flex plan and the Core plan.
- **Portion Control.** Innovative yet simple feature that provides pictures of normal portion sizes.

Weight Watchers offers an excellent product that works well in conjunction with online or offline meetings. If you are on the Weight Watchers program, you might find it helpful to use software that helps you track *POINTS* on a daily basis instead of using the other programs, which track calories. However, if you're not interested in tracking *POINTS* or using Weight Watchers' excellent support tools and features, then Weight Watchers might be overkill because it's one of the most expensive options available for food and exercise diaries.

Other Programs

There are many other software programs that will help you lose weight and keep fit. I've included some of the most popular ones in this chapter; Appendix B contains a more complete list. Although there are many choices, the important thing is to make *a* choice. Decide which software you'd like to use and use it. It will get you on the road to a more fit future. No matter what software you use, the steps are the same:

- **Fill in your personal information.** This includes your height, weight, age, gender, diet preferences, goal weight, and timeframe for meeting your goal.
- **Select a meal plan or manually enter your meals.** Meal plans will result in faster weight loss because you'll be eating fewer calories, and it's easier to eat what you're told to eat. However, it might be better in the long run to simply pick out your own foods and eat them. If you can lose weight on your own meal plans, you'll be more likely to keep that weight off after you've reached your goal.
- **Use your food and exercise diary.** Dutifully enter all of the food you eat, the water you drink, and the exercises you do each day. Be sure to measure and weigh your foods. These are the keys to weight loss.
- **Community.** Be a part of the weight loss community. You'll learn from others, and others will learn from you. You need support to succeed.
- **Reports.** Examine your reports and celebrate your accomplishments.

In Chapter 3, I'll take this to the next step. Assuming that you are using a food diary, where do you go for support and encouragement along the way? What sites help you learn more about diets and exercise? Who has the best message boards? And what sites have the best recipes and tips for weight loss and fitness?

Chapter 3

Support Sites

"I asked my wife, 'Where do you want to go for our anniversary?' She said, 'Somewhere I have never been!' I told her, 'How about the kitchen?'"

—Henny Youngman

Okay, so now you know some of the secrets of staying healthy. You've found your favorite food diary, but what to eat? And when? And how much? Plus, won't you get sick of eating the same things? There are some great Web sites that will help you achieve your goal of losing weight and eating more healthfully, and many have active user bases that will provide support and guidance along the way. Many provide information about diets, others have great recipes, and numerous provide the support that dieters need. In this chapter, we'll consider how these research and support sites can help you reach your goals.

Components of a Good Support Site

If you were building a Web site for business purposes, the site would need to have all of what we call the three Cs—content, community, and commerce. A site can't thrive without all three, because without content, no one would visit and form a community, and without commerce, no one would host it. Good support sites also need the three Cs to survive, albeit in somewhat different forms. Content comes from the information on the site, and it can be in many different forms, as discussed in this chapter. Same thing with community, which goes well beyond message boards. A site can often take on a life of its own with the support of the people who visit and participate. Commerce can come from subscriptions, advertising revenue, product sales, and one-time purchases, among other things.

You can't expect a site to be all things to all people. In fact, just like you don't only visit one site for a job search, a hobby, or your favorite pastime, you might regularly visit many sites in your quest for a healthier you. However, if there was a perfect support site, it would have the components listed in the following sections, in addition to a food and exercise diary. (The components are listed in alphabetical order, along with which of the three Cs each one belongs to.)

TURN POP-UPS ON!

On many Web sites, much of the support information, such as polls, message boards, and so on, works better if pop-ups are enabled for that Web site only. If you use the Google Toolbar to disable pop-ups, you can enable them one Web site at a time. That way, when you go to other Web sites, you'll still block those annoying pop-up ads.

Advertising (Commerce)

Advertising is a good source of revenue for the site, which is good for you because a lot of revenue will help the site stay in business. Also, the ads might be interesting and helpful to you. Some sites have ads for food products, health and medical devices, and items that might appeal to someone who is on a diet, such as books, magazines, or even dating services. Others, particularly sites with offline components, such as magazines, have many of the same ads that are in the magazine. A good Web site with a lot of traffic is appealing for advertisers because they get access to a community beyond the readers of the magazine. They also get an opportunity to appeal to the online audience for the Web site.

Conferences (Community)

An annual conference or convention is a great opportunity to meet offline others who share your interests. The conference might be a professional conference, such as Weight Loss Frontiers, or a personal conference that gets together a group of people who've lost weight, such as Dotti's Weight Loss Zone Conference (see Figure 3.1).

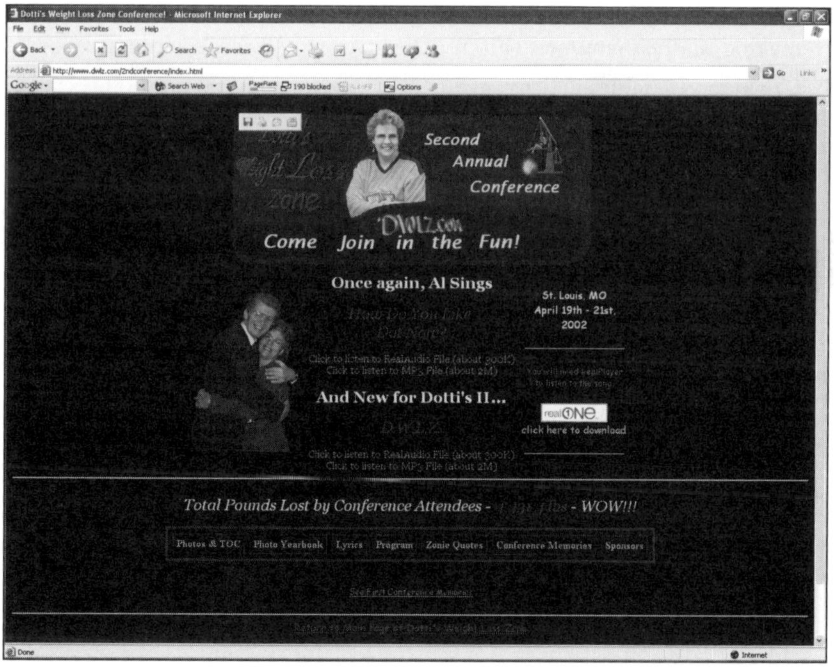

FIGURE 3.1 *Dotti's Weight Loss Zone Conference is an annual conference that celebrates the amount of weight lost by attendees.*

Cooking Tips (Content)

What's a weight loss site without cooking tips? After all, you've gotta eat, right? Many sites have a number of great cooking tips to help you reach your ultimate weight without giving up too much. We'll discuss this in much more detail when we examine some of the best cooking sites on the Internet in Chapter 4, "Healthy Cooking Online." Some of our favorite tips garnered online are

- **Cooking veggie packets on a grill.** Put a few ice cubes in the packets to keep the vegetables moist and protect them from overcooking. (From 3 Fat Chicks at http://www.3fatchicks.com.)
- **Substitute for heavy cream.** Use evaporated skim milk instead of heavy cream in sauces and soups. (From Ladies Home Journal Online at http://www.lhj.com.)
- **Stir-fry without oil.** Substitute broth, white wine, or water infused with herbs for oil when stir-frying vegetables. The vegetables will brown as the liquid reduces. Stir constantly. You can also use this approach for sautéing vegetables, such as onions, bell peppers, and garlic. (From Lowfat Lifestyle at http://www.lowfatlifestyle.com.)
- **Low-carb "mashed potatoes."** Substitute mashed cauliflower for potatoes when making mashed potatoes. (From eDiets at http://www.ediets.com.)
- **Cooking vegetables.** Microwave or steam vegetables; do not boil them. Either method retains nutrients better than boiling. (From Better Health Channel at http://www.betterhealth.vic.gov.au.)

Dieting Tips (Content)

When you are trying to change your lifestyle, you need tips to help you get to the next level. As a result, most support Web sites devote a lot of content to tips to help you get through some very difficult emotional times. Some of our favorite dieting tips follow.

- **Soup will help you cut calories.** Eating soup is always a good way to get a lot of nutrition for a small amount of calories. (But watch that sodium—soups are often high in salt.) Having a cup of soup before a meal is also effective in lowering the overall total calories of what you eat. (From About.com at http://www.about.com.)
- **Eat breakfast.** Think you're saving calories for later when you skip breakfast? Wrong! Studies show that people who eat breakfast regularly are thinner than those who don't. You tend to get hungrier throughout the day when you don't eat breakfast, so you eat many more calories than you would have if you had eaten breakfast instead. (From Shape Up America at http://www.shapeup.org.)
- **Get 30 minutes of physical activity per day.** Break it up into segments if you have to. Three 10-minute segments are beneficial as well. (From the National Institutes of Health at http://www.nih.gov.)
- **When cooking in a pan, use nonstick cooking spray instead of margarine or oil.** You'll save about 100 calories. (From FreeWeightLoss.com at http://www.freeweightloss.com.)
- **To lose body fat, increase your meal frequency.** Eat the same amount of calories as you normally would, but eat smaller meals more often throughout the day. This increases your metabolism and helps burn body fat. (From Diet & Body at http://www.dietandbody.com.)

KEEP YOUR HANDS OFF THE TRIGGER FOODS

All of us have weaknesses for certain foods. Mine tend to be snack foods, such as tortilla chips, pretzels, and dips. These foods tend to trigger bad eating behaviors for me because I start eating them, get hungry, and start eating more food. Occasionally, this can lead to a binge.

Foods that result in you eating more than you should, or foods for which you have a weakness, are called *trigger foods*. The best advice for dealing with trigger foods is to know which ones trigger bad eating behaviors in you and stop eating them. Or at least severely limit your consumption of them by eating very small portions. It's better to stop eating them, though. You'll be surprised by how little you miss them. For me, I've banished potato chips from my diet. I haven't had a potato chip in years, and I don't miss them at all.

Support for Specific Health, Gender, or Age Issues (Content)

The Internet is a marvelous source of information. Nearly all health-related maladies, rare or common, have Web sites devoted to them. There are also sites for seniors, men, women, and children. Many general support sites also include information about specific health, gender, and age issues. For example, eDiets has a newsletter about diabetes and another one about childhood obesity. We'll discuss age and gender issues in Chapter 5, "Healthy, Fit, and Well," and health issues in Appendix A, "Sites for Specific Diseases and Conditions."

Education (Content and Community)

It's difficult to be uninformed about health issues and still lead a healthy life. Our ancestors did it, but they didn't get to go to the grocery store and be tempted by all those processed foods that are high in calories, fats, trans-fats, and simple carbs.

Many sites have online learning areas devoted to helping people learn about a variety of health-related topics. Sometimes this is content in the form of educational materials, but often it includes online classes and lectures that you sign up for and take at a specific time or at your convenience. eDiets and Weight Watchers are two sites that offer online learning, but others do as well.

Events (Content and Community)

Attending an online discussion by an expert is an invaluable experience. You can often ask the expert questions and get answers in real time. Later, after the event, this discussion morphs into content because you can read the transcript online. These events could range from a discussion by an author of a popular book to a discussion by a health expert about a particular topic. Some sites also sponsor offline events, such as the traveling Mind, Body, Spirit Games by *Fitness* magazine and its Web site, http://www.fitnessmagazine.com (see Figure 3.2). These games include a four-mile run, a two-mile walk, massages, demonstrations, and more. In 2004, there were games held in New York, Chicago, and San Francisco.

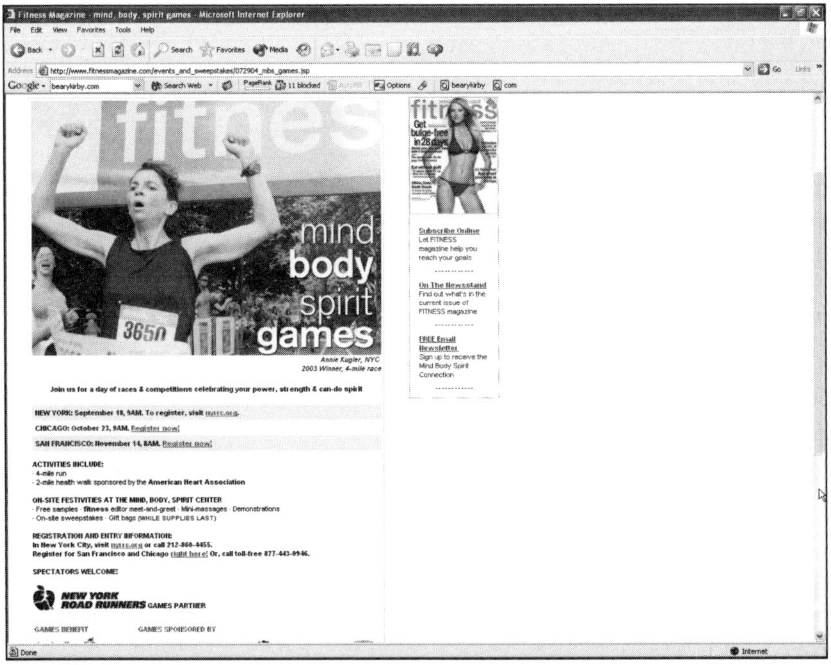

FIGURE 3.2 Fitness *magazine's Mind, Body, Spirit Games*

Fitness Tips (Content)

Fitness tips go hand in hand with cooking and eating tips. When you're trying to get into shape, it's best to take the advice of lots of people in planning your workout schedule. Here are a few fun fitness tips garnered from a number of Internet sites:

- **Do stomach crunches in bed.** Before you get out of bed in the morning, do 10 stomach crunches. Increase the number by one each day until you get to 100 per day. (From Health & Fitness Tips at http://www.health-fitness-tips.com.)
- **Cross-train to lose the last five or 10 pounds of a diet.** By cross-training, which means doing a variety of exercises, you'll get your body off of a diet plateau and start losing weight again. (From eDiets at http://www.ediets.com.)
- **Lift weights with your eyes closed.** By lifting weights with your eyes closed, your body will improve its proprioception, which will result in you using proper form and eventually lifting heavier weights. (From Men'sHealth at http://www.menshealth.com.)

- **Pushups will wake you up in the morning.** If you're really tired, do a few pushups each morning as soon as you wake up. (From Global Health & Fitness at http://www.global-fitness.com.)
- **To avoid crashes while biking, stay in the front part of the group.** Most accidents happen in the back half of the group. (From Bally Total Fitness at http://www.bally-fitness.com.)

Mentoring (Community)

Losing weight and getting into shape is very difficult, so some sites go out of their way to pair you with someone who has already achieved success in the areas on which you are focused. These mentors are usually anxious to help others and guide them through the pitfalls and difficulty of losing weight and getting fit. In some cases, this is informal, through message boards and other community-related topics. However, eDiets is one site that has a formal mentoring process and requires people who want to mentor others to qualify to be a mentor (see Figure 3.3). There is a training program to ensure that mentors truly can help others. Each mentor has a set of responsibilities and gets support and training as well.

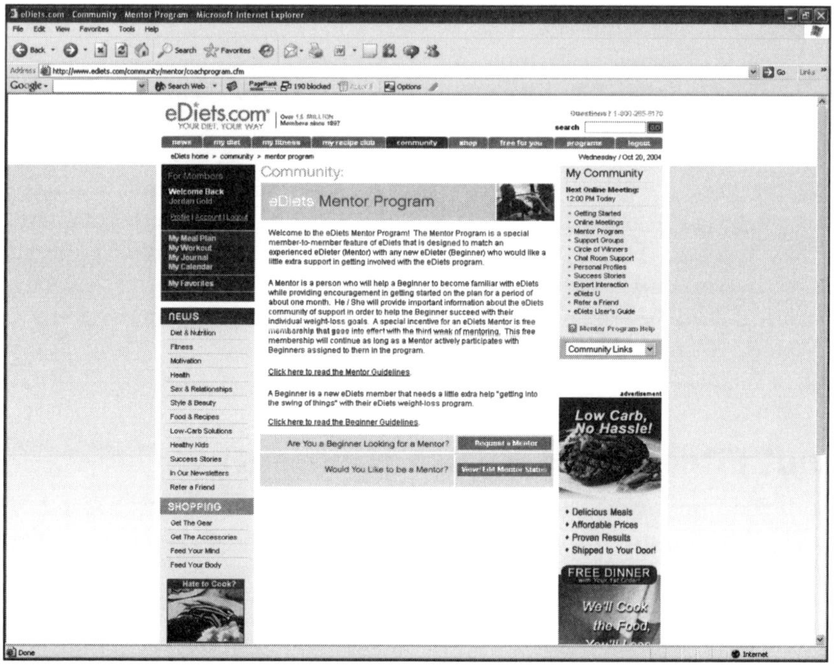

FIGURE 3.3 *eDiets' Mentor Program*

Message Boards (Community)

Some sites are a façade. Oh, sure, they might *look* like they are great community sites, but check under the hood to be sure. The heart of any support site is its message boards. These areas will tell you at a glance whether you want to join a site. Are the message boards interesting? Well trafficked? Lots of activity? Were there several posts today? Good answers? Good questions? If so, you have found a site with a great community, and one that will help you immensely in your search for a healthy lifestyle. If the site has little activity on the message boards, run away and go find a site with a community that you can learn from and participate in.

AGE IS NOT GOOD FOR MESSAGE BOARDS

A way to quickly judge the quality of a site's message boards is to look at the last dates that messages were posted in particular categories. If there has been a lot of activity over the last week, fine. If all of the postings are one or even several weeks old, stay away. This site is starting to collect dust.

Weight Watchers Online is an example of a site with great message boards and lots of activity on them (see Figure 3.4). They organize their mind-boggling 36 message boards into multiple categories, including a category for new members (The Lobby); a tip exchange area; boards organized by age group, by how many pounds you have to lose, by special interests (just married, guys, vegetarians, and so on); recipes; fitness and exercise; and motivation. In fact, there are so many message boards that it gets a little confusing. But that's better than some sites that have a few message boards, none of them well traveled. For example, Buzzle.com (http://www.buzzle.com) is a very nice site with lots of news and information about a number of subjects, including health and fitness, but its message boards are not well traveled by any means. Figure 3.5 shows Buzzle's health and fitness message boards. There clearly are only a few posts each day.

News about Fitness and Health (Content)

The health and fitness world is filled with lots of news about reports, research studies, new books, and other information. Some sites have news feeds that provide this information for their members. Also, news sites have health and fitness sections, as shown in Figure 3.6. CNN mimics their offline TV coverage with a comprehensive Health/Diet & Fitness news section that you can subscribe to so you receive it every day.

For example, clicking on the full story in an article about vending machines brings much more detail to the story, a poll asking whether you would use vending machines if the food got healthier, and an opportunity to subscribe to health and fitness alerts, which puts this information on your desktop as it changes. CNN also has a Health section that includes some of

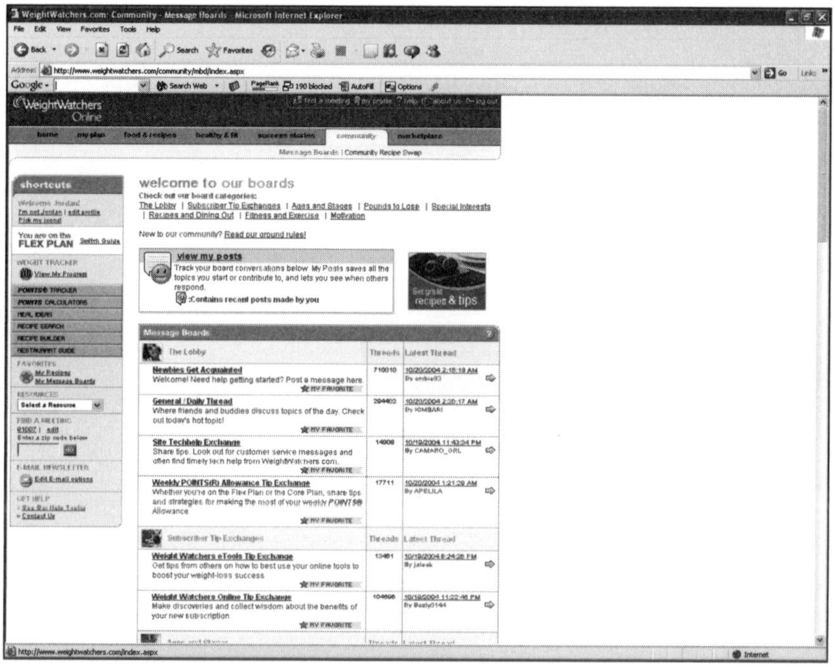

FIGURE 3.4 *Weight Watchers' message boards*

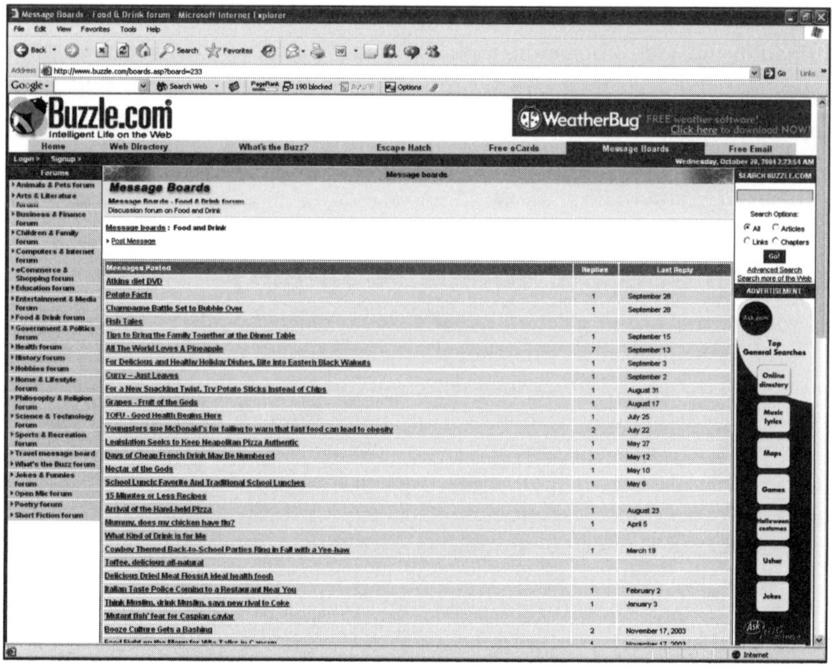

FIGURE 3.5 *Buzzle.com's message boards are not as well traveled as Weight Watchers' boards are.*

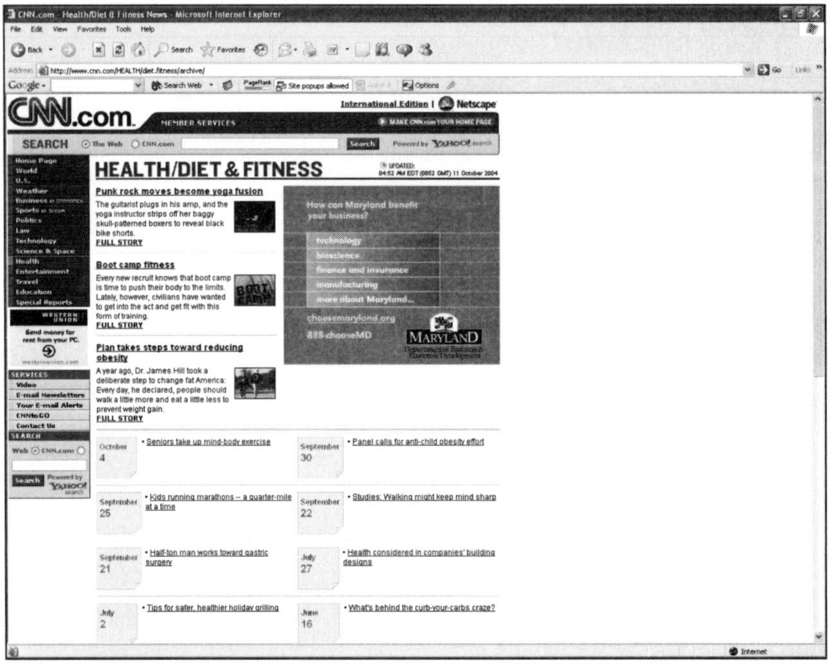

FIGURE 3.6 *CNN Health/Diet & Fitness news*

this information and adds other, more topical coverage, such as a story about a man who needed a liver transplant and developed a Web site and a billboard campaign for potential donors.

Many other sites include health and fitness news, including local and national newspapers (*Chicago Tribune, LA Times, USA Today*, and so on), magazines (*Fitness, Shape, Men's Health*, and so on), and TV and radio stations.

Newsletters on Specific Topics (Content)

In a way, you can think of newsletters as serialized message boards. Although they don't share the same content as message boards, they do share the same target market. You can subscribe to any number of health and fitness newsletters online and off. Nearly every health and fitness site has at least one interesting newsletter. Topics vary, from recipe ideas to fitness tips and specific newsletters for specific age groups. eDiets, for example, sends out 13 newsletters to a total of 12 million subscribers. They have newsletters for low-carb diets, diabetes, heart disease, fitness, and many other topics. About.com offers eight health- and fitness-related newsletters among the 80 that they offer on all subjects. Health and fitness newsletters offered include alternative medicine, healthy eating, diabetes, and pregnancy. Other helpful newsletters are offered by Bally Total Fitness (http://www.ballyfitness.com), The South Beach Diet Online (http://www.southbeachdiet.com) and Atkins (http://atkins.com), which offers a large monthly newsletter filled with advice, recipes, offers, and much more (see Figure 3.7).

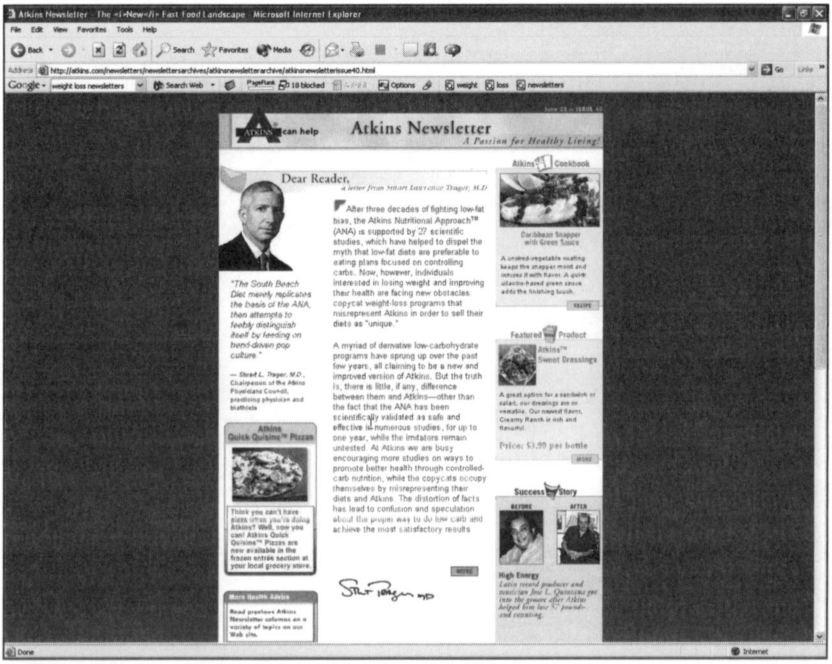

FIGURE 3.7 *Atkins Newsletter*

DON'T SUBSCRIBE TO TOO MANY NEWSLETTERS

If you subscribe to too many newsletters, your mailbox will be full of them and you'll likely not read any. It's better to pick a few that you like and subscribe to those. Then, unsubscribe to a newsletter if you're not reading it, and pick another. Pick newsletters from multiple Web sites, and don't get all of your health news from one source. This way, you'll get multiple points of view.

Online Meetings (Community)

If you're going to an online meeting, you don't have to worry about traffic, what you're wearing, or who else is going to be there; all you have to worry about is showing up on time. And if you do, you'll often have just as much fun as if you were there in person. Overeaters Anonymous has a large number of online meetings taking place every day. Through the Recovery Group, there are online meetings every three hours every day (see Figure 3.8).

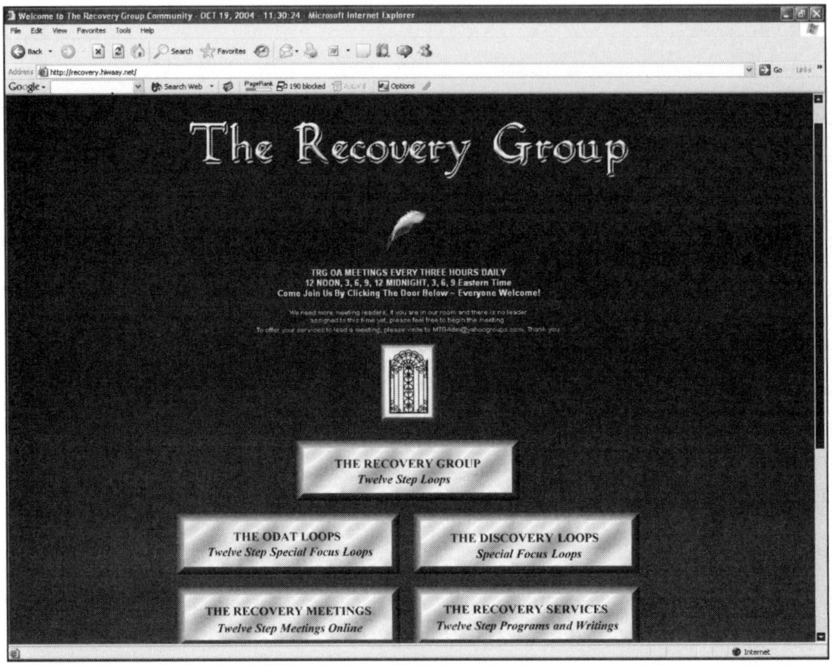

FIGURE 3.8 *The Recovery Group and Overeaters Anonymous have online meetings every three hours all day, every day.*

For an online meeting to be successful, it has to be as structured and orderly as an offline meeting. There have to be set rules in place, or chaos will result and the meetings will be a waste of time. HealthyPlace.com (http://www.healthyplace.com) has online meetings for a wide variety of support groups, ranging from domestic abuse to drug abuse, depression, and many other subjects (see Figure 3.9). They have devised a rule set for every type of online meeting, no matter what the subject.

They structure all meetings just like a face-to-face meeting, with a chairperson or host who calls the meeting to order, greets the attendees, introduces the speaker (if there is one), and closes the meeting for everyone at the end.

The speaker speaks (okay, types) uninterrupted. To raise their hands, listeners type an exclamation mark and are called on by the chairperson for questions. As a rule, speakers get up to 10 minutes of typing time, and listeners get up to three minutes. When someone has more to say, they type an ellipsis (…) and press Enter at the end of each line. When they are finished, they type "done" or "pass." Here's an example of an online weight loss meeting using HealthyPlace.com's format:

> I'd like to share what happened to me today… (Enter)
>
> I went for a long walk this morning… (Enter)

> Then, when I came home, I was very hungry and… (Enter)
> wanted to eat a sandwich and potato chips… (Enter)
> Instead, I drank a large glass of water and had a… (Enter)
> Salad… (Enter)
> I weighed myself later in the day, and I've lost two… (Enter)
> More pounds!… (Enter)
> Pass. (Enter)

HealthyPlace.com says this format keeps people under control so they don't go on long typing binges, leaving others wondering whether they are finished. They say that this is the smoothest way of running an online meeting. HealthyPlace.com also has specific rules for weight loss meetings, which basically revolve around using good manners. No screaming (typing in ALL CAPS), no insults, no profanity of any kind, no overt sexuality, and no personal attacks.

If someone doesn't follow the rules, he or she will be given a warning. If that person continues to behave in a way that is not constructive to the rest of the group, the host will kick him or her out of the meeting.

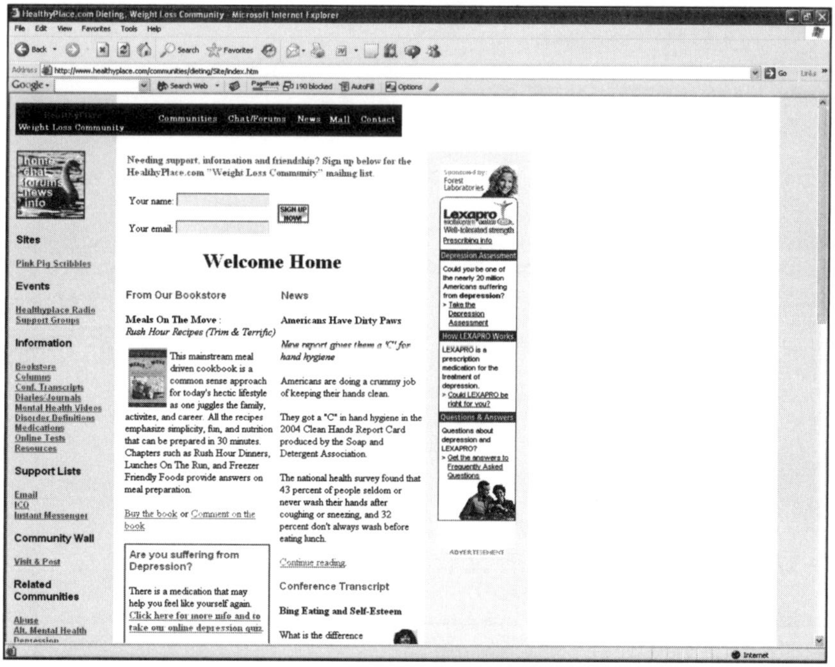

FIGURE 3.9 *HealthyPlace.com's weight loss community*

Polls (Community)

People love to give their opinions and see what others think as well. Many sites have polls that ask your opinions on various things—are you eating fewer carbs, how much weight have you lost, what's your favorite food, and so on. Once you give your answer, the poll generally takes you to the next page, which shows you how people have voted so far on this subject, and possibly links to other polls the site has done in the past.

A good poll question should be interesting, provocative, and related to the subject of the Web site. As a Webmaster, you know you're doing a good job if a lot of visitors vote in your polls. Good polling software should show the number of people who voted and the percentage who voted for each choice.

For example, Prevention.com's Web site (http://www.prevention.com), which is an offshoot of *Prevention* magazine, asked a poll question that probably generated a lot of interest: "What was your favorite movie this summer (2004)?" (see Figure 3.10). Although interesting, the topic is not related to the content of the site, and the software doesn't tell you how many people voted (just the percentage who voted for each choice).

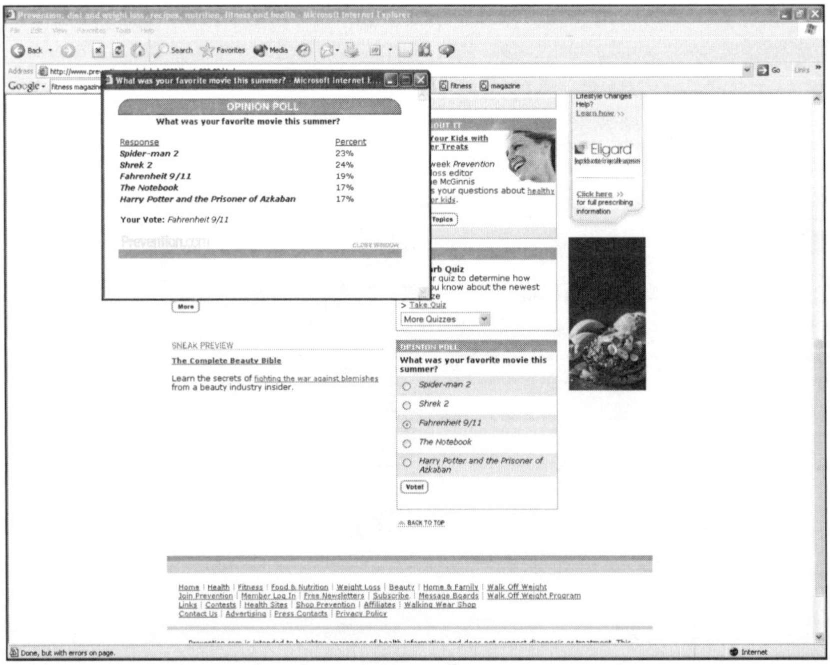
OPINION POLL
What was your favorite movie this summer?
Response
Percent
Spider-man 2
23%
Shrek 2
24%
Fahrenheit 9/11
19%
The Notebook
17%
Harry Potter and the Prisoner of Azkaban
17%
Your Vote: Fahrenheit 9/11

FIGURE 3.10 *Prevention.com poll results*

A much better poll is from CNN.com, which has a Quick Vote feature after certain articles. For example, after a story about healthy food in vending machines, CNN.com asked whether the reader would use vending machines more if products got healthier (see Figure 3.11). With more than 30,000 votes, 59% said yes. This is a very good measure of both readership and reader participation.

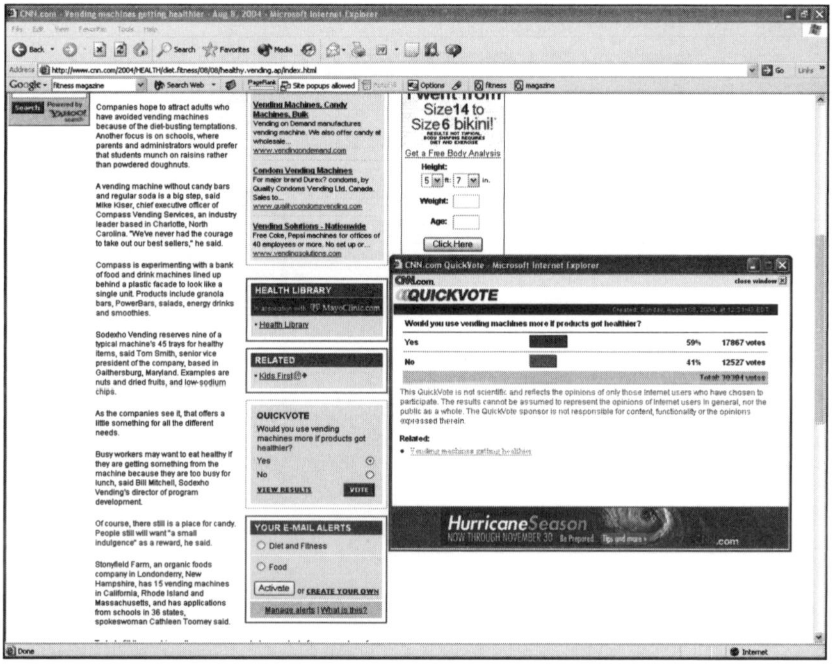

FIGURE 3.11 *CNN.com poll results*

Quizzes (Community)

How well do you think you know a subject? When a site gets you involved, you tend to be more engaged. Plus, it's fun to find out just how much you know (or don't know), and what you need to work on to get better at it. And if you like taking quizzes and a site has good ones, it will keep you coming back for more. *Prevention* magazine, whose parent company, Rodale Press, publishes the South Beach Diet books, has tons of quizzes on its Web site. The low-carb quiz is shown in Figure 3.12.

Prevention.com actually has more health-related quizzes than any site we've seen, with more than 30 quizzes available to take at the click of a mouse, testing your knowledge on a variety of subjects ranging from heart disease to relationships, diseases, fast food, and exercise.

Of course, the point of quizzes isn't to take them; it's to learn from them. So after you take a quiz, a good Web site will provide you with your results and an explanation of each question. Prevention.com does an excellent job of this, as shown in Figure 3.13.

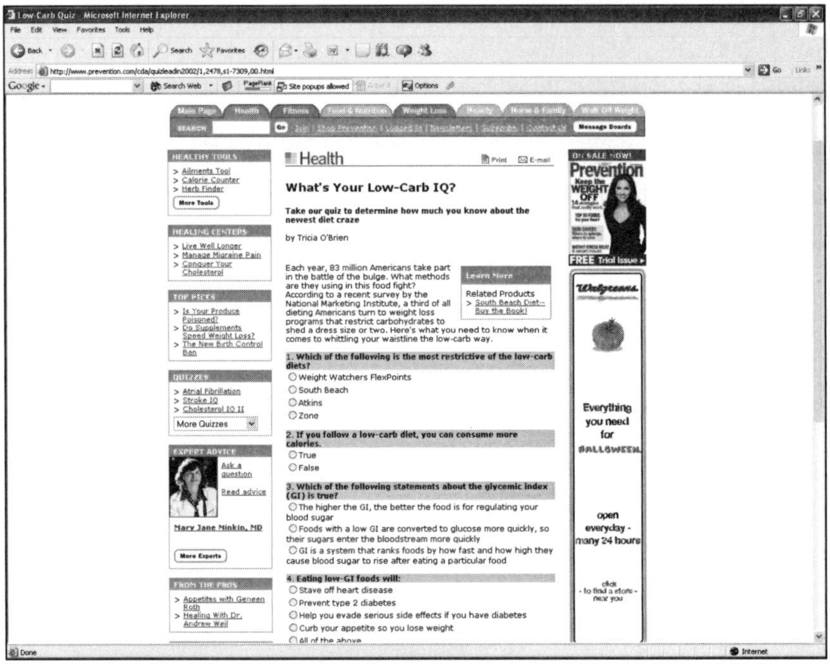

FIGURE 3.12 *Low-carb quiz on Prevention.com*

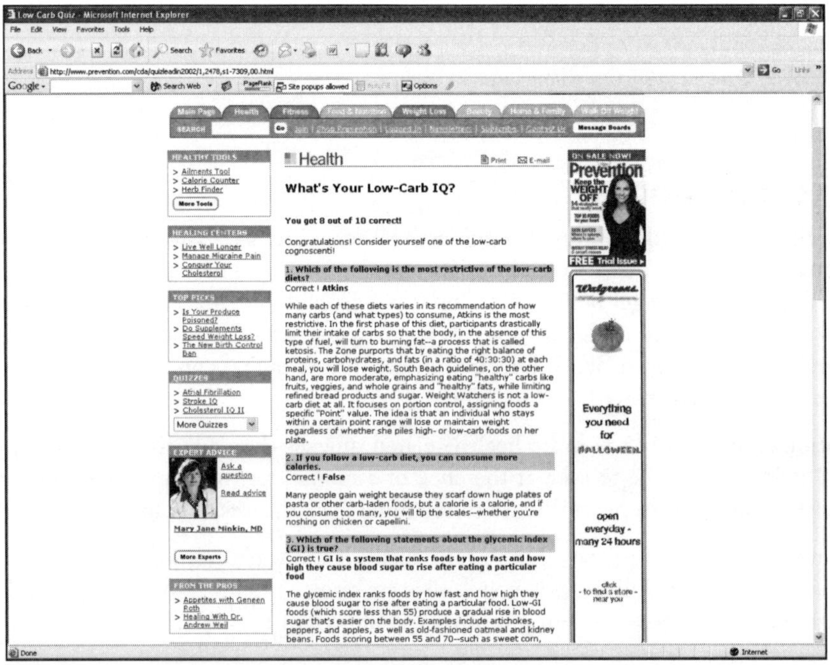

FIGURE 3.13 *Low-carb quiz results and explanations*

Recipes (Content)

You can have all the tips you need, but you often will need guidance about what to cook. Many sites have a large variety of recipes online, so you don't necessarily have to buy a cookbook to help you prepare healthy meals at home. Weight Watchers, eDiets, SparkPeople and many other sites offer great recipes. We'll cover this topic in more depth in Chapter 4, "Healthy Cooking Online."

One of my favorite recipe sites is the Cooking Thin site on FoodNetwork.com (http://www.foodnetwork.com), the online version of the hit show on the Food Network (see Figure 3.14). Chef Kathleen Daelemans helps someone improve their diet in each episode, sharing some recipes along the way. The Web site includes those delicious examples with step-by-step instructions.

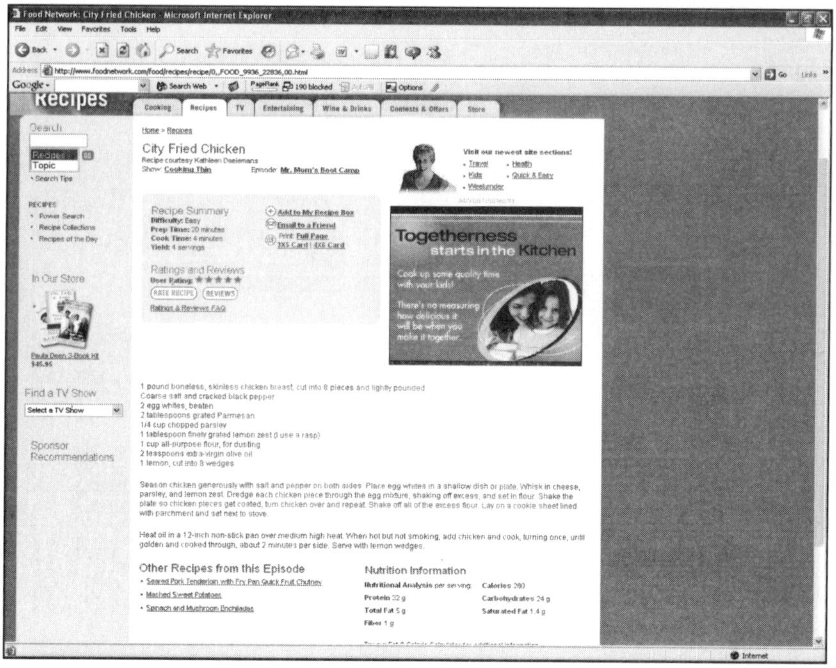

FIGURE 3.14 *Chef Kathleen's City Fried Chicken recipe*

Chef Kathleen rates all recipes by difficulty level, and includes prep time, cooking time, and yield. She also includes nutrition information; detailed instructions; and the ability to print, e-mail, and save recipes. The site also includes a community feature in the form of user ratings and reviews of each recipe. In the case of the recipe shown in Figure 3.14, there weren't very many ratings, but the people who tried it loved it—they gave it five stars out of five.

Store (Commerce)

An online store is a convenient addition to a Web site, and many sites include stores that offer discounts to members, including DietPower, eDiets, and Weight Watchers, among others (see Figure 3.15). These aren't often the best place to buy products online; specialized Web sites are often a better choice. However, they are convenient and sometimes do provide some excellent values. We'll cover online commerce in detail in Chapter 7, "Shop Naked."

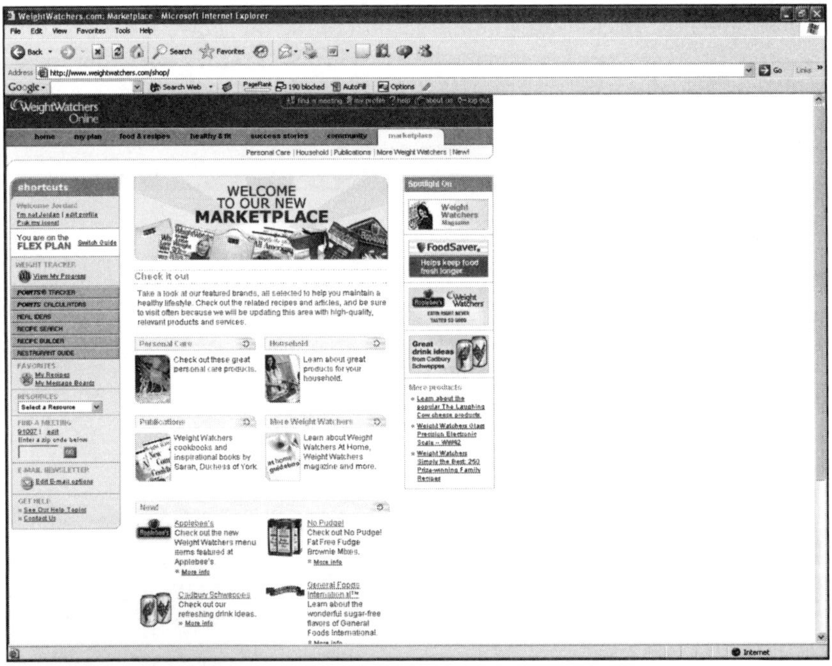

FIGURE 3.15 *Weight Watchers Online Marketplace*

Subscriptions (Commerce)

Many sites are subscription-based and derive most of their revenue from individual subscriptions. The rates range from inexpensive (SparkPeople costs $9.95 per year) to much higher (Weight Watchers and eDiets can cost hundreds of dollars each on an annual basis). Each Web site understands the importance of attracting qualified members who will stay and be successful in attaining their goals, because successful members create word of mouth that is better than anything advertising can buy.

Some sites, such as CalorieKing, offer users a trial period so they can check out the site first, and then pay to join (see Figure 3.16). Sites such as CalorieKing and eDiets offer users something for free as an enticement to join, such as a free diet profile. Other sites, such as Weight

Watchers, require upfront payment first. In all cases, however, the process must run smoothly or users will walk away. If the process proceeds in an unexpected way, most users will walk away and go somewhere else. Users have to feel as if they are being gently guided through the process, not pushed through it. All of the sites mentioned in this book have reasonable subscription processes that work well. Some of the processes are confusing, such as the many options that eDiets offers, but in most cases, the processes work well.

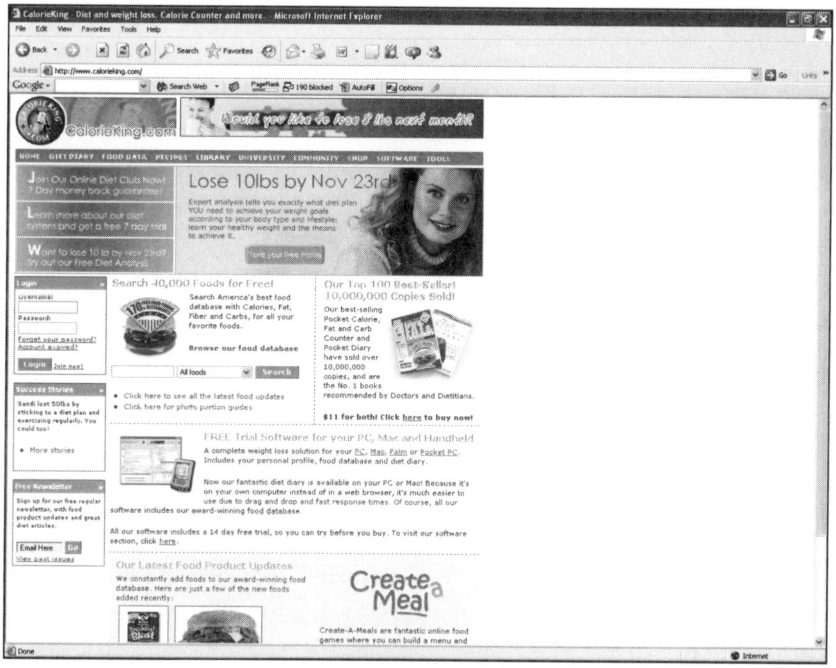

FIGURE 3.16 *CalorieKing.com offer page*

Some of the Best Support Sites on the Internet

There are many support sites on the Internet—many, many sites. We scoured the Internet for the best health and fitness support sites and picked a few to profile based on their breadth or uniqueness. While no site is perfect, there are many excellent choices to support you through your changing lifestyle. You'll probably use one for most of your needs and others for variety and different points of view.

MORE SPECIFIC INFO IN OTHER CHAPTERS

This chapter concentrates on relatively generic support sites. We'll cover more specific sites, such as sites for men only, women only, kids only, and so on, in Chapter 5, "Healthy, Fit, and Well." Appendix A, "Sites for Specific Diseases and Conditions," covers support for specific health issues, and Chapter 7 covers shopping sites for health and fitness equipment and diet products.

About.com

Free

http://www.about.com/food

http://www.about.com/health

Summary: Lots of content, good community, innovative features on its message boards

There is a lot of content on About.com. With more than 20 million visitors monthly, there had better be. Founded as the Mining Company in 1997 by Scott Kurnit, an early pioneer in the online world, About.com was renamed in 1999 and purchased by Primedia in 2000, toward the end of the dot-com boom.

There are 23 content channels, 475 content guides, and 50,000 topics on About.com, ranging from sports to politics to relationships to science. There are more than one million original content articles on About.com. Each category is organized in much the same way, with subcategories along the side of the page, a featured article along the top, resources in the middle, and ads along the side and bottom of the page. There's also a feature that shows the articles that are the most popular with readers on the site, but this hardly qualifies as community. You can also subscribe to a featured newsletter on your topic of interest.

Each area has a guide, hired by About.com to serve as the resident expert on the topic. Guides provide solutions, tips, and advice, as well as links to their favorite related Internet sites. There are also forums for members to discuss these topics. The forums are fairly well traveled, but there's not much more on About.com that relates to community.

Think of About.com as the *USA Today* of the reference world, offering quick tips and advice about a myriad of subjects. All of the content on About.com is free; the site generates its revenue from advertising.

Two of the categories relate directly to us—Food & Drink and Health & Fitness (see Figures 3.17 and 3.18). We'll concentrate on those here.

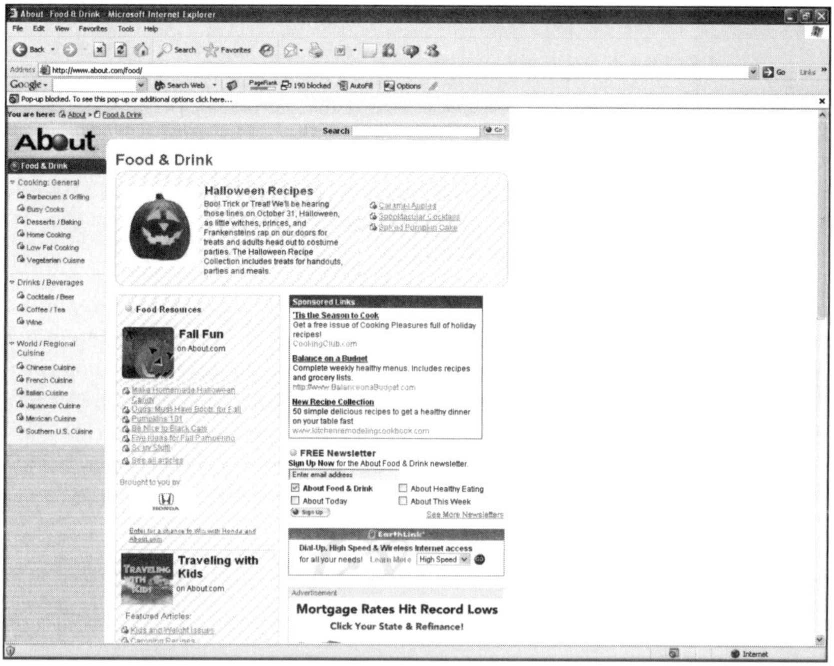

FIGURE 3.17 *About.com Food & Drink page*

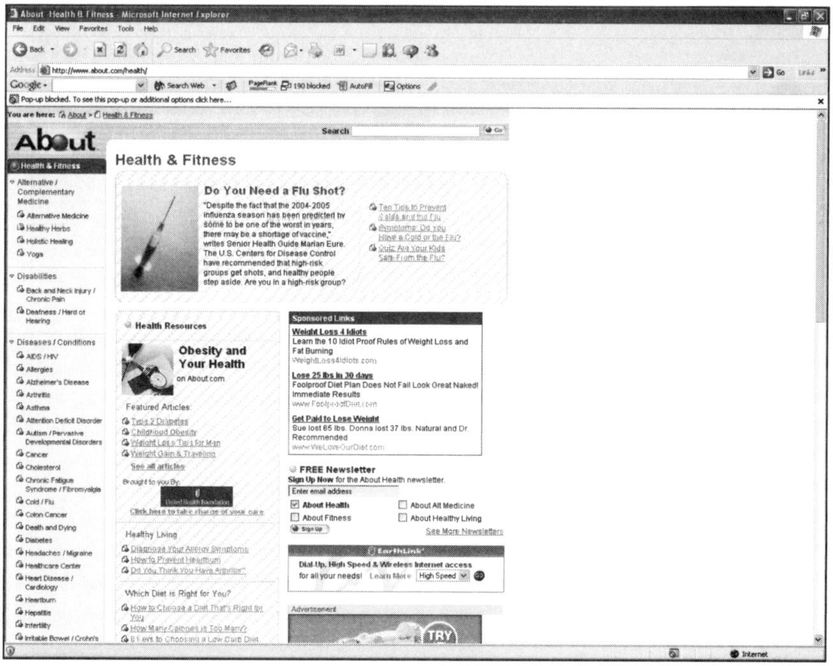

FIGURE 3.18 *About.com Health & Fitness page*

About.com Food & Drink

About.com's Food & Drink site is filled with easy-to-find information. A general cooking area divides information into types of cooking—barbequing and grilling, cooking for busy people, desserts and baking, home cooking, low-fat cooking, and vegetarian cooking. There are also areas for drinks and beverages and for world and regional cuisines. Each section includes a guide, who helps select the content for the area and provides overall editorial direction. In all, there are 15 separate sections in the Food & Drink area. The area home page is basically a "best of" compilation from all the other sections.

In Barbeques & Grilling, for example (see Figure 3.19), there are a lot of top and most popular lists, such as the top 10 smokers and the top 25 recipes. However, there are also helpful recipes of the week and a recipe archive; a FAQ about barbeques and grilling; lots of recipes, sauces, and secrets; grilling forums; a buyer's guide; special offers; and a resource library of articles and other information. There are also headings for most popular subjects and what's hot, which is determined by the section guide, as well as sponsored links that are purchased by advertisers. Each of the other general cooking sections is organized in a similar manner.

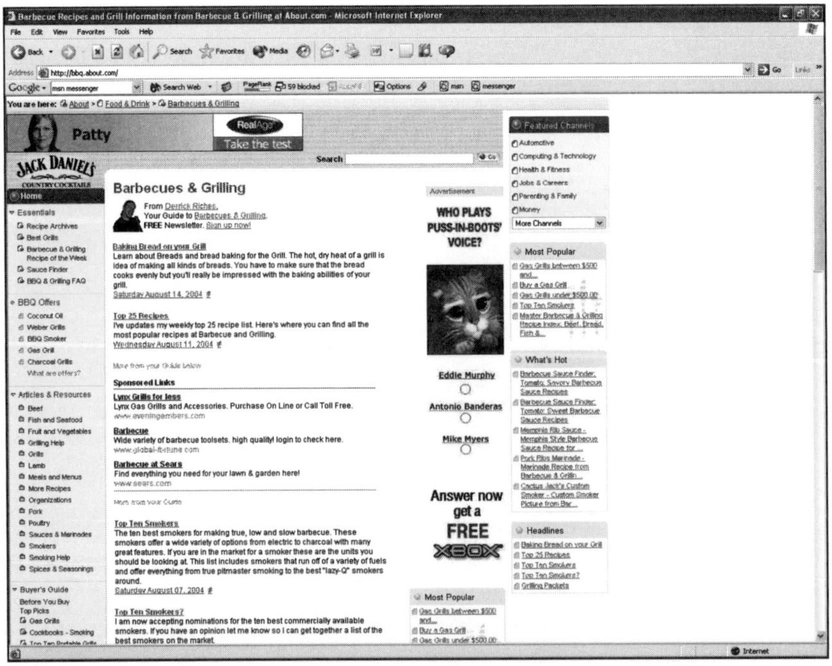

FIGURE 3.19 *About.com Barbeques & Grilling home page*

About.com Health & Fitness

While the Food & Drink area includes 15 sections, the Health & Fitness area is gigantic, with 67 separate sections on a dizzying array of topics. The main categories include Alternative & Complementary Medicine, Disabilities, Diseases & Conditions, Fitness & Wellness, Medicine & Allied Health, Mental Health, Recovery & Addiction, a Sponsored Section for PMDD, and a Women's Health area. The Health & Fitness area is extremely comprehensive, well trafficked, and popular. If you need support for something, it's probably here.

The Weight Loss area (see Figure 3.20) features tips on weight loss and dieting, lots of recipes, reviews of weight-loss products and books, a resource library, a buyer's guide, articles, lots of offers from sponsors, and a newsletter to which you can subscribe.

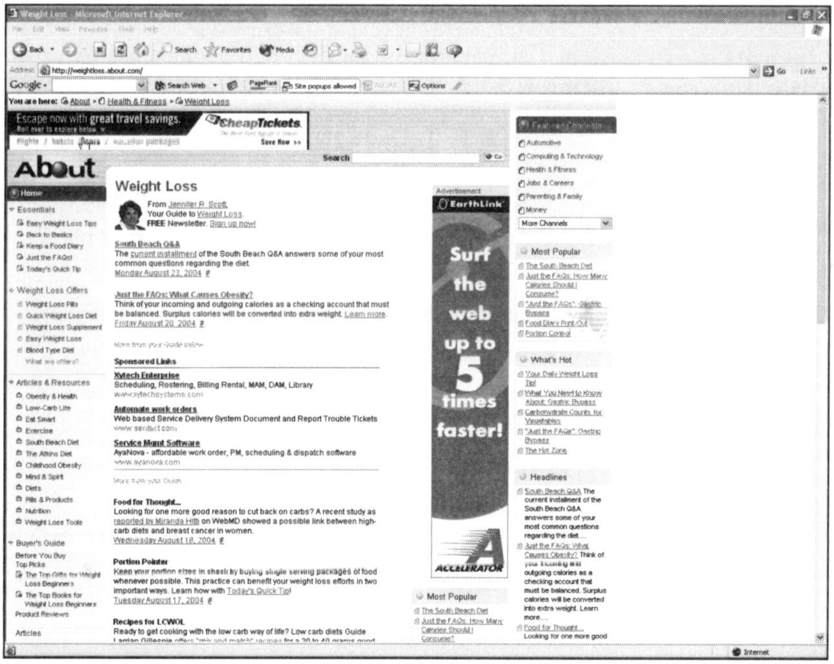

FIGURE 3.20 *About.com Weight Loss home page*

The message boards in the Weight Loss area are very active, with more than 60,000 messages in 15 message board categories when we visited (see Figure 3.21). The categories include:

- **General Discussion.** This category is fairly self explanatory. However, the more general an area is, the less helpful it's likely to be.
- **Journals.** This category allows users to share their thoughts and feelings during the process with others.

- **Ask & Answer.** This is a very active Q&A area.
- **Newbie Central.** This area is for those who are new to About.com.
- **Share Your Success.** This is a place for users to inspire each other with their accomplishments.
- **Good Eats.** This category includes favorite healthy foods, recipes, and other information.
- **Exercise Basics.** This category covers fitness in the weight loss process.
- **Commercial Archive.** This area contains ads for weight loss products.
- **Weight Loss Buddies.** Need a partner for your weight loss program? Find one here.
- **The Emotions Connection.** Are you an emotional eater? This section covers topics of interest to you.
- **Support & Motivation.** This category is for people who need a little extra push to help them stay on their diets.
- **The Crisis Line.** This category is for people who are having a lot of trouble staying motivated.
- **100 Pounds+.** This area is designed for those who have a lot of weight to lose.
- **Low-Fat/Reduced Calorie Diets.** This area covers all low-fat diet plans.

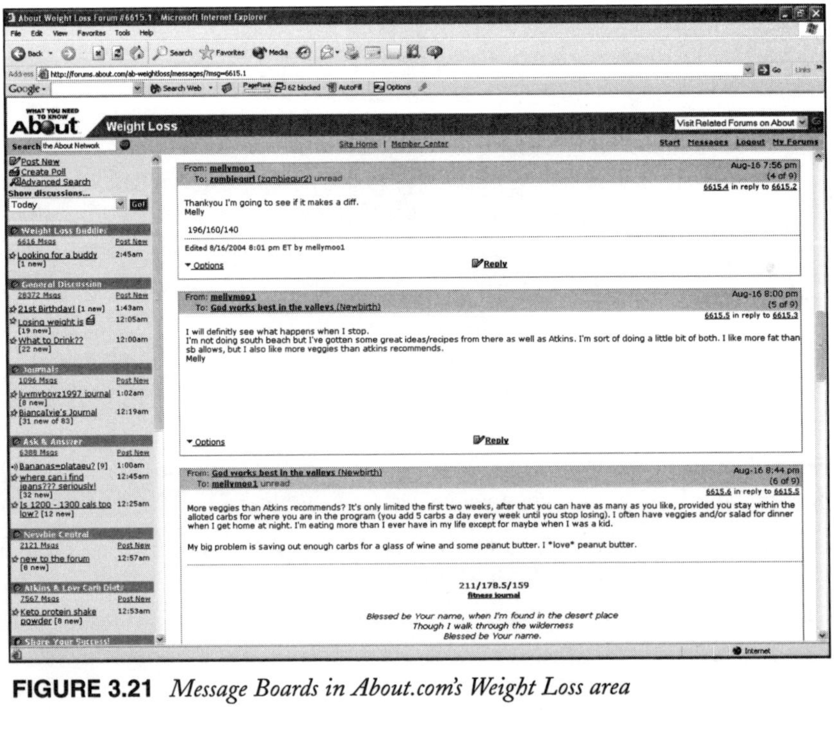

FIGURE 3.21 *Message Boards in About.com's Weight Loss area*

Note that ads and announcements are often interspersed with About.com's message boards. This is a unique way to get people who only go to the message boards to see other parts of the site. The idea is similar to the concept of pop-up ads for other programs that appear in the lower-left corner of the TV screen during TV shows.

One very innovative feature of About.com is its polling capabilities in the Message Boards area. You can create your own polls and set the parameters for them. We created a poll about weight loss (see Figure 3.22). We made the length of the poll seven days and got 50 responses. The results, shown in Figure 3.23, are surprising in that most people created their own diets and almost no one is on strictly a low-fat diet, although a lot of the folks who created their own said that a low-fat diet was part of their plan.

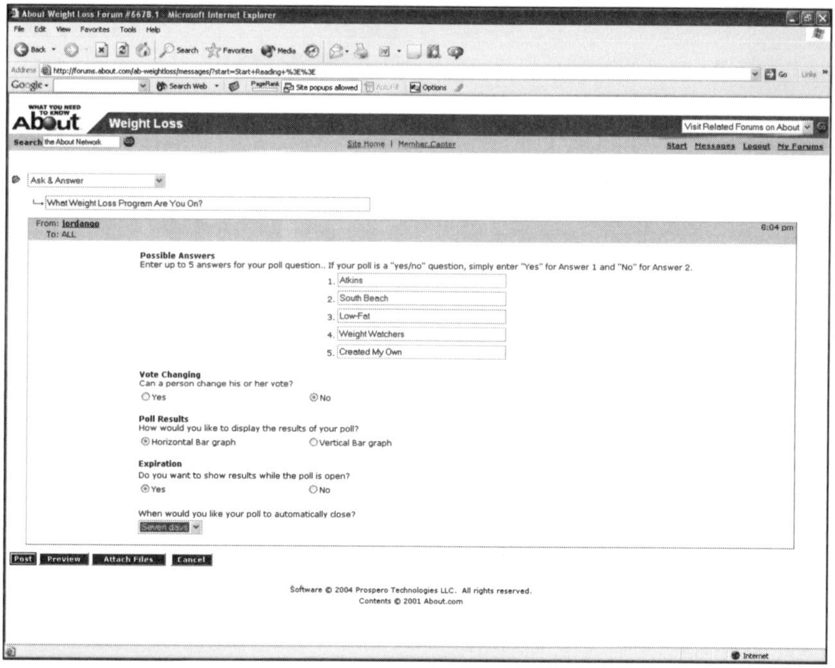

FIGURE 3.22 *Creating your own poll on About.com*

eDiets.com

$1.99 per week to $6.99 per week, depending on how many options you choose

http://www.eDiets.com

Summary: Tons of content and excellent community-building features make eDiets a great site for weight loss and healthy living.

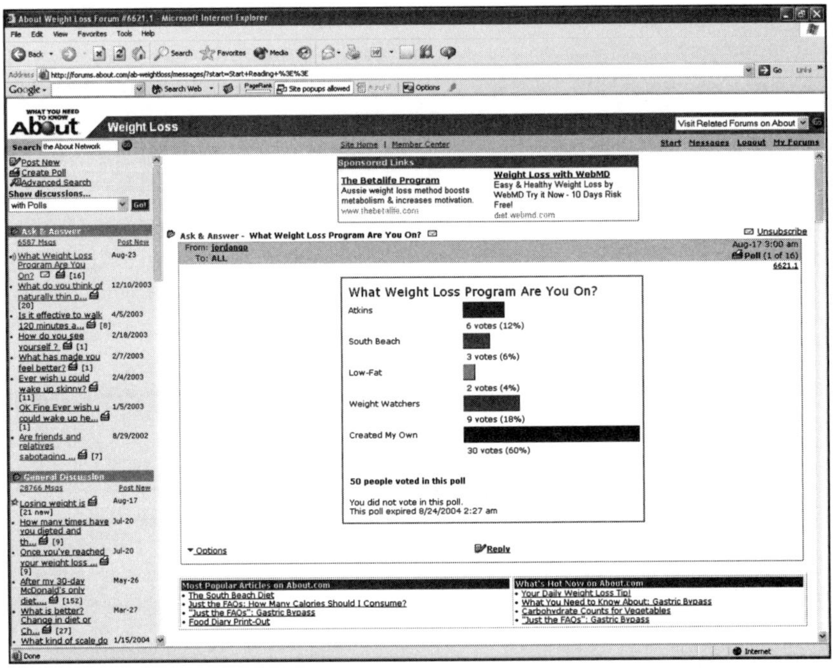

FIGURE 3.23 *Poll results on About.com*

eDiets.com is literally filled with support activities. It's easily one of the best support sites on the Internet. It features 13 newsletters, 20 diet plans, more than 100 message boards (eDiets calls them "Support Groups"), a mentoring program, a recipe club, a store, special offers, a fitness section, and much more. It is rich with content and community, although it lacks a little on the shopping side and it doesn't include a good food diary capability. But if you're interested in getting support for your weight loss efforts and learning as much as you possibly can, eDiets is the place to be.

The home page for eDiets support is eDiets Solutions, reached through http://www.ediets.com (see Figure 3.24). eDiets is supported by a large editorial and health and nutrition staff. As a result, there is a lot to choose from. On the content side, there are product reviews on the latest new foods (see Figure 3.25). Although they are not extensive, they include bite-sized (sorry) information about foods, including all relevant nutritional data and subjective opinions on taste and the overall healthiness of a food.

eDiets also includes articles from *Psychology Today* magazine and special health reports from Harvard Health Publications and Harvard Medical School. The *Psychology Today* articles are about topics such as motivation and the psychological factors in weight loss. The Harvard reports are more concrete, covering health issues such as weight loss, diabetes, healthy eating, stress, and heart disease (see Figure 3.26).

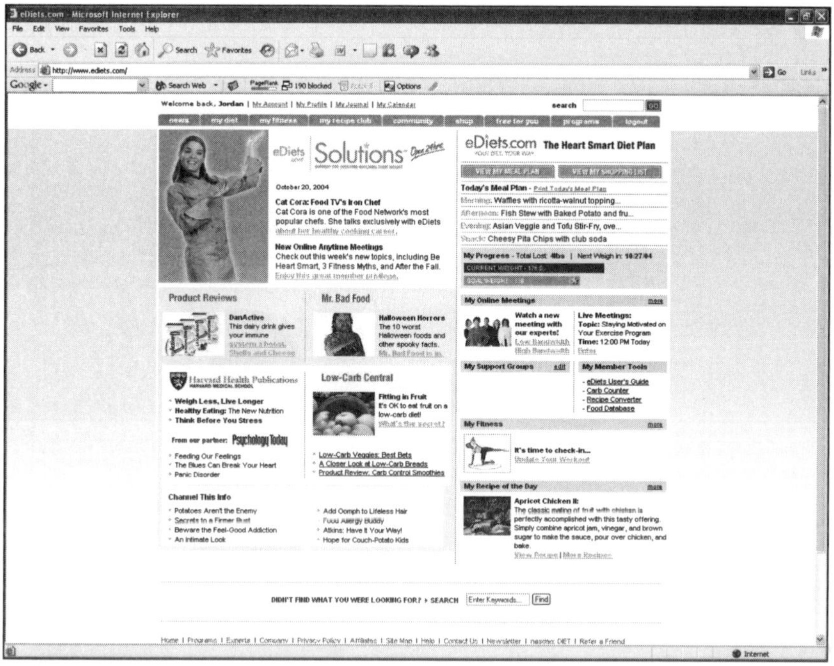

FIGURE 3.24 *eDiets Solutions home page*

ABOUT.COM'S 10 FOODS THAT SABOTAGE YOUR DIET

Although this list appeared in the low-carb section of About.com's Weight Loss area, these 10 foods will hurt you on any diet program.

- **Donuts.** We've mentioned these in other chapters already. There is nothing good about donuts. They are high in fat and simple carbohydrates, and they are loaded with trans-fats.
- **Margarine.** Thanks to trans-fats, most margarines are a bad choice. About.com suggests butter as an alternative. I suggest avoiding both whenever possible. Butter isn't called "the cow's revenge" for nothing.
- **Sugared cereals.** Simple carbs and trans-fats make for a bad combination.
- **Sports drinks.** Lots of sugar, plus they include some things that wind up in antifreeze!
- **Toaster pastries.** More trans-fats.
- **Chips.** Salt, trans-fats, and fats.
- **Sugared Sodas.** Lots of sugar and empty calories.
- **Bologna and hot dogs.** Lots of fat, sodium, and nitrites, with little nutritional value.
- **Crackers.** Lots of calories and trans-fats per cracker.

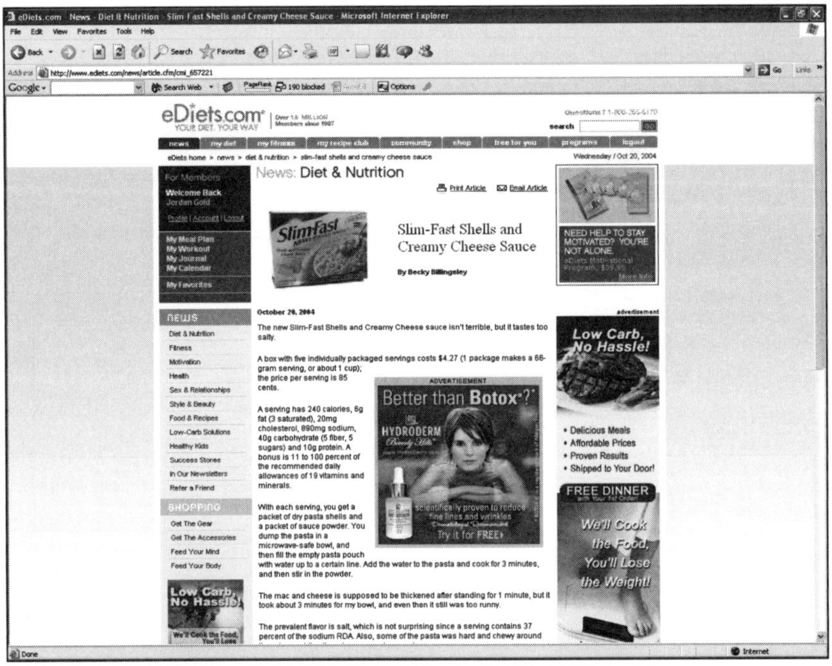

FIGURE 3.25 *An eDiets product review*

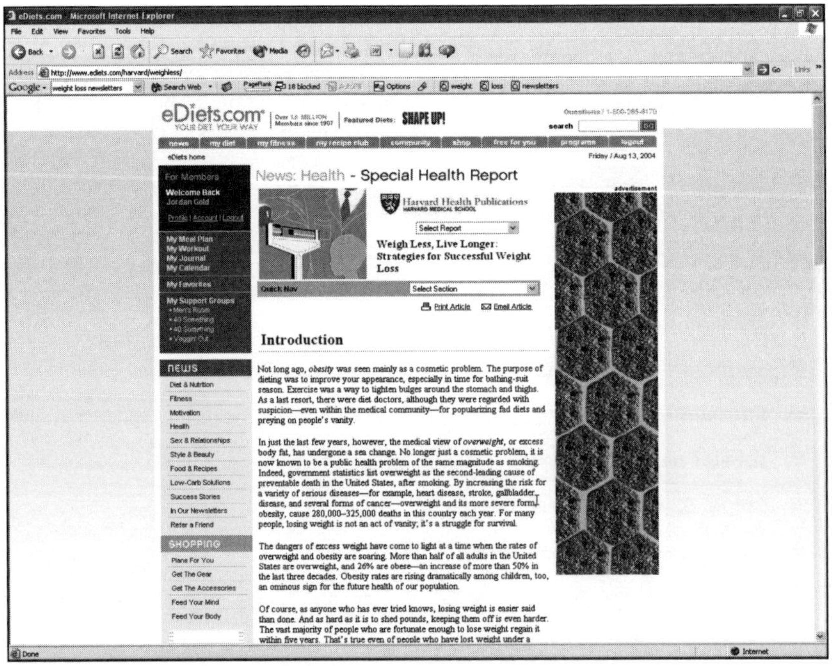

FIGURE 3.26 *Harvard Medical School health report on weight loss*

There are feature articles on celebrities who have lost weight or are involved in health and fitness in some way, polls, contests, and quizzes. There is also a news section that is really more of a collection of articles about various topics. It's broken into several channels, including Diet & Nutrition, Fitness, Motivation, Health, Sex & Relationships, Style & Beauty, Food & Recipes, Low-Carb Solutions, and Success Stories. Most of those channels have newsletters associated with them. Here's a description of each of eDiets.com's newsletters:

- **eDiets Extra! (Published twice per week).** Covers the latest trends in fitness and health, particularly focusing on fitness, healthy eating, and motivation. Free to anyone who completes a diet needs assessment (also free).
- **eDiets Exclusive (Published once per week).** A version of eDiets Extra! that's published once per week. It includes all of the information in Extra!, plus tips to help members get the most out of their eDiets membership.
- **Low-Carb Lifestyle (Published weekly).** Includes the latest information about low-carb diets, plus hints, tips, and recipes. Free to anyone.
- **Living with Diabetes (Published weekly).** Includes success stories, product reviews, recipes, and inspiration for people living with diabetes. Free to anyone.
- **eFitness Extra! (Published weekly).** Workout, nutrition, sex, and health advice from the folks at eFitness.com (which is owned by eDiets). Feature articles from fitness experts. Free to anyone.
- **Healthy Hearts (Published weekly).** Covers heart-related issues including hypertension, stress, cholesterol, and heart disease. Also includes recipes and product reviews.
- **Dr. Perricone's Beauty Secrets (Published every other week).** Beauty tips from dermatologist Dr. Nicholas Perricone, author of several best-selling books about dermatology and looking and feeling younger. Free to anyone.
- **Healthy Kids (Published weekly).** Tackles the issues related to childhood obesity with weight-management strategies, exercises, and recipes designed for children. Free to anyone.
- **Psyched for Success (Published every other week).** Motivational newsletter designed to help people achieve their goals. Published in conjunction with *Psychology Today.*
- **Worst Foods (Published weekly).** Concentrates on the foods you shouldn't eat. Describes them in detail and explains why they're bad for you. Free to anyone.
- **eDiets Sex Factor (Published every other week).** Features sex and relationship tips from Laura Corn, a self-described sexpert. Free to anyone.
- **Daily Horoscope (Published daily).** Astrological data for everyone. Free to anyone.
- **Daily Bytes (Published daily).** Diet and fitness tips plus a recipe of the day. Free to anyone.

The community features on eDiets are excellent, with online meetings, a mentor program, message boards, chat rooms, profiles of other members, and help from experts. Other support features include a wide-ranging fitness program and a customizable and powerful recipe database called the Recipe Club.

Online Meetings

eDiets is serious about online meetings. The Web site hosts six or seven online meetings each day, with either experts in the field or the nutrition support team at eDiets leading the meetings. Each of the major eDiets channels hosts these meetings on topics ranging from staying motivated to primers on various diets to fitness to current events.

Users can either attend meetings in real time or watch them later; eDiets archives selected meetings for later viewing by members (see Figure 3.27). A scheduling feature allows members to add meetings of interest to their daily calendar to ensure that they don't miss something they really want to attend.

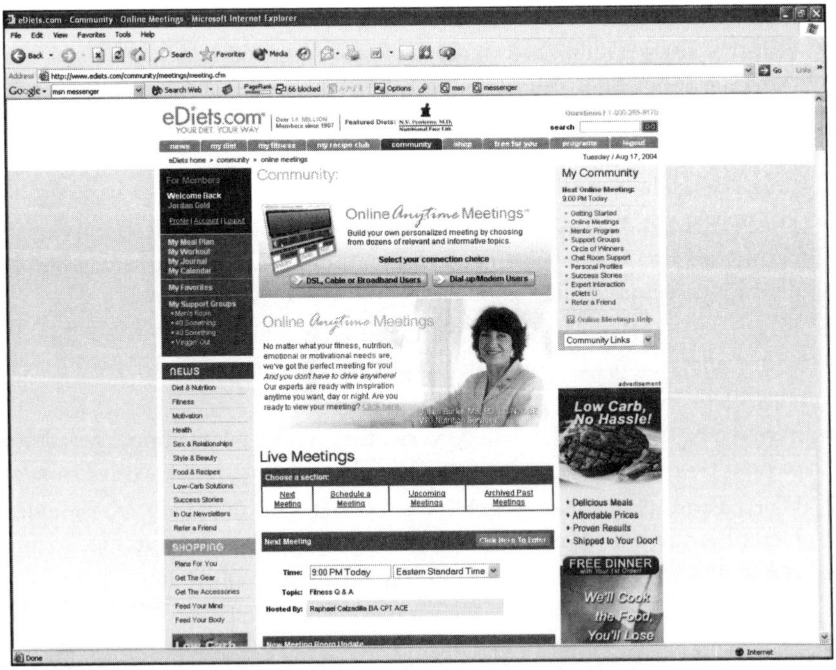

FIGURE 3.27 *Online meetings*

Mentor Program

eDiets' mentor program helps both the mentor and the beginner being mentored. For one thing, it's quite a compliment to become a mentor because it tells the person that he or she has succeeded and is now ready to help others. For another, mentors get a free membership in eDiets beginning with their third week of mentoring and lasting as long they are mentors.

To be a mentor, an eDiets member has to follow very specific guidelines (see Figure 3.28). For example, mentors must have been part of the program for at least six weeks and have weighed in four times in that span. They have to contact their assigned beginner at least once in the first 24 hours, send supportive e-mails several times per week, protect their privacy, and keep the relationship to eDiets only, not allowing it to get too personal.

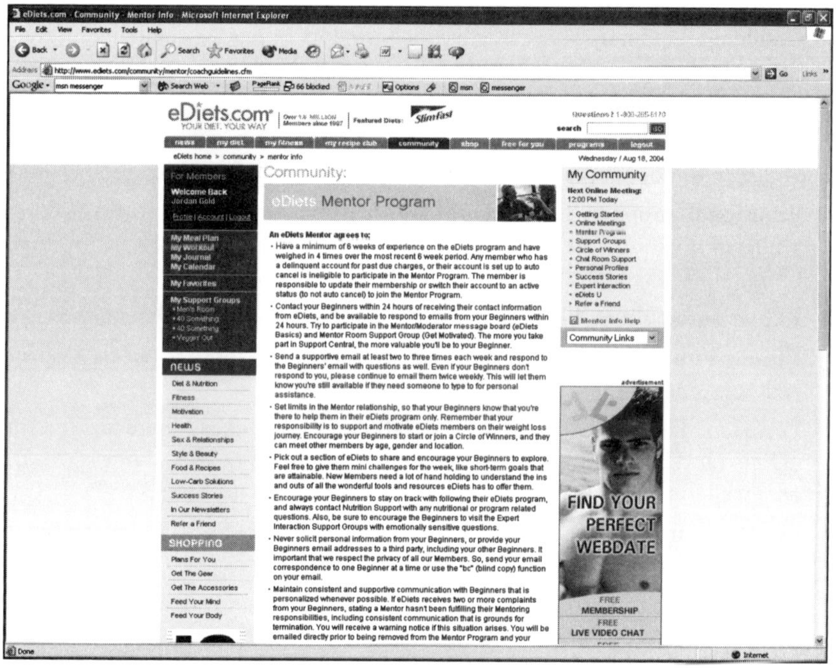

FIGURE 3.28 *eDiets mentor program guidelines*

On the flip side, beginners also have responsibilities. They, too, have to limit the relationship to eDiets topics only, and not allow the relationship to get too personal. They have to protect the mentor's privacy. And, for the month they are being mentored, they have to communicate and ask questions about features of the program that they don't understand.

Support Groups

Most other sites call them message boards or forums, but eDiets calls them Support Groups. Whatever the name, there are a ton of them online (see Figure 3.29), ranging from general topics (eDiets 101) to specific ones (there are 29 different Support Groups for nearly all major diets, regardless of whether they are offered on eDiets). Each Support Group has a moderator who keeps things under control, guides conversations, and comes up with topics when necessary.

The more than 100 Support Groups are organized into 14 categories:

- **Diet Support Groups.** The diet plans on eDiets each have their own support group, as do plans that aren't unique to eDiets, such as South Beach, Dr. Dean Ornish, Slim-Fast, Weight Watchers, and Jenny Craig.
- **Age-Related.** These are forums for 20-, 30-, 40-, and 50-year-olds, plus seniors.
- **Around the World.** These are Support Groups for Canadians, Europeans, Spanish-speakers, and other international groups. There are more of these groups to come as eDiets expands its membership base.
- **Challenge Yourself.** This category includes lots of fitness challenges. (See the sidebar for more details on the Ultimate Challenge, a 21-day event that is based on eating well and exercising.)
- **eDiets Basics.** This category provides support for basic issues, such as beginners getting started, people trying to maintain their weight, and veterans, among others.
- **Emotional Support.** These boards provide help for people fighting addictions of all kinds, motivational help, and help for those who are trying to get back on the weight-loss wagon.
- **Expert Interaction.** This area provides a little help from eDiets experts.
- **Fitness Fun.** This category contains several boards about a variety of fitness activities, including walking and running.
- **For Men.** There's even a board that talks sports! Because there aren't many men on eDiets (and because there are much better message boards about sports), this isn't a very well-traveled message board; it gets almost no activity.
- **For Women.** This is a much more active group of boards, including boards for new moms, brides-to-be, career women, and more.
- **Get Motivated.** Boards here help you find a diet buddy, reach your goals, get motivated, and improve your spirituality. There's also a Support Group for mentors in this section.
- **Group Headquarters.** Several companies have adopted eDiets as their weight loss program of choice. Message boards for those companies are located here.
- **Just For Me.** This is where the most specialized Support Groups reside. There are groups for people looking to lose 100 pounds or more, people looking to lose 50 pounds, singles, students, gays and lesbians, and a wide variety of other options. Some boards, such as the 50 Plus Club, even have their own Web sites with pictures and profiles of the active members.
- **Miscellaneous.** Then there are the Support Groups that don't fit into any of the aforementioned categories, including groups for people who are trying to reduce clutter, people interested in crafts, folks who want to learn HTML, and others.

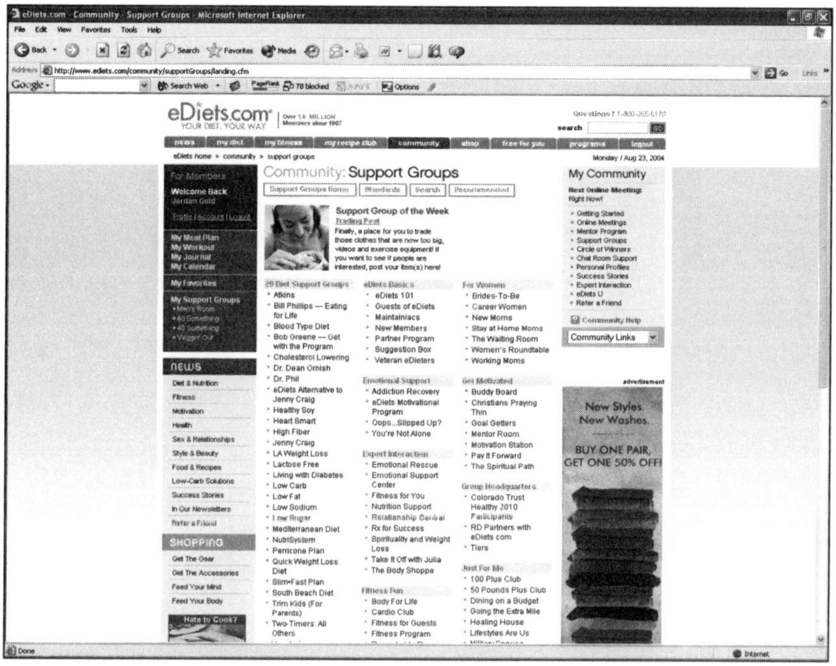

FIGURE 3.29 *eDiets Support Groups*

THE ULTIMATE CHALLENGE

In the Ultimate Challenge, members pledge to lose a certain number of pounds over a 21-day period (eDiets recommends losing only 1–2 pounds per week), combined with a certain amount of exercise (eDiets recommends 150 minutes per week for beginners). The idea is to teach members new life skills and to help them develop habits that result in a healthier lifestyle.

There are several rules that must be followed: Members must drink at least 64 ounces of water daily, stay on their meal plans daily, and have 21 days in a row of making their calorie allotment (see Figure 3.30). If they don't, they have to start over. After all, it takes about 21 days to create habits that will stay with you for a lifetime.

Members join the challenge in teams of eight. Each team has a captain. The idea is to motivate users and to support each other. At the end of the challenge, each team selects its Most Valuable Player (MVP). Winners are chosen based on the percentage of pounds lost versus pledged, percent of exercise done versus pledged, and the overall percentage.

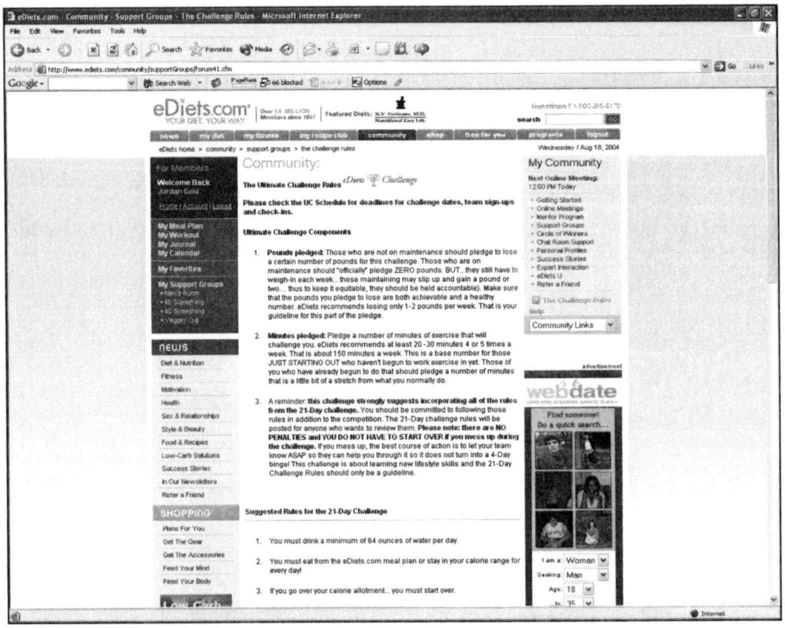

FIGURE 3.30 *The Ultimate Challenge*

Chat Rooms

As shown in Figure 3.31, a variety of chat rooms are available on eDiets at all times. Some are intended for specialized groups, such as 100+ members or mentors, while others are focused on general chats, such as motivation, fitness, or community.

Fitness Programs

eDiets' fitness program includes a workout diary, suggested workouts, links to fitness tools, a virtual trainer, guidelines for exercise, and a store where you can buy products. The virtual fitness trainer shows you how to do a wide variety of exercises (see Figure 3.32). You tell the program which exercise you're doing and which part of your body you're working on, and it shows you how to do it, with very specific instructions for each step. An animation shows the proper way to exercise.

Recipe Club

eDiets' Recipe Club is a powerful product that lets users exchange recipes and find new ones (see Figure 3.33). A helpful feature lets you find recipes that meet certain nutritional requirements, such as finding all sandwiches with 400 calories per serving that have less than 25% of their calories from fat (see Figure 3.34). After trying these recipes, users can rate and review them (see Figure 3.35).

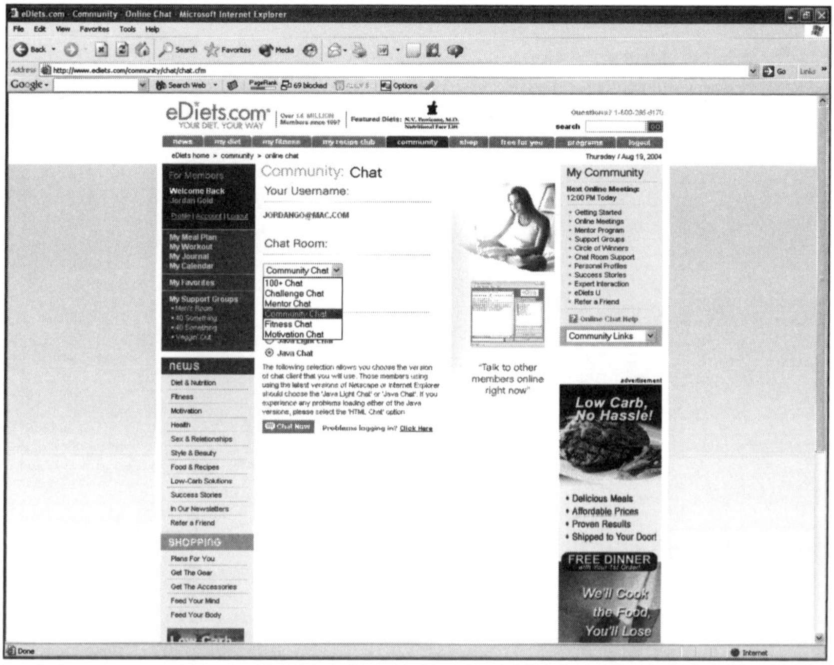

FIGURE 3.31 *Chat rooms*

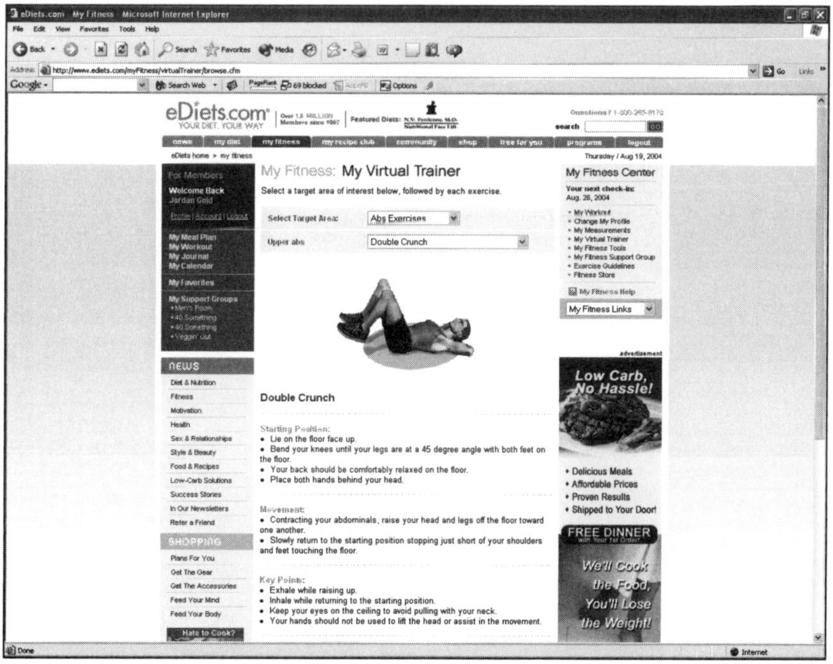

FIGURE 3.32 *Virtual fitness trainer*

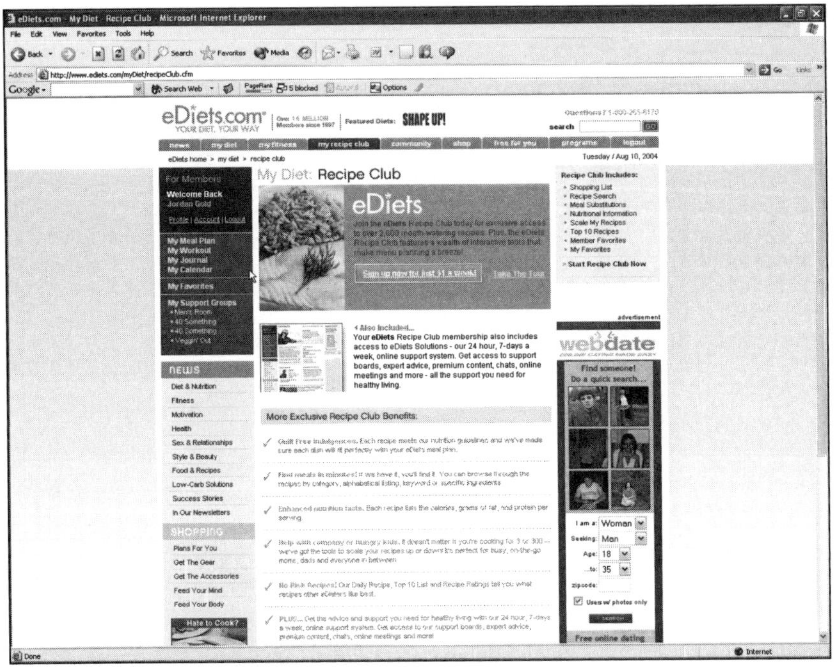

FIGURE 3.33 *Recipe Club*

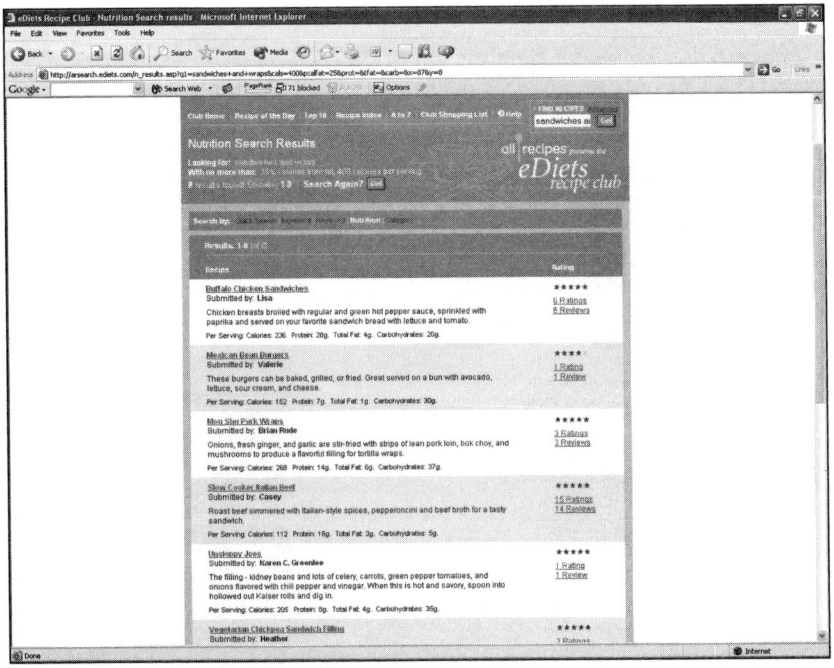

FIGURE 3.34 *Recipe Club search results for sandwiches and wraps*

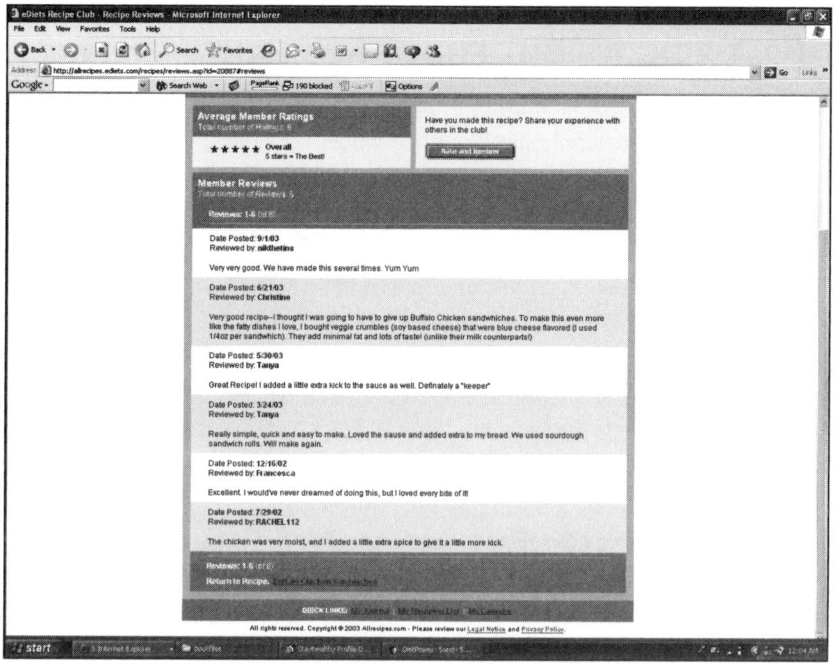

FIGURE 3.35 *A Recipe Club review*

LOSING WEIGHT FROM THE HEART

On September 3, 2002, Lynn Key of Oklahoma City thought something was wrong. She was having chest pains and felt funny, so she decided she was having a heart attack. Key's weight was at an all-time high at this point. At 48 years old and 5'6", she weighed 314 pounds.

After waiting a few days, with the symptoms still persisting, Key went to the doctor and had him do an EKG. It turned out to be heartburn. After she read that heartburn is often a sign of heart problems, Key decided to make some drastic changes in her life.

Key had tried many ways to lose weight and had failed each time. After leaving her doctor's office, she was determined to never experience such feelings again, and she decided that losing weight was the key to this.

She prayed for the Lord to lead her in the right direction. "When I turned on the computer, there was an ad for eDiets on it," she says. She took this as a sign from above. "I liked this idea because it was private and no one had to know that I was going to give it another attempt."

Key chose a standard eDiets plan, nothing based on any special program. "I wanted a generic plan," she says. "I wanted to eat based on portion control."

LOSING WEIGHT FROM THE HEART *(CONTINUED)*

After starting eDiets, Key learned to eat in moderation and began her journey to 150 pounds, which is her goal. She thought it would take her a year. So far, she has lost 97 pounds, getting her weight down to 217. It's taken her nearly two years to lose 100 pounds, and she still has another 67 to go. She is somewhat impatient with the results.

"I thought it would take me less time than it has," she says. "However, I see that taking it off this slowly really makes it harder to put back on."

Besides changing her diet, Key has increased her exercise level dramatically. She is planning to ride in the "Hotter 'N Hell Hundred," a bicycle race in Wichita Falls, Texas, that takes place each August. She rides about 170 miles per week on a regular basis, an activity that really helps burn those calories.

Key has been an active user of the support features of eDiets. "At first, I read everything on the site," she says. She looked at everything she could to inspire her, including message boards, success stories, and before and after pictures. She also took many of the exercise challenges.

In addition to eDiets, Key likes FitDay. She likes the educational areas on FitDay, particularly the graphs and charts that teach the finer points of weight loss. "I learned to keep trying through FitDay," she says. "Too many people try and give up after a bad day or two," she says. "I learned that one or two bad days isn't going to derail a weight loss plan. I've learned to never give up."

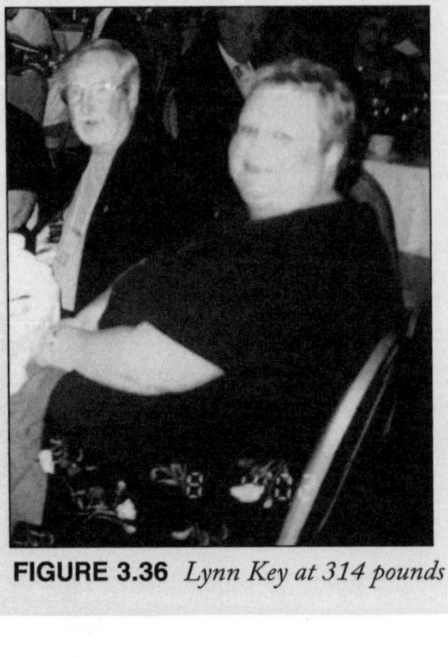

FIGURE 3.36 *Lynn Key at 314 pounds*

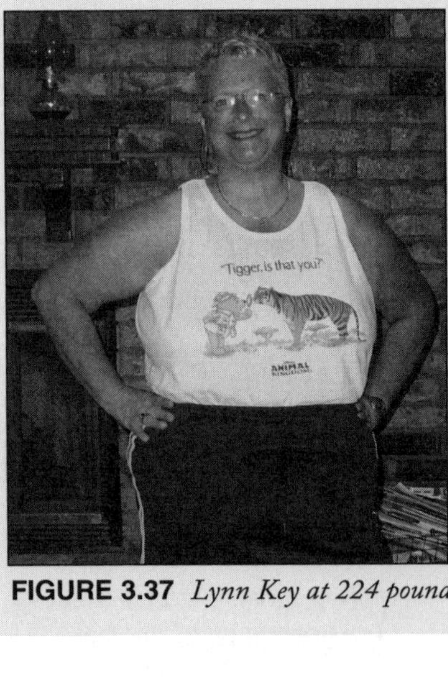

FIGURE 3.37 *Lynn Key at 224 pounds*

Prevention.com

Free support site, except for Walk Off Weight area, which costs $5.95 per month for a minimum of three months, or $69.95 per year

http://www.prevention.com

Summary: The quizzes alone make this an interesting site; the South Beach diet area is one of the busiest message boards on the Internet

Prevention magazine has a great online site that goes well beyond what's offered in the magazine (see Figure 3.38). The magazine and Web site both have the same mission statement—"Smart Ways to Live Well"—and the site fulfills its purpose. Prevention.com features articles from the magazine, news tips, recipes, expert advice, message boards, quizzes, and polls. There's also a store, but it only sells books from Prevention's parent company, Rodale. Rodale hit the jackpot with the South Beach diet series, and Prevention.com is home to the most trafficked South Beach diet message boards and a special site devoted to the diet. There's a lot here, and a lot to explore.

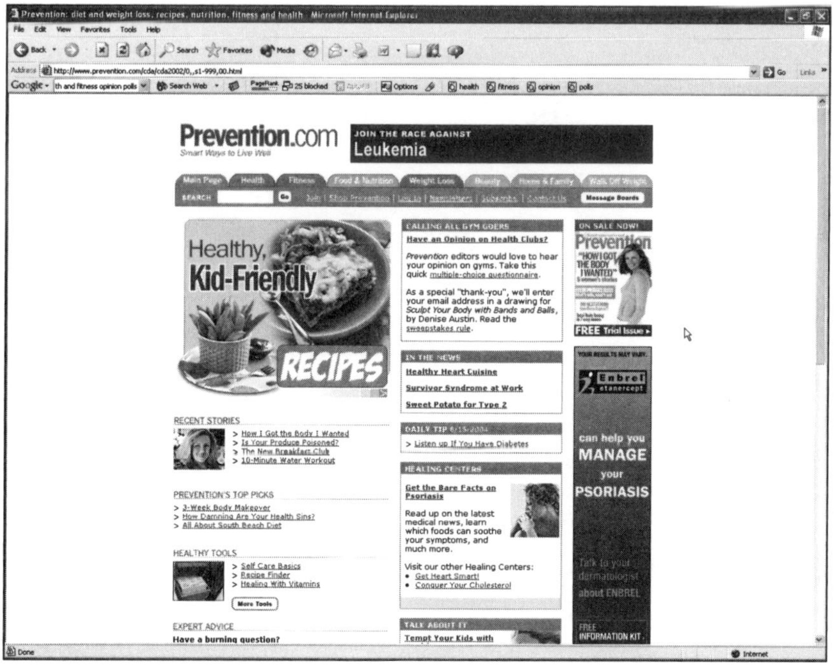

FIGURE 3.38 *Prevention.com*

Celebrating its 55th birthday in 2005, *Prevention* magazine has undergone a renaissance of sorts over the last few years and claims a monthly readership of nearly 12 million. The magazine was redesigned in January, 2004, and is focused on health issues primarily pertaining to women and children. Although it's not strictly a "for women" magazine, women make up just over 80% of the readership.

Much like the offline magazine, Prevention.com is organized into seven sections—Health, Fitness, Food & Nutrition, Weight Loss, Beauty, Home & Family, and Walk Off Weight (see Figure 3.39). Each section features news, articles, tools, top picks, quizzes, and expert advice. Prevention.com features experts on a number of topics, from senior health to women's health, to fitness, weight loss, and beauty.

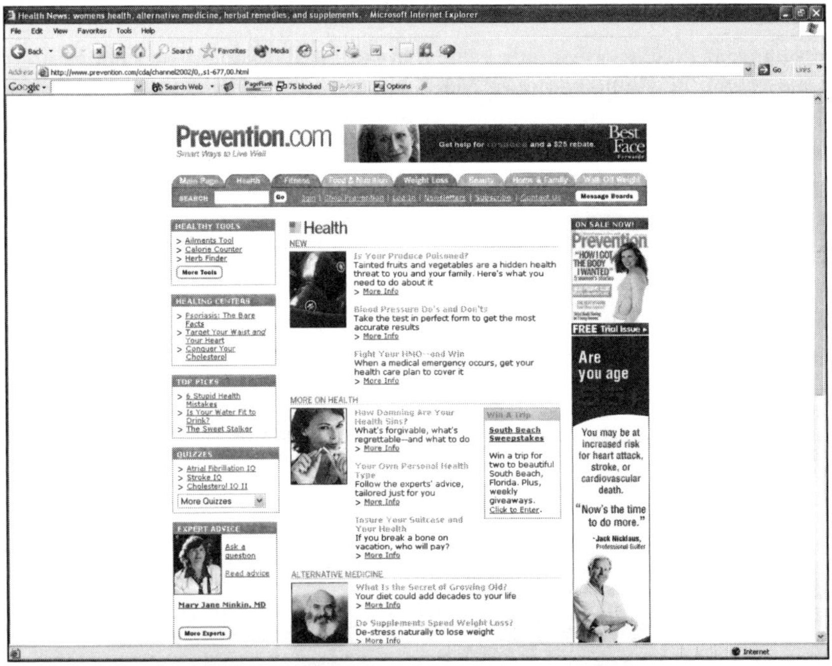

FIGURE 3.39 *Prevention.com Health page*

There is also a store where you can buy Rodale Press books and subscribe to *Prevention* magazine or any of 29 newsletters. And, there are message boards on a variety of topics.

Message Boards

One of the most extraordinary things you'll see when visiting Prevention.com's home page for message boards is the traffic (see Figure 3.40). Most of the sites are fairly well traveled, but one site completely dwarfs all others. As of August, 2004, Prevention.com's South Beach Diet forum was one of the busiest on the Internet, with 46,643 topics and 671,519 messages. The other nine categories combined had 5,893 topics and 50,397 messages, so about 90% of the traffic on Prevention.com's 10 message boards is on one.

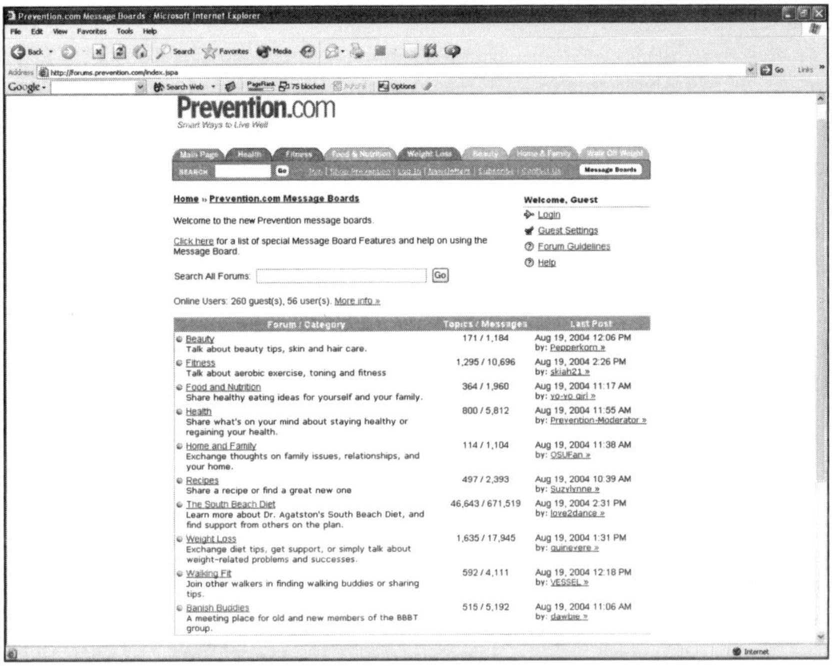

FIGURE 3.40 *Prevention.com's message boards home page*

If you are following the South Beach diet, it's a great place to go. Although South Beach Diet Online (http://www.southbeachdiet.com) offers more in the way of meal plans, Prevention.com provides a tremendous amount of support. There are message threads for people who started the diet the same day you did, so you can each share in the issues associated with Phase One of South Beach. There are also threads for people on each phase of the diet and a variety of other South Beach diet topics (see Figure 3.41).

In addition to the message boards, Prevention.com devotes part of its Weight Loss section to the South Beach diet, with news, articles, FAQs, and recipes (see Figure 3.42). There are also food guides and the transcripts of chats with Dr. Arthur Agatston, the founder of the diet and the author of the mega-selling books.

Newsletters

Prevention.com publishes 25 free newsletters, many on unique topics such as macular degeneration, lung issues, and Alzheimer's and other diseases. We'll provide more details on this in Appendix A, "Sites for Specific Diseases and Conditions." Other newsletters are more general, focusing on weight loss, skin care, recipes, and overall site news (see Figure 3.43).

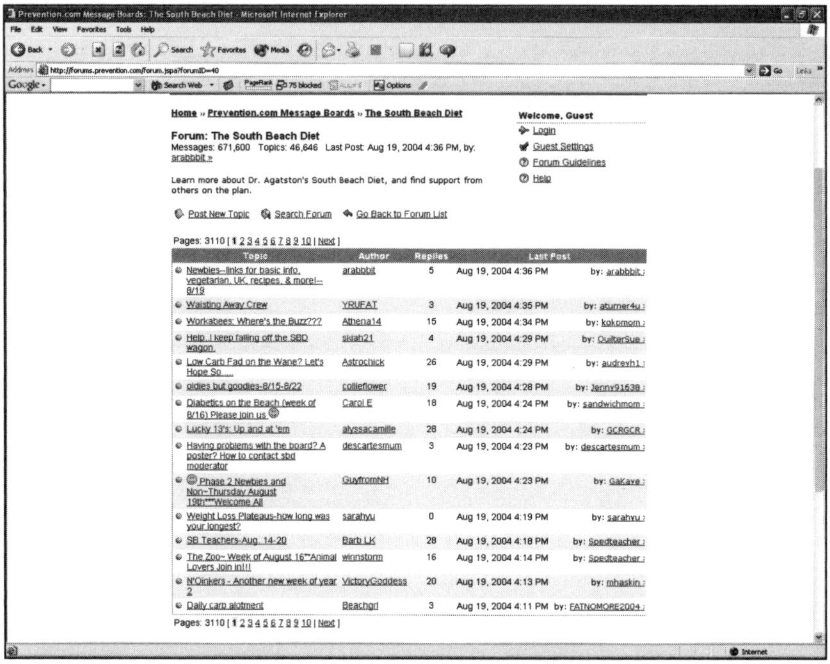

FIGURE 3.41 *The South Beach Diet forum on Prevention.com*

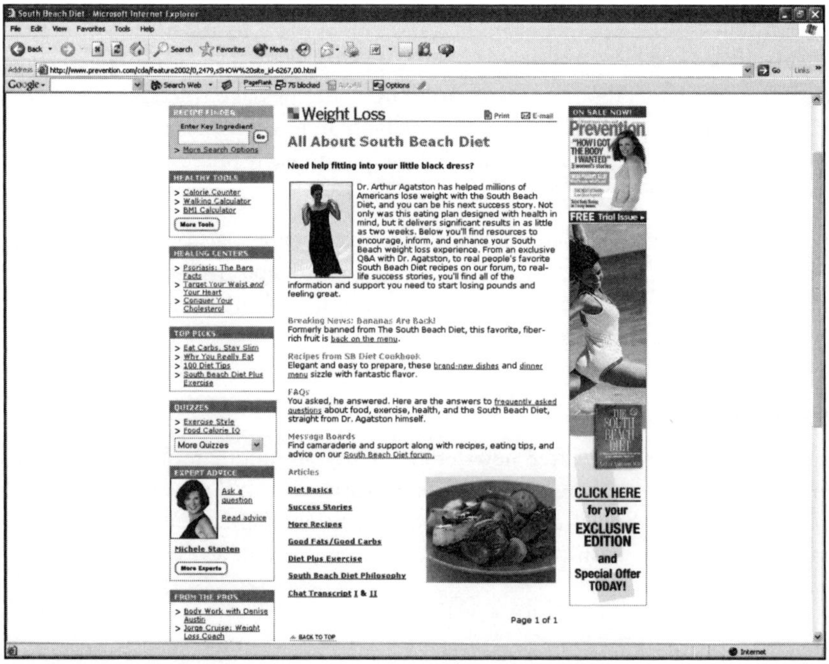

FIGURE 3.42 *All about the South Beach diet on Prevention.com*

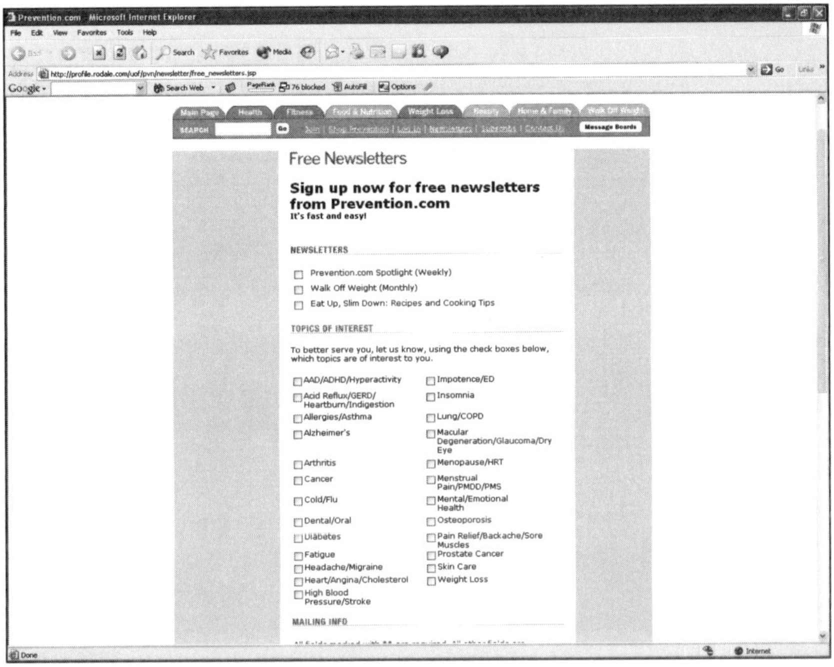

FIGURE 3.43 *Prevention.com newsletter list*

Walk Off Weight Program

Prevention.com features a program called Walk Off Weight that helps people lose weight by exercising (see Figure 3.44). The site includes product reviews, tips and techniques, FAQs, inspirational stories, quizzes, a walking calculator, and a calorie counter, among other things. Joining the program gets you customized walking plans that gradually increase your fitness activities to as many as 15,000 steps per day. As you progress, the program introduces strength training and other exercises in addition to walking, and also includes a personalized nutrition program. The cost of the program is either $5.95 per month or $69.95 per year.

Shape Up America!

Free sponsored membership

http://www.shapeup.org

Summary: Great nonprofit site with lots of content in a no-frills package

In 1994, former surgeon general C. Everett Koop founded Shape Up America!, a nonprofit Web site dedicated to raising awareness about the health effects of obesity and providing responsible information about weight management to the public, as well as health care professionals (see Figure 3.45).

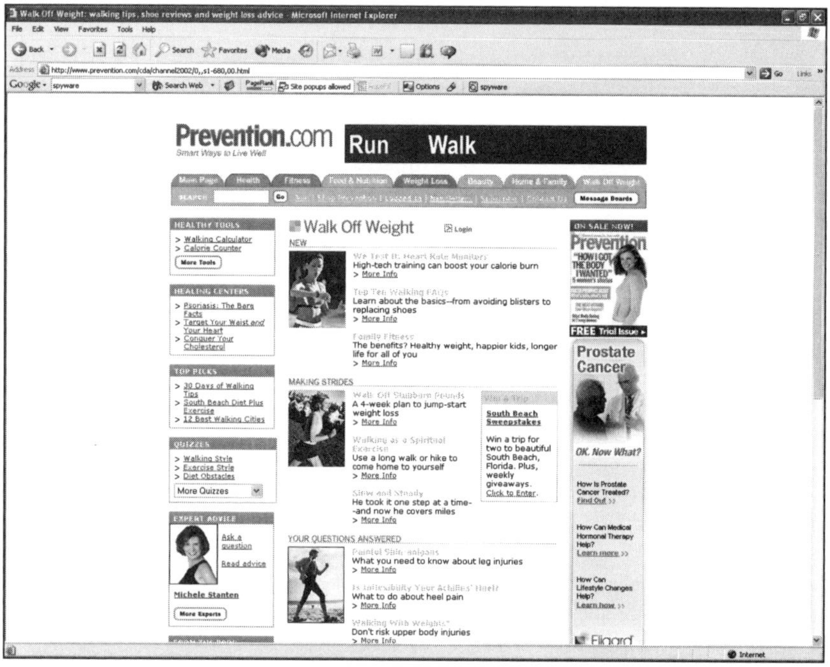

FIGURE 3.44 *Walk off Weight home page*

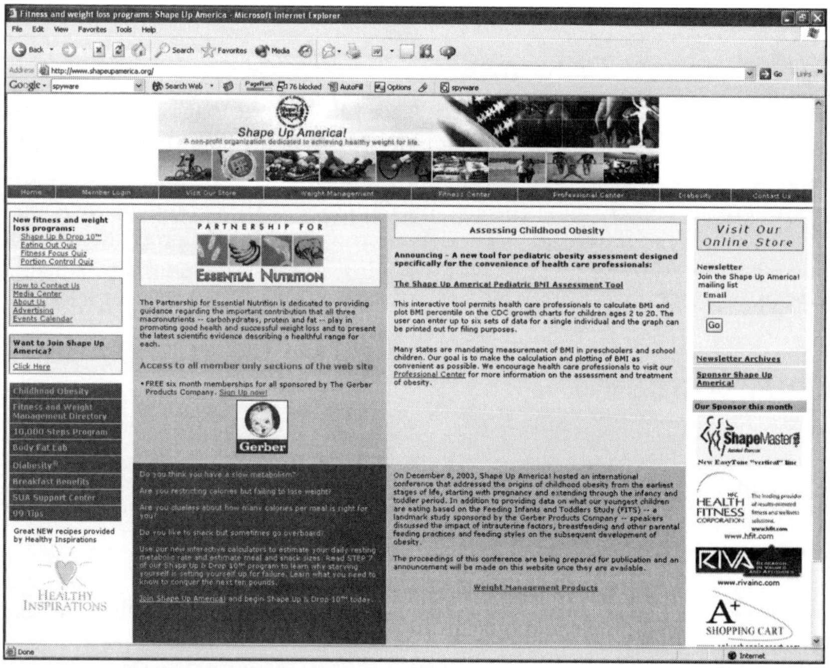

FIGURE 3.45 *Shape Up America! home page*

Shape Up America! is a phenomenal reference for fitness and health information. Although it has no real community features, it offers a wealth of highly accessible content about diet and exercise, including weight management and fitness areas, a variety of quizzes to test your knowledge about fitness and health, a store, and an area for professionals. There's also a regular newsletter.

At this writing, free six-month memberships to Shape Up America! were being offered by the Gerber Corporation to anyone who wanted one. The membership section includes two calculators—a meal and snack calculator and a metabolism calculator—plus a recipe section and a support area.

Shape Up America! bills itself as "A non-profit organization dedicated to achieving healthy weight for life." As a result, Shape Up America! is against dieting and in favor of changing eating habits. It has a point of view that the really healthy way to eat is to control portions, limit fats, and eat plenty of fresh fruits, whole grains, and vegetables. It also believes that physical activity is essential. It does not believe that low-carb diets are healthy or that any program in which you lose a lot of weight quickly is a good idea.

Shape Up America! is not a fancy Web site; it just has a lot of good information. The Cyberkitchen, for example, is a simple meal-planning system that helps you lose as much as one pound per week through a variety of meal plans. You select the foods for the meal plans, and Cyberkitchen does the calculating as far as calories are concerned. The program does not let you choose a plan that limits your calories to more than 500 fewer than your daily allotment, thereby forcing you to lose weight slowly. At the end of the day, it shows you how many calories you've consumed versus your goal (see Figure 3.46). The program automatically creates recipes and a shopping list for your daily foods.

Fitness Center

The Fitness Center is an ingenious place that provides a clear picture of your fitness level (see Figure 3.47). After you answer a series of short questionnaires, the Web site assesses your activity level. Then, after you time yourself in a 1.5-mile run, the Web site assesses your fitness level. You then take this information to determine how many calories you should consume each day. The Fitness Center includes areas that provide tips for improving your fitness level, with suggestions for gradually increasing your fitness activities. It helps you overcome your own barriers to fitness by suggesting solutions to your issues. For example, if one of your issues for not exercising enough is that you don't have enough time, the Web site suggests working out three times per day for ten minutes each time, because research shows that this is as good as one 30-minute workout per day.

Shape Up America! also includes a table to help you understand how hard you are working out. Called the *Borg scale*, it measures your perception of your physical exertion. Your goal is to exercise hard enough to be at 13 on the scale; the ratings are perceived exertions and are listed in Table 3.1.

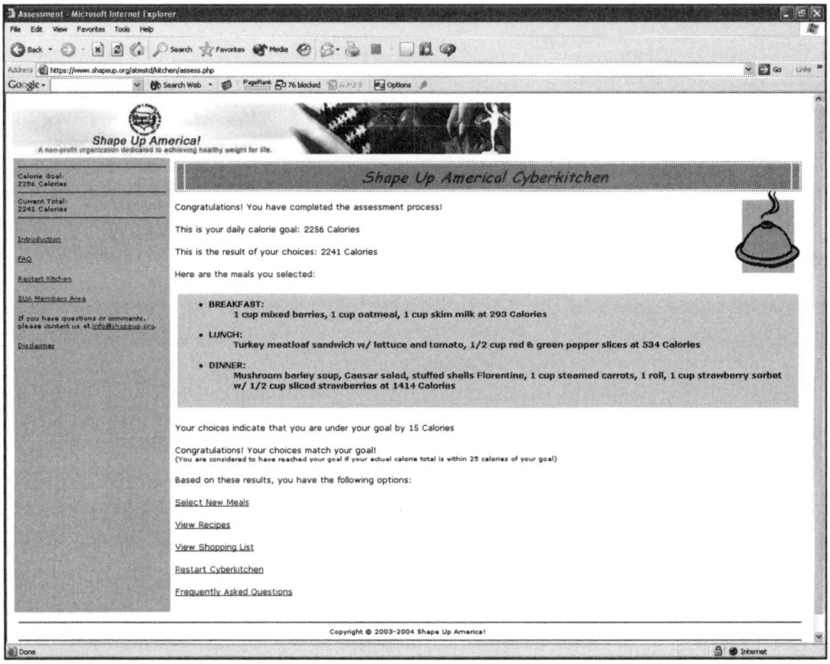

FIGURE 3.46 *Cyberkitchen meal plan for a day*

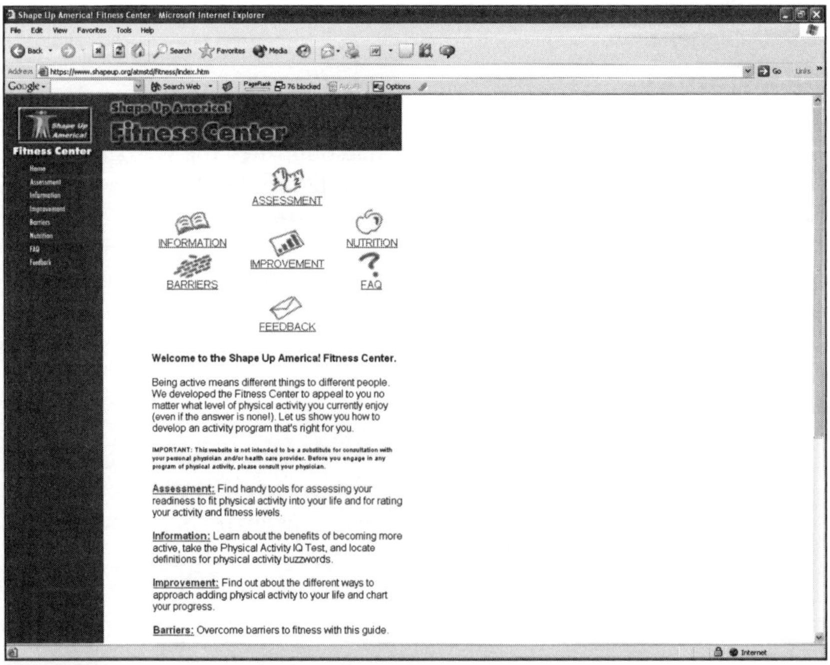

FIGURE 3.47 *Shape Up America! Fitness Center*

Table 3.1 The Borg Scale of Perceived Physical Exertion

Rating	Perceived Exertion
6, 7, 8	Extremely light
9, 10	Very light
11, 12	Fairly light
13, 14	Somewhat hard
15, 16	Hard
17, 18	Very hard
19	Extremely hard

Tutorials

A series of tutorials about eating and fitness provide essential information about eating and exercise. There are tutorials on portion control, eating in restaurants, childhood obesity, proper exercise, and other topics. They are available as free downloads to members. Following are some highlights from these tutorials.

- **When eating in restaurants, choose items that are lower in fat.** Choose baked, grilled, poached, steamed, or stir-fried over breaded, buttered, fried, crispy, and scalloped.
- **Eat slowly and enjoy the meal and surroundings.** You'll eat less if you pause between bites.
- **Half a cup of cooked pasta is about the size of an ice cream scoop; half a bagel is about the size of a hockey puck.** Most of us go for several scoops of pasta, and some bagels are getting to be the size of a softball.
- **One tablespoon of salad dressing is about the size of your thumb.** Given that the dressing can be the vast majority of calories in a salad, it's a good idea to order salads with dressing on the side.
- **Don't eat snacks out of the box or bag.** Pre-measure portions in advance and put them in individual snack bags.
- **Put servings on your plate before you get to the dinner table.** Immediately refrigerate the extras.
- **At restaurants, choose fruit for dessert.** Ignore the dessert tray and be strong!
- **Visit the buffet table only once.** Or use my rule: Don't go to buffets!

NO CALORIE COUNTING FOR OLYMPIC ATHLETES

You think you're in shape? Or you see someone at the gym who looks like he or she is perfect? None of us compare to the physical specimens who are Olympic or world-class athletes, who train so hard that they don't have to bother to count calories.

Most people who are fit regularly do cardiovascular exercise and strength-training activities. World-class athletes use those as a starting point and add coordination, balance, and skills specific to their sporting event.

The difference between a world-class athlete and an average fit person starts with exercise. The average fit person exercises for 30 to 45 minutes per day, four to five times per week. The Olympic athlete exercises for four hours or more, six times per week.

When it comes to calories, the average fit person eats somewhere between 1,500 and 3,000 per day. Olympic athletes take in somewhere around 6,000 per day, depending on their sport and gender. They don't drink alcohol at all.

While most of us eat every three to four hours, a world-class athlete who is burning a lot of calories eats every two hours.

Sleep? World-class athletes take a series of short naps throughout the day before their workouts. The rest of us sleep six to eight hours per night.

The type of sport in which an athlete is engaged is key to his or her lifestyle. For example, weightlifters eat tremendous amounts of protein before events. And swimmers and runners eat more before events, while gymnasts eat very little before events.

Weight Watchers Online

$1.99 per week to $7.97 per week, depending on how many options you choose. There's also an all-inclusive plan for $5 per week if you pay for three months at a time.

http://www.weightwatchers.com

Summary: The mother of all community sites

In 1964, when Weight Watchers founder Jean Nidetch invited people into her house in Queens, New York, each week to discuss weight loss, she scarcely could have imagined the worldwide phenomenon that Weight Watchers would become. More than one million people attend 46,000 weekly meetings in 30 countries. And the potential for the online world is much greater.

When you have a market-leading brand and product offline, it's not always the easiest thing to move it online. However, Weight Watchers has done this successfully with Weight Watchers Online. Its community and support options are as strong online as they are off; Weight Watchers boasts some of the most well-trafficked message boards on the Internet, and a host of community and support features that enhance the program's reputation online.

Weight Watchers' Community home page is a good example of this (see Figure 3.48). Features abound and are usually one click away on a well-designed, uncluttered page that features message boards, a recipe swap feature, polls, advertising, and much more. Plus, there are links to the other main parts of the Weight Watchers site, the *POINTS* tracker, food and recipes, fitness, success stories, and the online marketplace. The heart of the community, however, is the message boards.

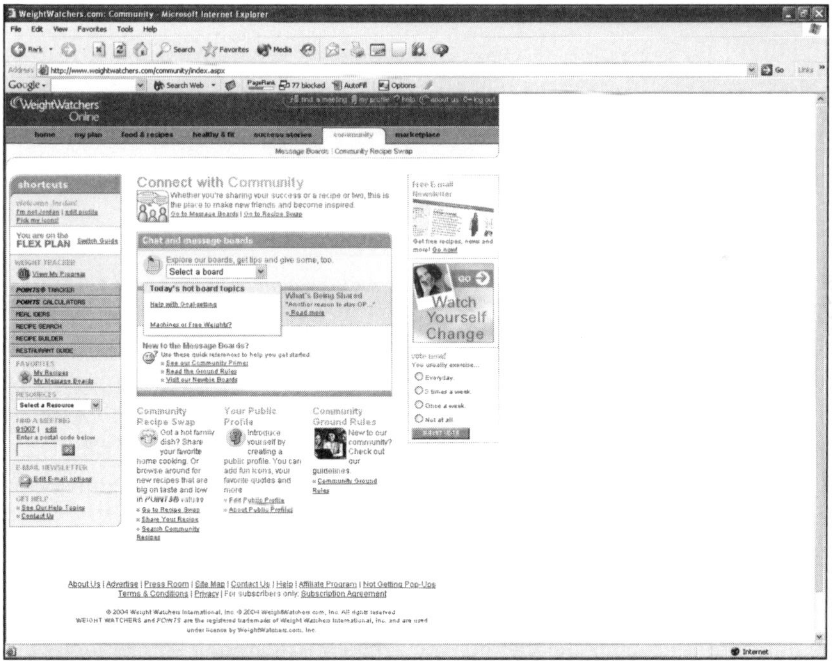

FIGURE 3.48 *Weight Watchers Community home page*

Message Boards

As discussed earlier in this chapter, Weight Watchers has 36 well-organized message boards (refer to Figure 3.4). Most of these boards boast very high traffic levels that approach Prevention.com's South Beach diet board. In fact, looking at just the total number of threads in each board provides a snapshot of the Weight Watchers Online community.

- **The new members board is the highest trafficked.** It's the place everyone starts, so that makes sense (see Figure 3.49).

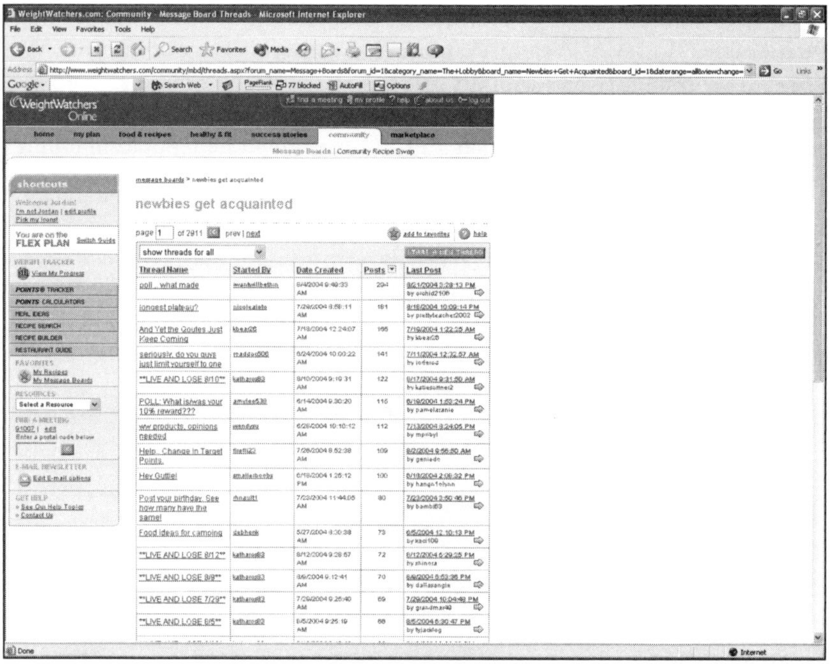

FIGURE 3.49 *Newbies Get Acquainted is the most popular message board on Weight Watchers Online.*

- **The twentysomething board is by far the highest trafficked among the age groups.** This probably speaks more to the technical savvy of this group than anything else.
- **The 100+ pounds to lose board gets the heaviest traffic of the pounds to lose boards.** It appears that, overall, the less weight you have to lose overall, the less support you think you need. But the 200+ pounds to lose board gets much less traffic, probably because there are a lot fewer people in that range than the folks trying to lose 50 or 100 pounds.
- **The moms group is the highest-trafficked board among special interests.** Most likely this is because women are more likely to share their feelings about weight loss than men are.
- **Challenges are very popular on Weight Watchers.** Everyone needs extra motivation. Challenge Central provides it, with lots of different weight loss and fitness challenges.

Success Stories

Hearing about someone else who does well on a diet or exercise program is motivating. That's why most health and fitness Web sites provide forums for their members to post success stories. After all, a weight-loss Web site with no success stories is probably not one that will provide you with much motivation. Weight Watchers Online devotes as much, if not more, space to success stories than any other site (see Figure 3.50). They have several message boards, an easy way for you to post your successes, lots of before and after pictures, and interesting articles about people who have lost weight.

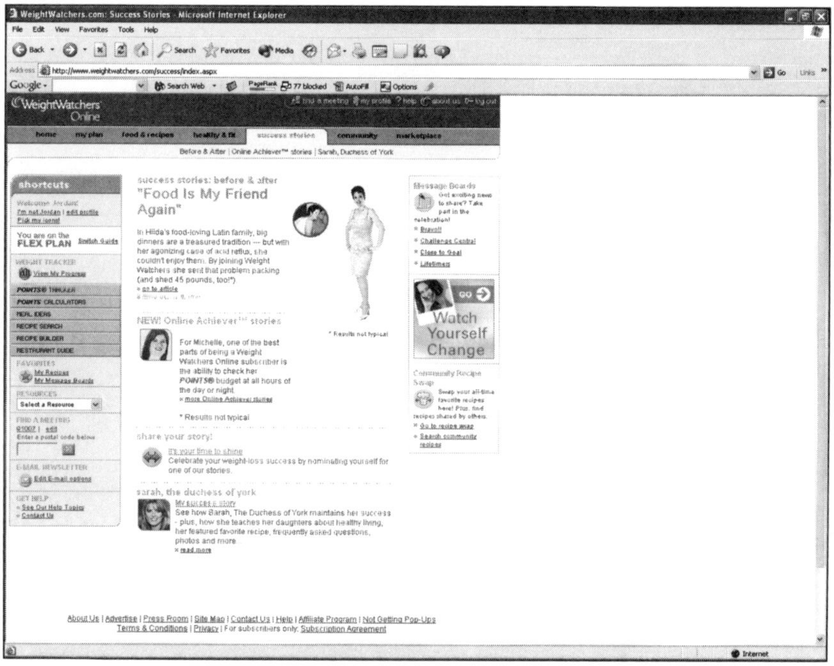

FIGURE 3.50 *Weight Watchers success stories*

Although many of these success stories are about people who achieved their weight loss primarily offline through Weight Watchers meetings, a growing section of Weight Watchers Online is for Online Achievers, or people who have lost weight through the online programs at Weight Watchers.

Healthy & Fit

The Healthy & Fit section on Weight Watchers Online includes a number of assessment tools, articles about health and fitness, better-living guides for helping you through particular times of the year, quizzes, motivation, and fitness Q&As (see Figure 3.51). Although it's not as comprehensive as fitness-oriented sites, it does provide a wealth of information. For example, the assessments and quizzes provide a wide variety of data, letting you know your BMI and your readiness for exercise while testing your knowledge of particular foods, such as summer fruits and fast foods. And Fitness Q&As answer questions about when to exercise, how much to exercise, what machines to use, and what shoes to wear, among many others.

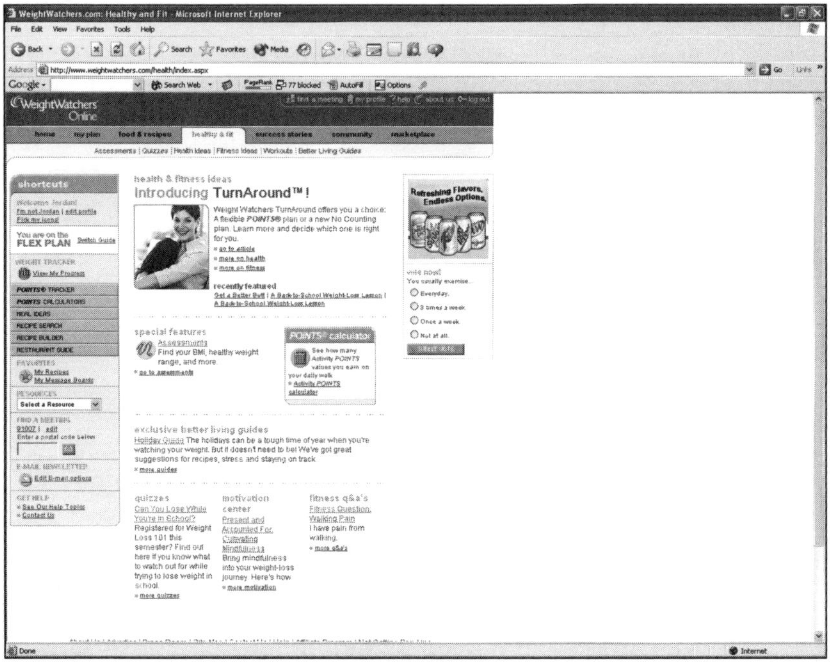

FIGURE 3.51 *Weight Watchers Healthy & Fit section*

BUSY MOM LOSES 50 POUNDS ON WEIGHT WATCHERS ONLINE

Before she got married, Michelle B. lost 40 pounds on Weight Watchers the traditional way, by attending meetings in person. However, after having two kids, she gained all of that weight back plus another 20 pounds over the next seven years. She attributes the weight gain to her two pregnancies, plus the fact that she didn't integrate a permanent healthy eating process into her life. "Once I lost the weight the first time, I stopped dieting," she says. "[This time] I realized that I needed to make a change in my lifestyle."

Her job as a consultant didn't allow her to go to Weight Watchers meetings in person, so she enrolled in Weight Watchers Online. "Weight Watchers Online provided a great way for me to accomplish my goals," she says. "As an avid computer user, I found it easy to keep the WW window open all day and refer to it at any time."

Michelle particularly likes the 24-hour availability of the online community and the many resources at Weight Watchers Online, which "met or surpassed" her needs. "The online community is extremely supportive," she says. "I felt that I could benefit from the experiences of many meetings and gather information at any moment, any time of the day."

BUSY MOM LOSES 50 POUNDS ON WEIGHT WATCHERS ONLINE

Thanks to Weight Watchers Online, Michelle lost 50 pounds from her 5'4" frame. The 40-year-old started the program at 185 pounds, lost 50 pounds in the first seven months, then went into maintenance mode and lost two more pounds in the next 18 months (see Figures 3.52 and 3.53).

Michelle credits two factors for helping her drop her weight—motivation and the ease and availability of Weight Watchers Online. "I'm always on my computer, so it's easy to input and track my ***POINTS***," she says.

Michelle uses the community features of Weight Watchers and participates in the exercise challenges. She learned about an exercise video called *The Firm* on the Weight Watchers message boards, and that got her so into the habit of exercising that she bought an elliptical trainer. She also bikes with her husband and two daughters.

Her tips for success—portion control, writing down (or entering online) what she eats, and leaving room in her ***POINTS*** budget for the foods she loves (in her case, chocolate). "Weight Watchers works, but don't do it until you're ready," she advises. "If you are going to begin a weight loss program, you need to be ready to make changes in your lifestyle. That includes planning a program that you can integrate into your existing lifestyle." For Michelle, that means being able to keep the Weight Watchers window open at all times!

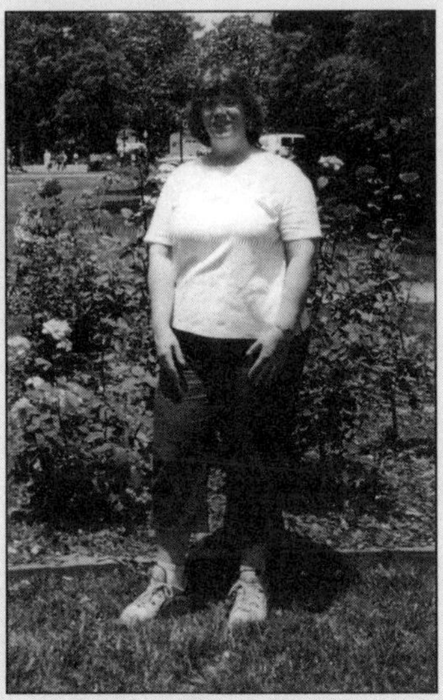

FIGURE 3.52 *Michelle B. at 185 pounds*

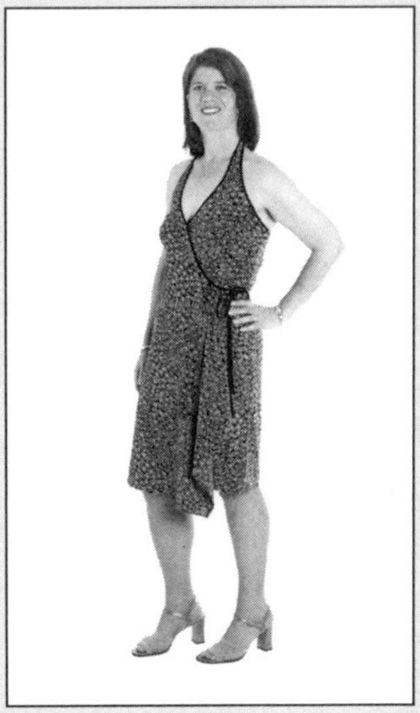

FIGURE 3.53 *Michelle B. at 135 pounds*

Other Support Sites

As mentioned, there are many other sites that provide health and fitness support. In this chapter, we've examined some of the best sites and provided you with a lot of tips and information about evaluating sites for their levels of support. The important thing isn't that you use one of the sites in this chapter; it's that you get support for your efforts so you are motivated to reach your goals.

In Chapter 4, "Healthy Cooking Online," we'll look at the best cooking sites on the Internet, so that you will be healthy while eating well and not get bored in the process.

Chapter 4

Healthy Cooking Online

"I was thirty-two when I started cooking. Up until then, I just ate."

—Julia Child

The Internet is nothing if not the world's largest reference library. Exchanging healthy recipes and cooking tips is a great way to get healthy. It can get boring eating the same foods day after day, and sites that offer a lot of healthy recipes and choices are in abundance online. This chapter will examine some of the best sites.

RECIPE FOR RUM CAKE

1 or 2 quarts rum

1 cup butter

1 tbsp. sugar

2 large eggs

1 cup dried fruit

Baking powder

1 tbsp. soda

1/2 cup cocoa

Lemon juice

Brown sugar

Nuts

Flour

Before you start, sample the rum to check its quality. Good, isn't it?

Now go ahead. Select a large mixing bowl, measuring cup, etc. Check the rum again. It must be just right. To be sure the rum is of the highest quality, pour 1 level cup of rum into a glass and drink it as fast as you can. Repeat. With electric mixer, beat 1 cup of buetter in a large, fluffy bowl. Add 1 sheespoon of thugar and beat again. Meanwhile, continue to ensure rum stays at room temperature. Try another cup. Open the second bottle if necessary.

Add 2 arge legs, 2 cups fried druit, and beat till high. If druit gets struck in the beaters, just pry it loose with a drewscriver. Rample the sum again, check for tonscisticity. Next sift 3 cups of perrepper or salt (it doesn't matter)—(sampletherrum). Shift 1/2 pint of lemon juice and fold in chopped butter and strained nuts. Add 1 babblespoon of brown thugar, or whatever colour you find. Wix mel.

Grease oven and turn the cake pan 350 gredees. Now pour the whol mess into the boven and cake.

Check the rum again and bo to ged.

And memrember, when you bake…dron't div.

Okay, so that's not one of the best recipes, but it's one of the funniest. If you look hard enough, you'll find lots of funny recipes online, and you'll also find scores of useful ones.

What Makes a Good Cooking Site?

As we mentioned in Chapter 3, the rules for a good site are that it has large helpings of each of the three Cs—content, community, and commerce. That applies to all Web sites, not just cooking or support ones. When it comes to cooking sites, however, content (in the form of recipes) is king. And community (in the form of submitted recipes, reviews and ratings of recipes, and comments from others) is queen. Commerce is a nice plus; having a good store is an important addition for many cooking sites.

Some things to look for when evaluating cooking sites include the following:

- Are there enough recipes in the database?
- Are they easy to access?
- Are there reviews?
- Is there a lot of activity on the message boards?
- How about articles and other content?
- Is there expert advice?

More than anything, a cooking site needs to be a community where cooks and aspiring cooks gather to give and get advice and share and exchange recipes. Good cooking sites are places where you'll spend lots of time. Just as you need support on your quest for a healthier lifestyle, you need help to cook a variety of foods so you don't get bored.

LOOK FOR HEALTHY ALTERNATIVES TO ETHNIC FOODS

Love Mexican and Italian foods? No problem. Just visit one of the many sites mentioned in this chapter and pick healthy alternatives to traditional dishes. Many sites include low-calorie versions of classic favorites. It's okay to have pasta with Alfredo sauce, for example, as long as the pasta is whole wheat, the Alfredo sauce is low-fat, and the portions are pre-measured.

Of course, having a large recipe database is essential. Many sites have thousands of recipes and reviews of those recipes. This helps make the user experience better. If a site has lots of reviews, you'll feel more comfortable that these are recipes you can trust. Reviews don't have to be anything in depth, just comments about a recipe, a sentence or two: "I liked it, but adding cilantro made it way better," for example.

Recipes have to be varied and interesting. Of course, if all you want are specialized recipes for vegetarian, kosher, diabetic, or other types of food, there are sites for that (http://www.kosher-cooking.com, http://www.vegweb.com, and http://www.diabetic-recipes.com, to name a few). However, many of the comprehensive sites mentioned in this chapter include sections for special categories of food.

When it comes to community in a cooking site, it all revolves around recipes. Don't expect to see very active message boards on any of these sites. The community comes from submitting, exchanging, and reviewing recipes, not from talking about recipes with each other.

Another key ingredient is searching. It's one thing to have a lot of recipes, but if you don't have flexible and powerful search capabilities, all that results is a frustrated user base. The search capabilities have to let you search through recipes by a variety of criteria—main dish, type of meat, special category, key ingredients, excluded ingredients, how much time it takes to cook, and many other factors.

A store is also a nice addition to a cooking site. Why not offer the ability to buy the equipment, ingredients, and other cooking-related products to a market that is interested in them? We'll cover online shopping in much greater detail in Chapter 7, "Shop Naked," but we cover it briefly here as well.

What follows is an examination of some of the best cooking sites on the Internet, with comments about what makes each one unique and popular.

Allrecipes.com

http://www.allrecipes.com

Summary: With more than 23,000 recipes in 37 categories, Allrecipes.com more than lives up to its name.

Allrecipes.com bills itself as the worldwide community cookbook (see Figure 4.1). It's no wonder—they feature more than 23,000 recipes from cooks around the world, including home cooks, corporate cooks, and professional cooks and dieticians.

Allrecipes.com is actually a compilation of sites. It began as cookierecipe.com in 1997, added appetizers, vegetarian recipes, and a store, and eventually merged into one site with 37 categories of recipes, including recipes for people on special diets. The site claims more than two million visitors per month and more than 45 million page views per month.

Recipes come from end users, corporate partners, and nutrition experts. All recipes are reviewed by others on the site and ranked in order of user preference, as well as by the number of reviews. Finding recipes is very easy; you can search by type of food, meal, keyword, or by choosing one of the 37 categories and narrowing your search from there. You can also find the hottest and top-rated recipes very easily.

Each recipe includes step-by-step directions for preparation, nutritional facts, and a shopping list for ingredients. It also includes user rankings and the number of reviews.

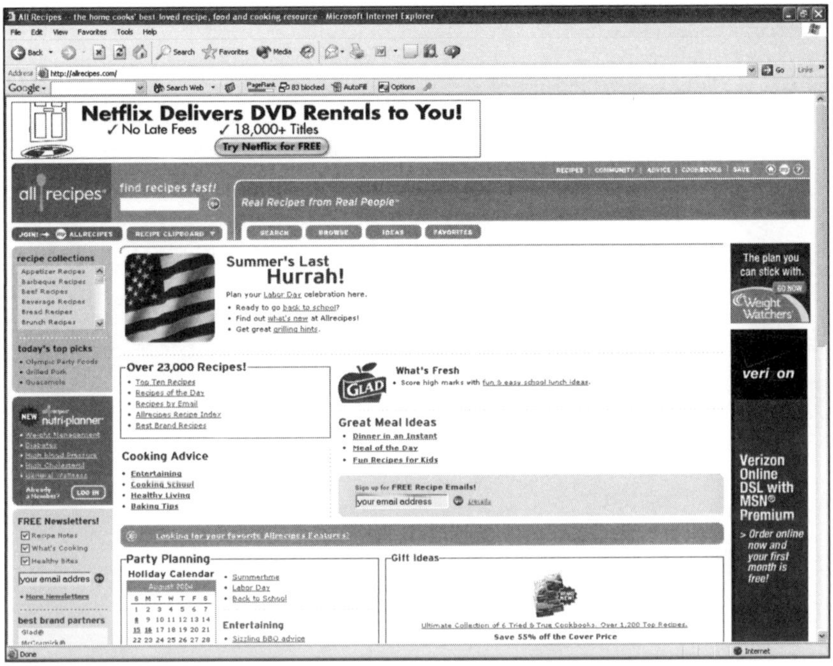

FIGURE 4.1 *Allrecipes.com home page*

Registered users (it's free to register) can create their own personalized recipe section called My Allrecipes (see Figure 4.2). This lets users store, organize, rank, review, and share their recipes and print them on 3×5 or 4×6 recipe cards or on full sheets of paper. Users also can scale recipes from one to 100 servings, making it easier to use a recipe for small or large groups.

The Tried & True recipe series is a series of cookbooks that are available for purchase on the site. Many of the recipes are available in the Recipe Collections area of the site, as shown in Figure 4.3. This area offers tried-and-true recipes in more than 40 categories, including by magazine (*Cooking Light, Southern Living*, and *Sunset*), holiday, or type of meal (dessert, appetizer, brunch, main course, and so on), plus other categories such as barbeque, chicken, beef, vegetarian, and kid-friendly. Each category is searchable and includes a top 10 list of the most popular recipes in the category.

Although there is a powerful search feature on Allrecipes.com, searching by nutritional information is not available for free. It costs $6 per month as part of the site's Nutri-Planner feature. There are several areas on the site that are available for a monthly fee. According to Allrecipes.com, at least 95% of the recipes on the site are free. However, the ability to search them by nutritional information is not free.

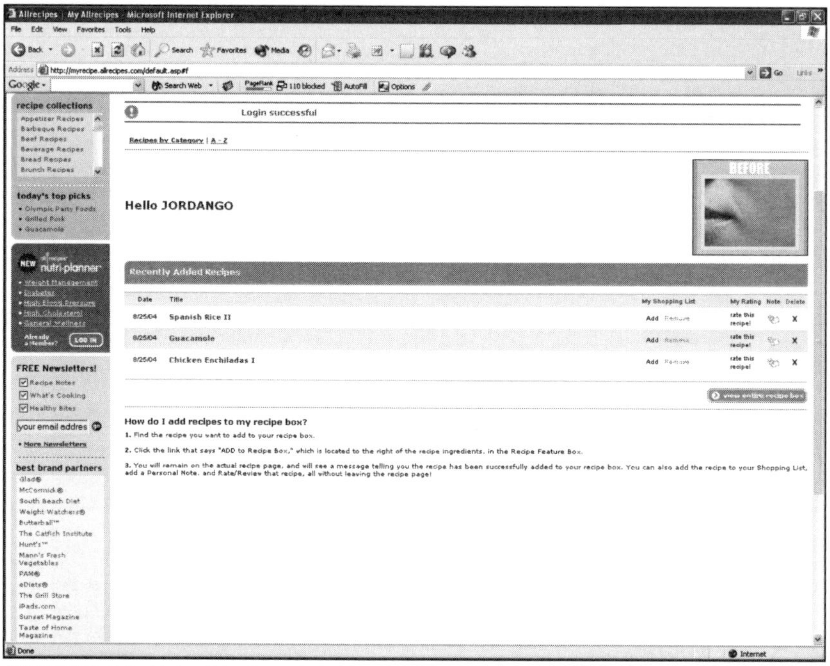

FIGURE 4.2 *My Allrecipes site*

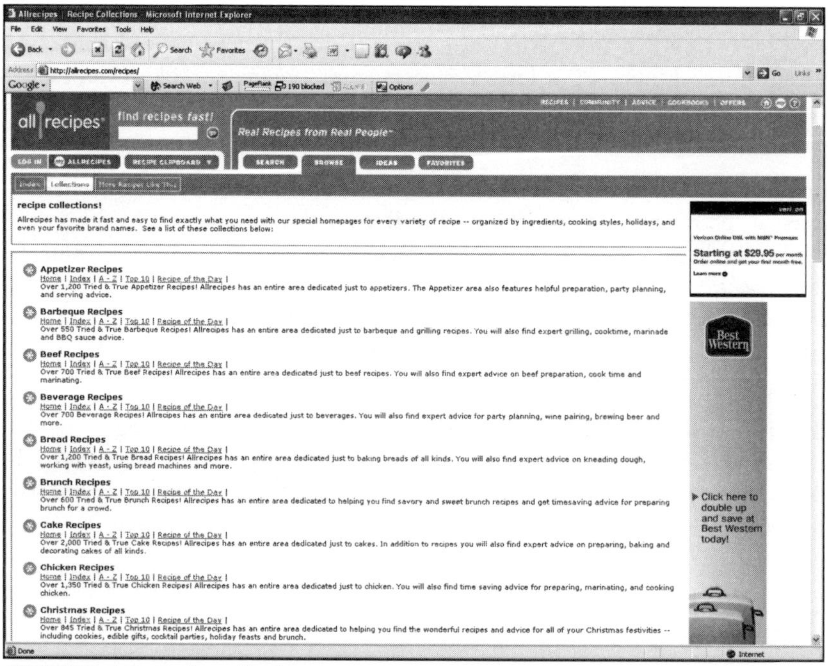

FIGURE 4.3 *Recipe collections*

The Web site features seven newsletters for a variety of purposes, including Recipe Notes, a free biweekly newsletter with more than 600,000 subscribers; What's Cooking, a weekly guide to what's new on the site; The Allrecipes Daily Dish, a daily newsletter with a recipe of the day; and Healthy Bites, which features the most healthy ideas and recipes.

The five percent of the site that is not free is called the Premium Quick-Smart Collections; it includes collections of recipes in a wide variety of categories, each available for $6.95 to $9.95 per month (see Figure 4.4). Each collection is actually an online cookbook developed by an expert in food and nutrition. Topics include light favorites, which are slimmed-down versions of traditional recipes, online cookbooks from *Cooking Light* and *Taste of Home* magazines, a low-carb recipe area, and a low-fat area, as well as recipes optimized for people with diabetes.

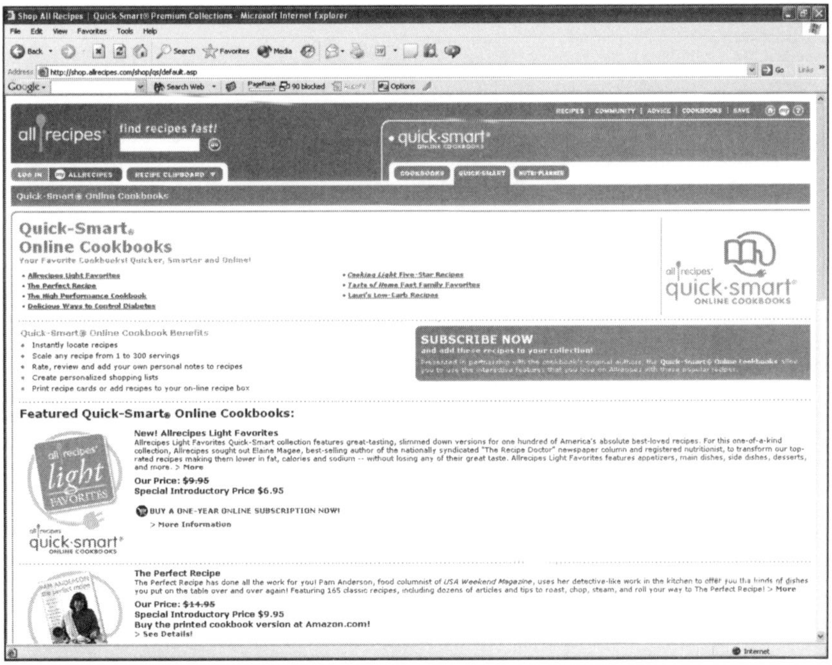

FIGURE 4.4 *The Premium Recipe Collections*

The Nutri-Planner program includes four options—weight loss, diabetes management, blood pressure and cholesterol reduction, and general wellness. Each program includes a food diary, advice from experts, meal plans, and support to help optimize a wellness program. The cost is $36 for six months, or an average of $6 per month. Free health assessment tests are available for anyone (see Figure 4.5).

Allrecipes.com features a lively community, billed as the world's largest community of home cooks. There are no message boards; the community includes recipes, requests for recipes, reviews, ratings of reviews, and home pages of reviewers. Users can review, submit, or request recipes and rate reviews.

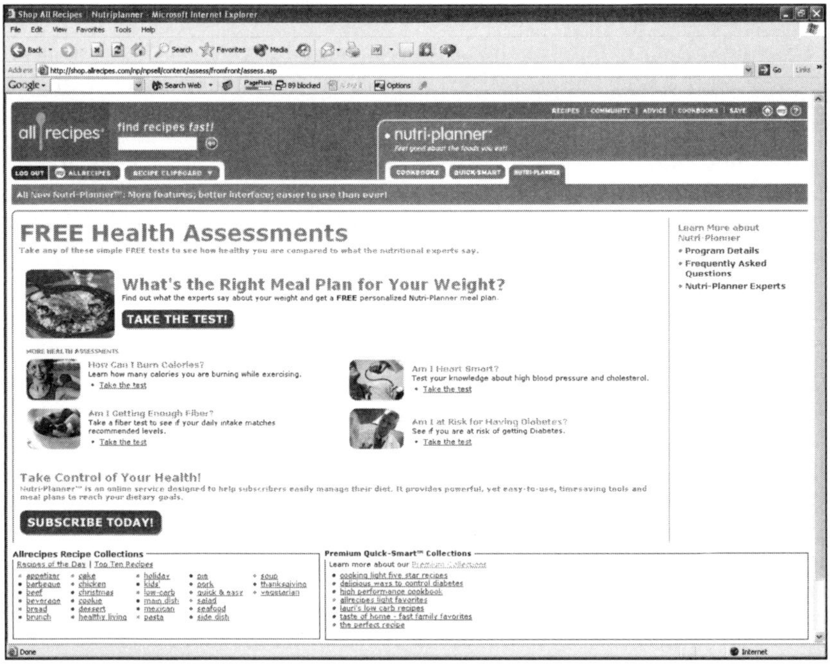

FIGURE 4.5 *Nutri-Planner*

Membership is free, and each reviewer gets to create a home page that tells everyone about himself or herself, including a short bio, what he or she likes to cook, cooking traditions, and kitchen disasters and triumphs.

The top 10 reviewers, by number of recipes they've reviewed, are highlighted on the site. Reviews aren't very long, and that's a good thing. Who wants to read a long review of a recipe? Most reviews say something like, "I liked this very much. The potatoes in particular are delicious." Users then rate the reviews as helpful, not helpful, or most helpful.

CookingLight.com

http://www.cookinglight.com

Summary: An active community and magazine content make this an interesting site.

CookingLight.com takes content from the popular magazine of the same name, adds one of the most active cooking communities on the Internet, throws in healthy living tips, and adds some cooking tips to result in one of the most interesting online cooking sites (see Figure 4.6). The site includes five main sections—Food, Menus & Planning, Cooking 101, Healthy Life, and Community. There is also a Market, where you can buy a wide variety of food-related products.

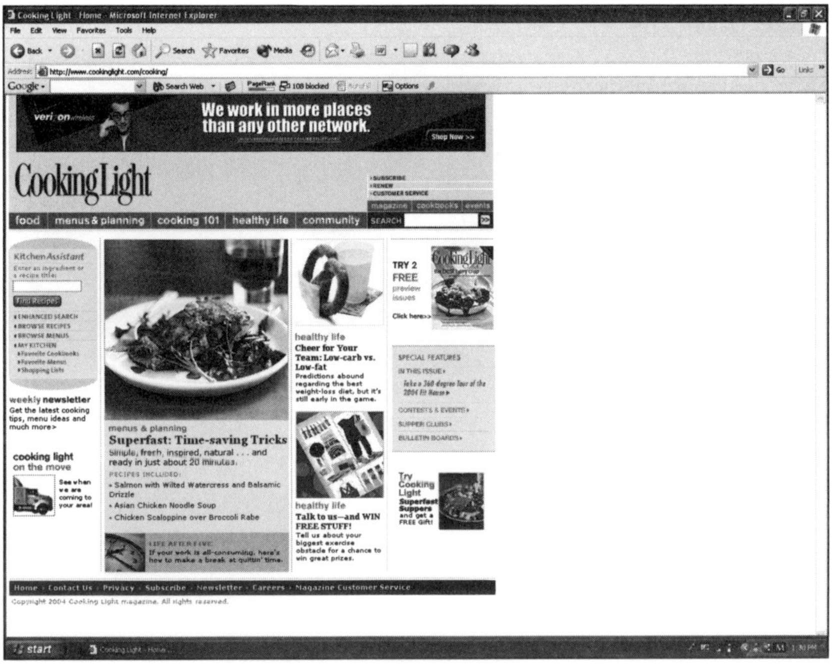

FIGURE 4.6 *CookingLight.com is free to subscribers and AOL members.*

JUST DESSERTS

Chocoholic's Revenge (http://www.chocoholicsrevenge.com) is a great site for those of us who love chocolate and don't want to give it up while we're losing weight (see Figure 4.7). The site provides more than 50 recipes for chocolate desserts using less sugar, fat, and simple carbs than traditional versions of the same desserts. Nutrition information, including Weight Watchers ***POINTS***, is provided. A sample recipe is shown in Figure 4.8. You can even send someone a chocolate-themed e-card for free.

There's an article on the site about the healthy benefits of chocolate (flavonoids are powerful antioxidants contained most heavily in dark chocolate) and they almost, but not quite, stretch the point of how healthy chocolate is. (It's not, but in moderation it's fine.)

Moderation is, of course, the key. The site points out that you could have 10 M&Ms for 33 calories and 1.5 grams of fat, or one Hershey's kiss for 25 calories and 1.5 grams of fat.

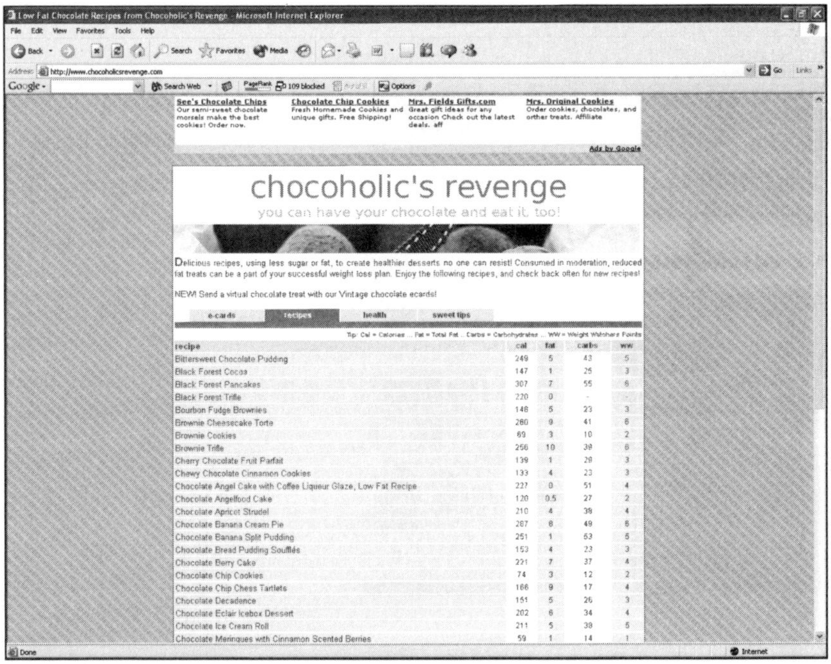

FIGURE 4.7 *Chocoholic's Revenge home page*

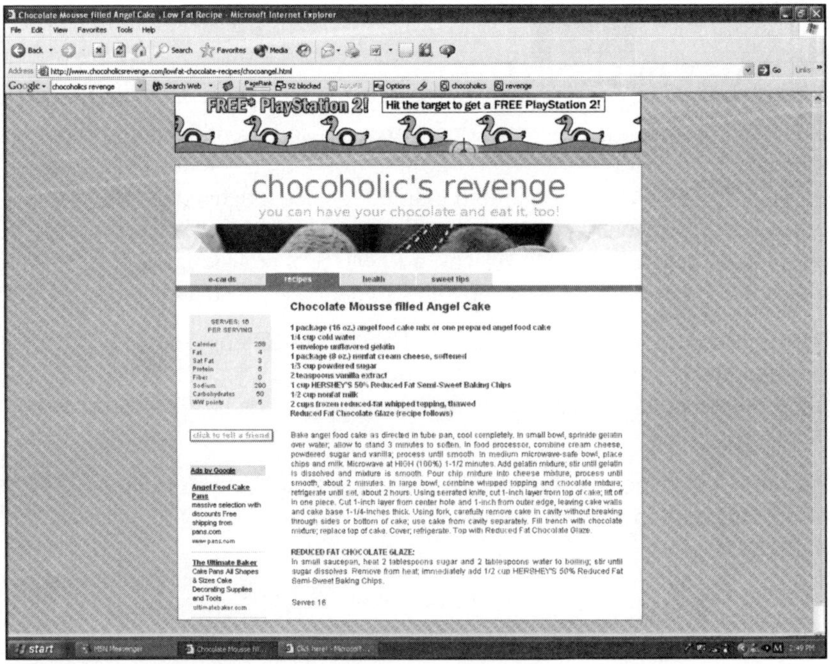

FIGURE 4.8 *A sample chocolate recipe*

Perhaps the reason why the community is the most active feature is because it's the one area that's free to all. For everything else, you have to be a subscriber to the magazine, an AOL member, or a newsstand buyer. Once you do qualify, there's a lot more content on hand.

The community feature includes a supper club area where people can hook up with others for outings, a healthy living area for discussions about a variety of healthful topics (including Weight Watchers; biking, hiking, and running groups; workout support groups; support for new moms; and support for folks on low-carb diets), and a variety of other areas (see Figure 4.9).

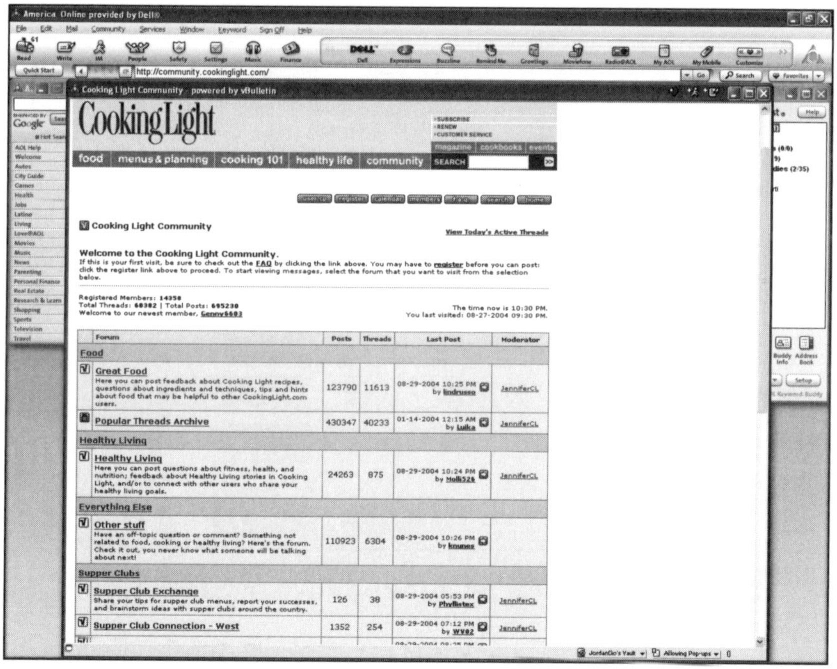

FIGURE 4.9 *CookingLight.com has one of the most active cooking communities on the Internet.*

A nice feature of the message boards is the most popular threads archive, a kind of "greatest hits" of the CookingLight.com message boards. These are boards with the greatest number of viewings on topics, including food gifts, nostalgia foods, most popular recipes, and—as people try to get to know each other better—what people do for a living.

The Food area is highlighted by articles from the magazine; the Clueless Gourmet column, which is basically a column for beginning cooks; and of course, recipes. Many of the recipes come from the magazine. Recipe searches are powerful and plentiful; you can search using a wide variety of parameters, including main courses, excluded foods, occasions, types of cuisine, conveniences (entertaining, kid friendly, and so on), and preparation method (slow cook, grill, steam, and so on). You can even search for meatless recipes.

Recipe results are organized in alphabetical order, and include ratings and the dates they were published in the magazine. Actual recipes include instructions and nutritional information (see Figure 4.10). Users can rate and review recipes; print them in full-page, 3×5, or 4×6 format; add notes; and put them into their cookbooks, menus, and shopping lists.

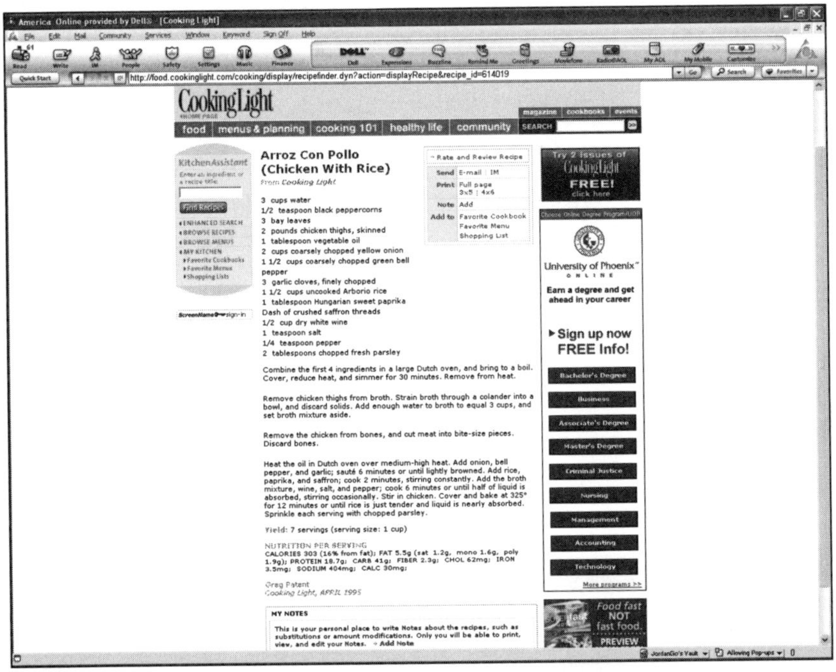

FIGURE 4.10 *Arroz Con Pollo (Chicken With Rice) recipe from CookingLight.com*

Menus & Planning concentrates on a variety of cooking situations—quick and easy menus, family food, outdoor dining, wines, and vegetarian cooking. There are also tips for creating the best menus, which are essentially several recipes that work together to make a meal—main course, side dishes, salads, and possibly dessert. A very helpful feature includes 31 days of dinner menus, which gives those of us who have a hard time deciding what to make each night a number of choices from which to select. You can select a week's worth of menus at a time, and then generate a shopping list. Our favorites in this area were some spicy healthy menus to substitute for one of the days (see Figure 4.11).

The Cooking 101 area on CookingLight.com is a really nice place to learn the basics about cooking (see Figure 4.12). It includes techniques, tips, and basic information about different types of cooking, such as baking, broiling, and grilling. It's an excellent resource for aspiring chefs as well as those of us who need a refresher.

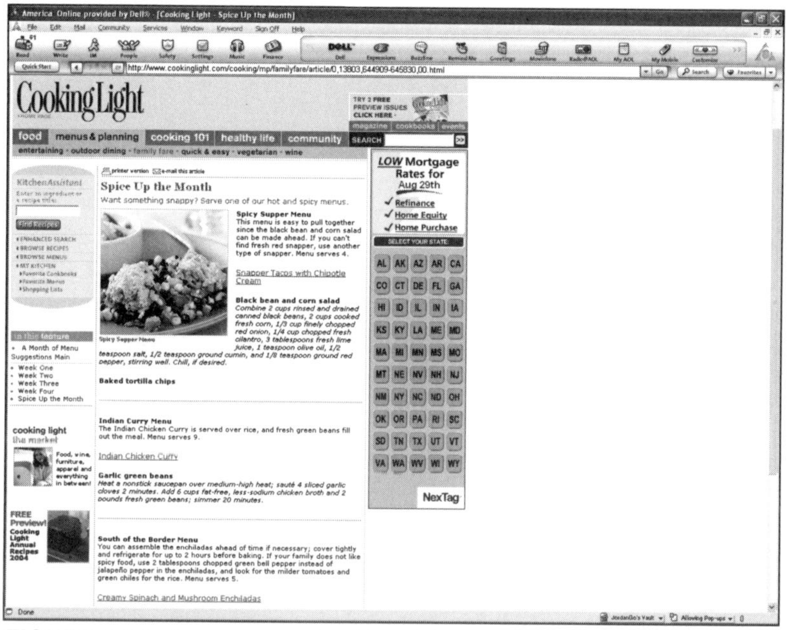

FIGURE 4.11 *Spicy menu on CookingLight.com*

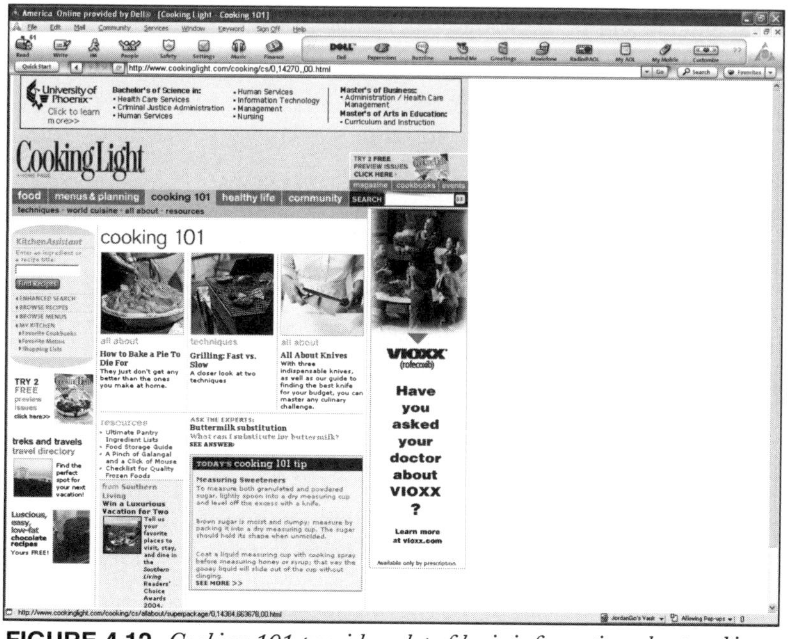

FIGURE 4.12 *Cooking 101 provides a lot of basic information about cooking, as well as tips and techniques.*

Healthy Life is a place that isn't about cooking. It's about the other ingredients to a healthy life, including beauty secrets, attitudes, travel, nutrition, and fitness and exercise. It includes a calorie calculator to measure calories burned during activities, as well as ways to determine your body mass index.

ITALIAN FOOD FOREVER

Most of us love pasta. And while eating it is not the best way to lose weight, the folks at Italian Food Forever (http://www.italianfoodforever.com) have created a site that celebrates Italian food while providing an outlet for those of us who want to eat Italian food without consuming too many calories (see Figure 4.13).

Italian Food Forever includes a wide variety of recipes, as well as forums and articles about Italian food. There is also essential information about Italian cooking, a glossary, a conversion calculator, suggested ingredient substitutions, and even tips for traveling to Italy!

Although nutrition information is not included, there are low-fat and low-calorie entrees. And there are great pictures of each recipe, an amazing accomplishment for a site without a food stylist.

Most of the recipes come from the Web master of the site, Deborah Mele, who lived in Italy for a time. Mele's philosophy is to make the best recipes possible with few shortcuts. And judging by the Forum comments on the site, she has succeeded; many people love this site.

Mele uses the freshest ingredients possible when cooking. She visits the grocery store each day to get inspiration for that night's meal.

The recipes on the site are great. Remember, however, that if you are cooking pasta, try to use whole-grain pasta. There are a lot of great whole-wheat pastas available.

Cooks.com

http://www.cooks.com

Summary: Lots of recipes, lots of advice, no frills.

When visiting Cooks.com, think of lots of information and no frills (see Figure 4.14). The folks at Cooks.com got a great URL and added lots of content, but didn't put any frosting on the cake. No matter; Cooks.com is a great site loaded with content. As a result, it consistently ranks as one of the most popular online cooking sites.

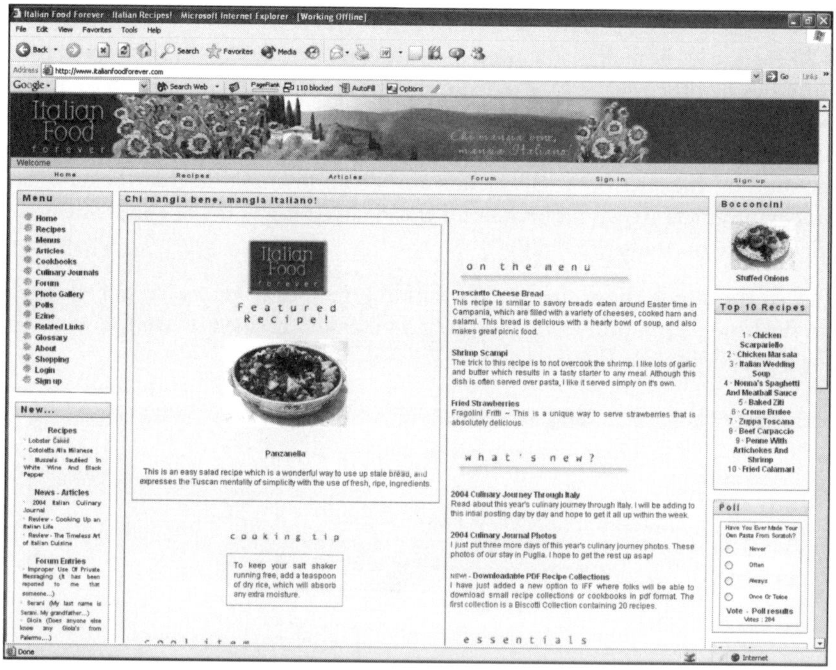

FIGURE 4.13 *Italian Food Forever*

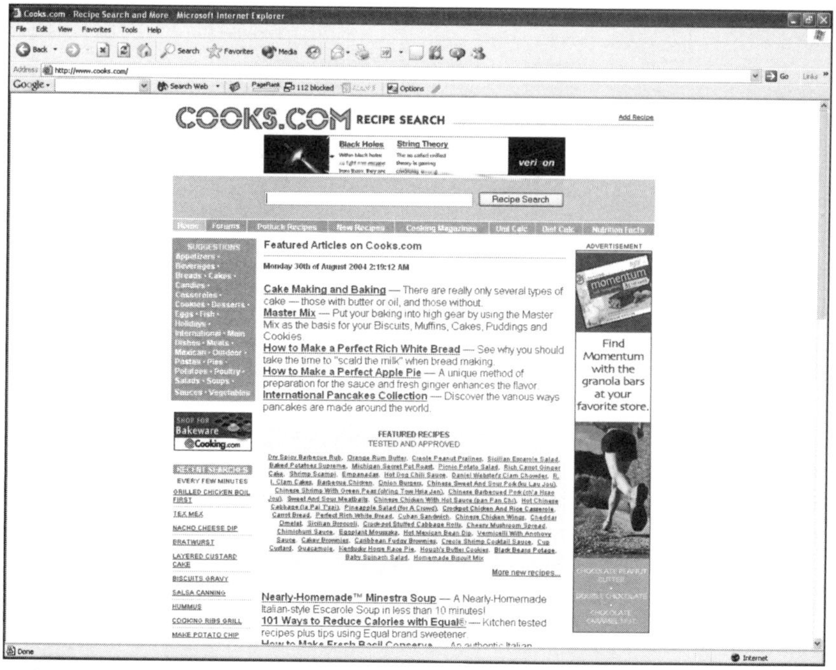

FIGURE 4.14 *Cooks.com home page*

The home page features popular articles that provide lots of basic information at a glance; links to 23 categories of recipes; featured recipes, which are tested and approved by Cooks.com; recent searches by other visitors (updated every few minutes); and links to a variety of calculators, cooking magazines, and specialty recipes. There's also a community area where users can discuss recipes and cooking techniques. There are almost no graphics except for advertisements, which abound on the site. Some of the ads are the annoying kind that flicker your screen and are for tacky products. It would be helpful if Cooks.com got rid of those advertisers, because they reflect badly on the site.

The heart of the site is the recipe search. Finding recipes is very easy. Searching for chicken, for example, brings up a mind-boggling 67,554 chicken recipes, as well as what appears to be an ad for a cookbook (see Figure 4.15).

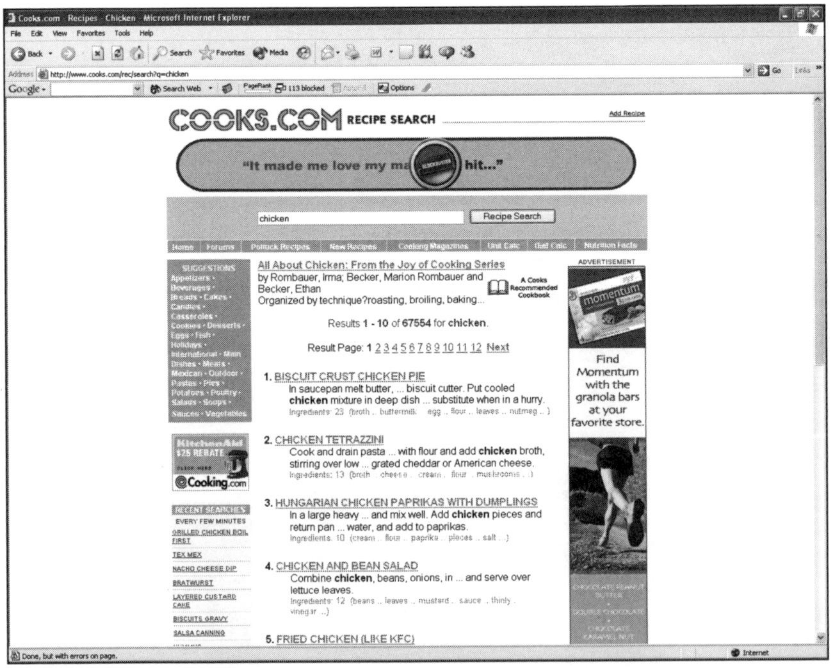

FIGURE 4.15 *Chicken recipe search results on Cooks.com*

Clicking on a recipe brings up instructions, as well as the number of servings for the recipe (see Figure 4.16). However, unlike on Allrecipes.com, there are no reviews and no nutrition information. Remember, this is a no-frills site. However, there is a copy of the USDA Nutrition Facts database on the site, so you can get information from that.

Aside from the recipes, probably the most useful feature on the site is the unit calculator area, which is simply loaded with information about weights and measures (see Table 4.1), temperature conversions, how to measure, how to weigh, and how to convert one measure to another.

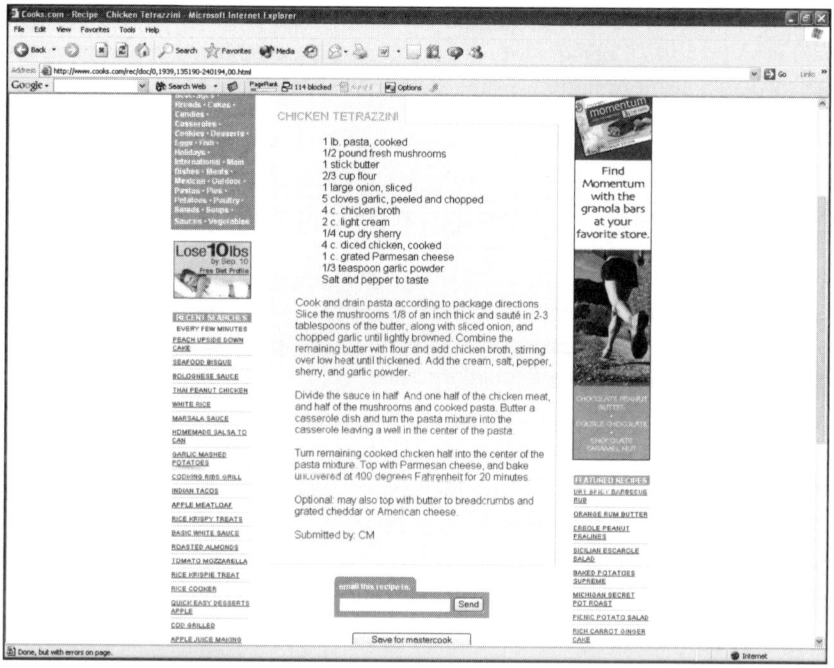

FIGURE 4.16 *Chicken tetrazzini*

Table 4.1 Cooks.com Table of Weights and Measures

3 teaspoons	equal	1 tablespoon
1 tablespoon	equals	½ ounce
2 tablespoons	equal	1 fluid ounce
4 tablespoons	equal	¼ cup
1 cup	equals	8 fluid ounces
2 cups	equal	1 pint
2 pints	equal	1 quart
4 quarts	equal	1 gallon
9 large eggs	equal	1 pound
4 cups flour	equal	1 pound
2 cups butter	equal	1 pound
2 cups sugar	equal	1 pound

There are other features on Cooks.com, but the main thing that makes this site stand out from the others is its breadth. Lots and lots of recipes and good editorial content make Cooks.com a fun site to visit. The community forums are not the best, but who cares? If you're looking for a chicken recipe, it's nice to have 67,000 choices!

MANUFACTURERS GET IN ON THE ACT

Food manufacturers have always had lots of recipes available, and many have published cookbooks featuring them (such as Betty Crocker, for example). Many manufacturers have very impressive Web sites that offer product information, recipes, tips, coupons, and other very helpful information.

One very nice and well-trafficked site is Kraft Foods (http://www.kraftfoods.com), home to such brands as A1 Steak Sauce, Breakstone's Cottage Cheese, Breyers, KOOL-AID, Kraft cheese, JELL-O, Maxwell House, Miracle Whip, Post Cereal, and Stove Top Stuffing, among others.

The Kraft Foods site includes recipes, recipe exchanges, an online version of the company's free *Food & Family* magazine, cooking tips and videos, nutritional information, and promotions.

More interesting is the Healthy Living area of the site, which features a wide variety of advice about weight management and weight loss, calorie and exercise calculators, meal planners, tips, and expert advice (see Figure 4.17). It even includes a guide for diabetics. Of course, many of the recipes and meal plans feature Kraft foods, but that's okay. All of the information on the site is free. Kraft has built a very nice site with a lot of information about healthy living.

Epicurious.com

http://www.epicurious.com

Summary: Flashy site with lots of sizzle and steak.

Epicurious.com (http://www.epicurious.com) is one of the oldest cooking sites on the Internet, first launched way back in 1994 (see Figure 4.18). Owned by Condé Nast, the publisher of both *Bon Appétit* and *Gourmet* magazines, Epicurious has a lot of content from which to draw. Much of the content comes from the two magazines, and some content comes from other Condé Nast publications, such as *Self* and *House & Garden*. But there's a lot more to Epicurious than that. The site bills itself as the world's greatest recipe collection, and it does have a good collection—more than 17,000 recipes. But it also includes a cooking site with articles, cooking tips, and dictionaries; a guide to wines; feature articles; restaurant reviews; and a very large cooking store. Plus, there are three newsletters—a weekly recipe guide, monthly wine reviews, and specials and features in the Epicurious shopping area.

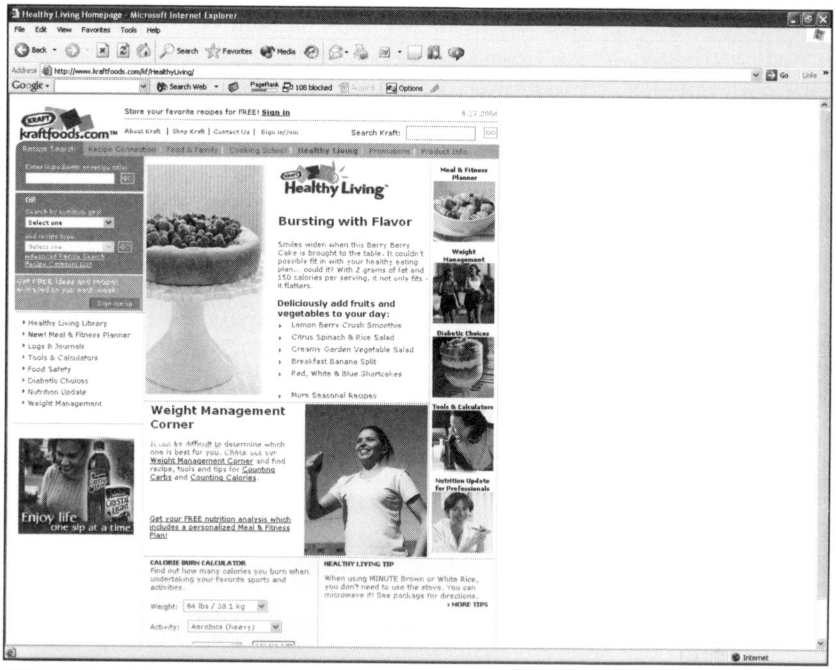

FIGURE 4.17 *Kraft Foods Healthy Living*

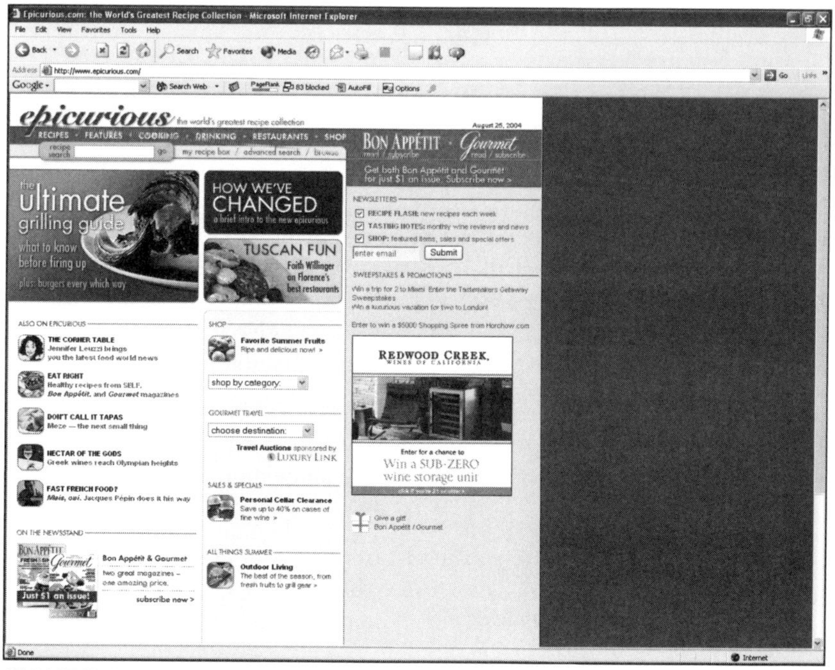

FIGURE 4.18 *Epicurious.com home page*

The recipe collection is impressive and easily navigable (see Figure 4.19). It includes a powerful search feature that pairs foods with wines, and offers menu suggestions, slideshows that demonstrate cooking techniques, a wide variety of topic-based recipe collections, and much more. Readers can save recipes in their recipe box, review others' recipes, and swap recipes in the Recipe Swap forum.

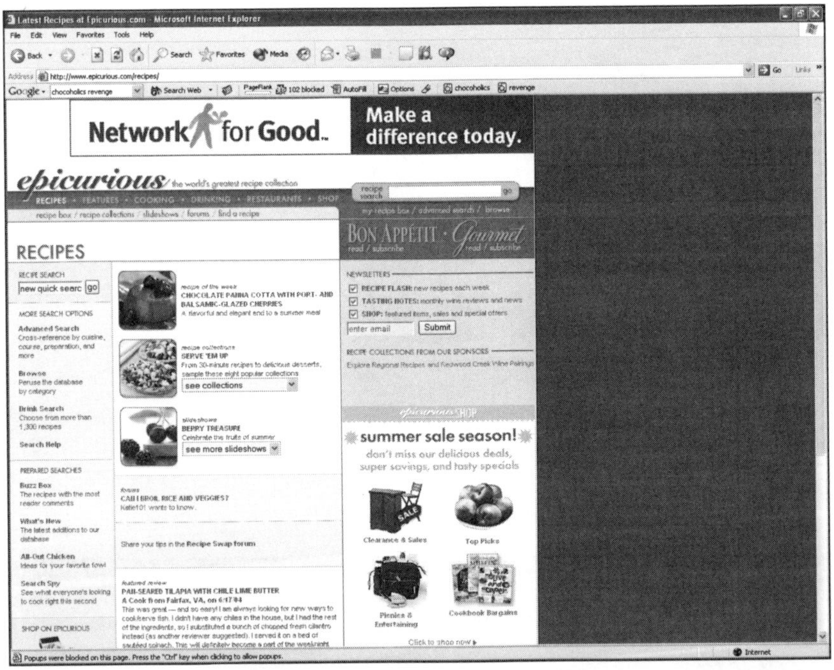

FIGURE 4.19 *The recipe collection on Epicurious.com lets users search more than 17,000 recipes.*

The advanced search feature is one of the most powerful we've seen, letting users search by many different parameters to select their meals, including low-fat, low-carb, and vegetarian options, and by course, cuisine, occasion, and main ingredient (see Figure 4.20). You also can specifically exclude ingredients from the search. One negative is that the recipes don't include nutrition information, so you have to figure that out for yourself.

The Features section includes a variety of articles from both magazines, as well as original content (see Figure 4.21). It includes cookbook reviews, expert advice, visual guides to foods, and a guide to Epicurious TV, the Web site's weekly TV show on the Travel Channel.

The Cooking page features cooking tips and articles, feature articles, videos that show you how to cook or handle a wide variety of foods, from eggs to poultry to fish to meat to fruits and vegetables. It also includes videos for entertaining, such as how to fold napkins and add garnishes. There are more than 50 helpful videos on the site, none more than a few minutes long.

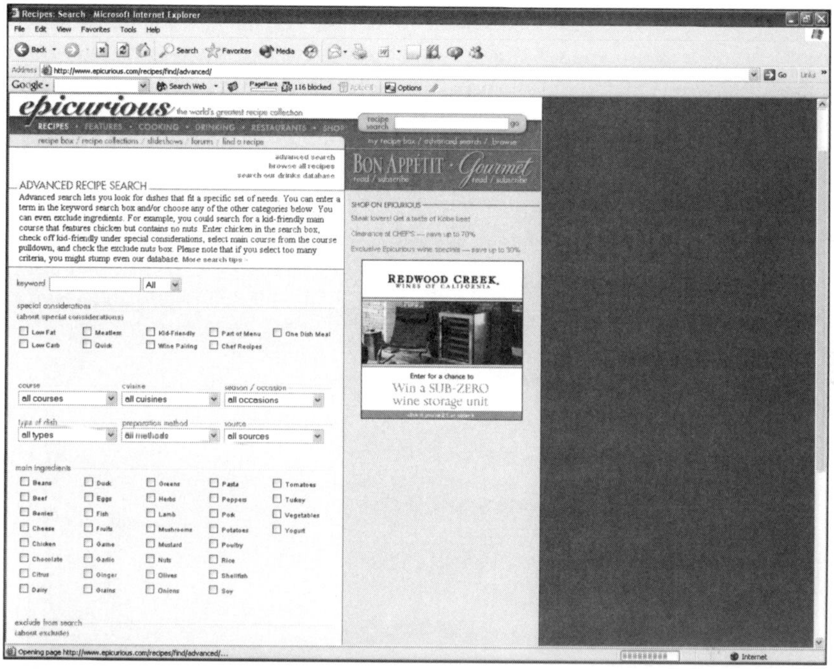

FIGURE 4.20 *The recipe search feature on Epicurious.com is extremely powerful.*

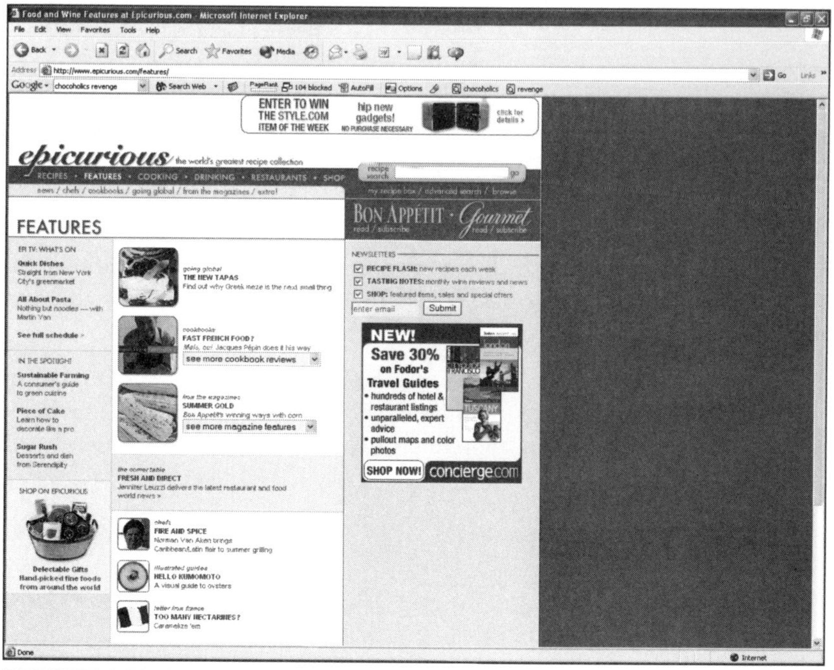

FIGURE 4.21 *The Epicurious Features page*

Two very interesting and helpful features on the Cooking page are the dictionaries. The Food Dictionary includes more than 4,000 culinary terms, while the Wine Dictionary includes more than 3,500 wine-related definitions. The definitions in the Food Dictionary come from *The Food Lover's Companion*, a food dictionary published in 1995 (see Figure 4.22). The Wine Dictionary, which covers all manner of wine terminology, comes from *The Wine Lover's Companion*, also published in 1995.

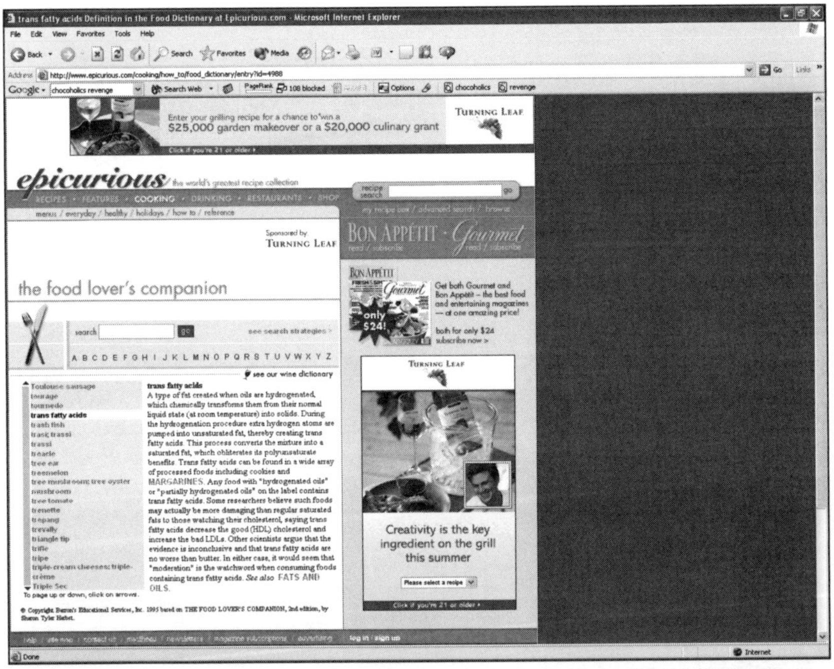

FIGURE 4.22 *The Epicurious Food Dictionary includes more than 4,000 culinary terms.*

The drinking area on Epicurious includes recipes for more than 1,300 drinks, from wine to beer to spirits to non-alcoholic drinks. It also includes shopping guides and features about drinks. The Wine Dictionary, of course, is also included here.

Epicurious Shop is one of the most impressive food-related cooking sites on the Internet (see Figure 4.23). It includes wines, gourmet foods, books, cookware, and a number of specialty shops. We'll discuss the Epicurious Shop in greater detail when we examine shopping sites in Chapter 7.

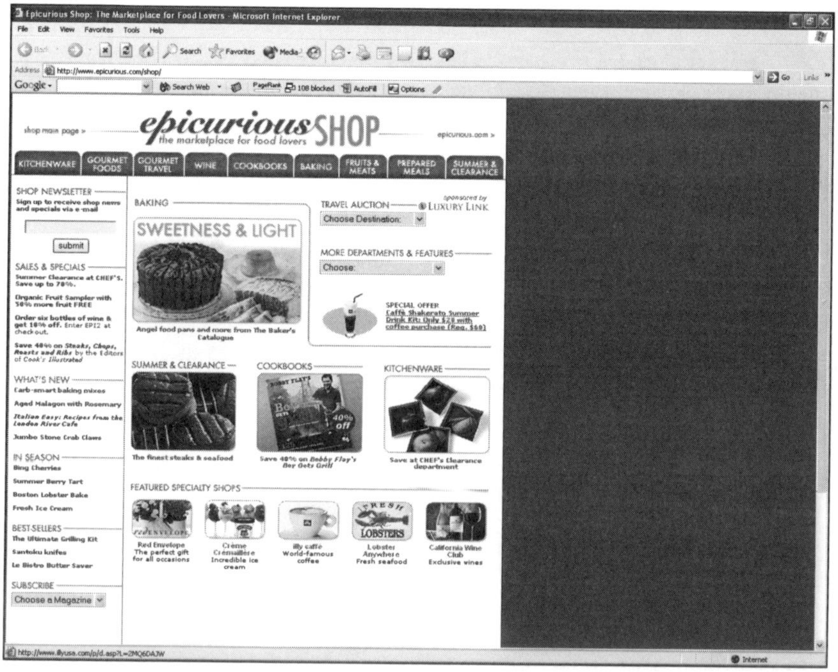

FIGURE 4.23 *The Epicurious Shop includes food, cooking, travel, and other products, making it one of the most impressive food-related cooking sites on the Internet.*

Other Cooking Sites

You can get recipes on a wide variety of sites, well beyond those mentioned in this chapter. We didn't include others because they don't add any discernible value over the ones that we chose. A number of cooking and home magazines include excellent recipes databases, including *Better Homes and Gardens, Cook's Illustrated, Country Living, Good Housekeeping, Redbook, Southern Living*, and *Sunset*.

Plus, many of the Web sites mentioned in earlier chapters (such as eDiets and Weight Watchers) have nice recipe areas, although none as extensive as the cooking sites in this chapter.

In Chapter 5, "Healthy, Fit, and Well," we'll start looking at ways that the Internet can help you improve your fitness and overall health. Plus, we'll look at the sites that help you get answers to health-related questions.

WHAT'S FOR BREAKFAST?

They say that breakfast is the most important meal of the day. That's where Mr. Breakfast comes in, with one of the most entertaining food-related sites on the Internet (http://www.mrbreakfast.com). The site is comprehensive, with more than 1,000 recipes for breakfast, reviews of scores of breakfasts at restaurants around the U.S., a breakfast shop, and lots of breakfast-related content (see Figure 4.24).

Mr. Breakfast is Eddy Chavey, an author and a graduate of the Los Angeles New School of Cooking. "Breakfast is more than a meal; it's a feeling," he says. "That smell of the morning and the first smile of the day." Chavey tries to instill that smile on his Web site, which is as enjoyable as it is informative.

He started the site to instill the importance of eating breakfast while showing how varied a breakfast menu can be. He also started a food charity for those in need, called The Breakfast of Love Miracle Network.

The site started in 2001, and traffic really took off when Chavey added the capability for users to submit their own breakfast and restaurant reviews. It currently gets approximately 10,000 unique visitors per day, according to Chavey.

Chavey, who lives in Los Angeles, has two favorite local restaurants for breakfast. He likes Duke's on Sunset Boulevard in Los Angeles for the food, and the Silver Spoon in Hollywood for the atmosphere.

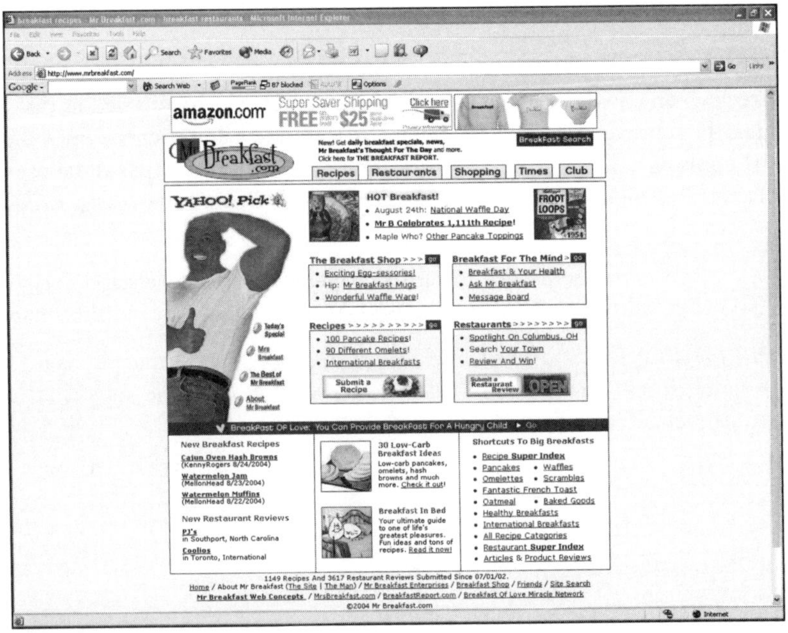

FIGURE 4.24 *Mr. Breakfast*

Chapter 5

Healthy, Fit, and Well

"The only way to keep your health is to eat what you don't want, drink what you don't like, and do what you'd rather not."

—Mark Twain

Maybe that was accurate (or not) in Mark Twain's time, but a lot of people still agree with him. Living a healthy life is not easy. For many of us, it would be easier to sit on the couch, eat junk food, and live in denial. However, if you felt that way, you wouldn't have bought this book.

In this chapter, we're going to look at sites that give you advice to keep you healthy and that help you when you don't feel so good. Although this chapter isn't entirely about losing weight, many of the general health and wellness sites and the gender- and age-specific sites that we'll look at later in this chapter include excellent nutrition, fitness, and weight loss sections.

General Health and Wellness Sites

The Internet has always been a great place to research general health information. You can find detailed information about any disease, sneeze, or sore throat, as well as specific information to help you get through issues specifically pertaining to you. There are many comprehensive health and wellness sites on the Internet. In general, those sites provide the following:

- **Age-, gender-, and topic-specific support groups and information centers.** Most sites have information centers, complete with articles, message boards, and other information for age-, gender-, and disease-specific categories. In general, this includes separate areas for men's issues, women's issues, seniors, babies, and children, as well as topics for AIDS, cancer, diabetes, fitness, food, nutrition, and weight loss, among others. Some sites have hundreds of categories such as these.
- **Disease-specific information.** The Internet covers it all, from allergies to women's conditions and everything in between.
- **Dictionaries.** From drugs to health conditions, the Internet has you covered with some fabulous jargon-free medical dictionaries intended to be read by non-doctors.
- **First-aid.** Complete instructions for dealing with wounds, broken limbs, and other maladies abound online.
- **Health articles.** Many sites include excellent, up-to-the-minute articles about health-related topics. For example, when former president Bill Clinton had heart bypass surgery, many health sites posted articles about bypass surgery, explaining what it is and what it resolves.
- **Prevention.** How do you prevent bad things from happening in the first place? Reading this book is a good step in the right direction. Sites provide even more information.
- **Quizzes.** One of the best ways to teach is to provide quizzes that let users see just what they know or don't know about a subject, and then provide them with answers.
- **Self-care.** Many sites feature extensive information about how to treat certain maladies or afflictions yourself.

- **Symptom finder.** Some sites provide flowcharts and questions and answers aimed at helping you get to the bottom of an illness from which you or someone in your family is suffering.
- **Tips.** Everyone likes them, not just waiters. Health-related tips provide useful information in bite-sized portions. Many sites include hundreds of tip-related articles.
- **Treatment.** When it comes to treating an illness, injury, or condition, what are your options? When should you seek medical care? Many sites provide advice on this as well.

This chapter focuses on a few health-related sites and some gender- and age-specific sites, and highlights others that provide interesting and unique information. As always, try to get your data from more than one site. We picked the two best health sites in the U.S., then found a few others around the world and highlighted some government sites as well. Then we picked a few gender- and age-specific sites based on the quality of information provided by the scores available online.

DON'T (NECESSARILY) TRY THIS AT HOME

Many sites include disclaimers that expressly warn readers that they are providing health information, but not prescribing anything or giving medical advice. When visiting health and wellness sites, keep this in mind. As is the case with anything that is medical-related, it's always a good idea to check with your doctor first before following the advice of anything that you read on a Web site.

MayoClinic.com

http://www.mayoclinic.com

Summary: Content-rich site that does its namesake proud with a wealth of health-related information presented in a well-organized and easy-to-understand fashion.

The Mayo Clinic has been world-renowned for nearly a century, first as the Mayo's Clinic, as it was called when it opened its doors in 1907. MayoClinic.com is a great Web site with lots of health-related content that does its namesake proud. Loaded with content, MayoClinic.com is a great place to go when you want to research health-related information (see Figure 5.1).

The site is filled with tips, quizzes, articles, recipes, and expert advice. There are 26 health centers and four main categories on the site, including Diseases & Conditions, Healthy Living, Drugs & Supplements, and Health Tools. There's also a store where you can buy books and subscribe to newsletters, and an area that includes only the subjects you're interested in, called My Health Interests.

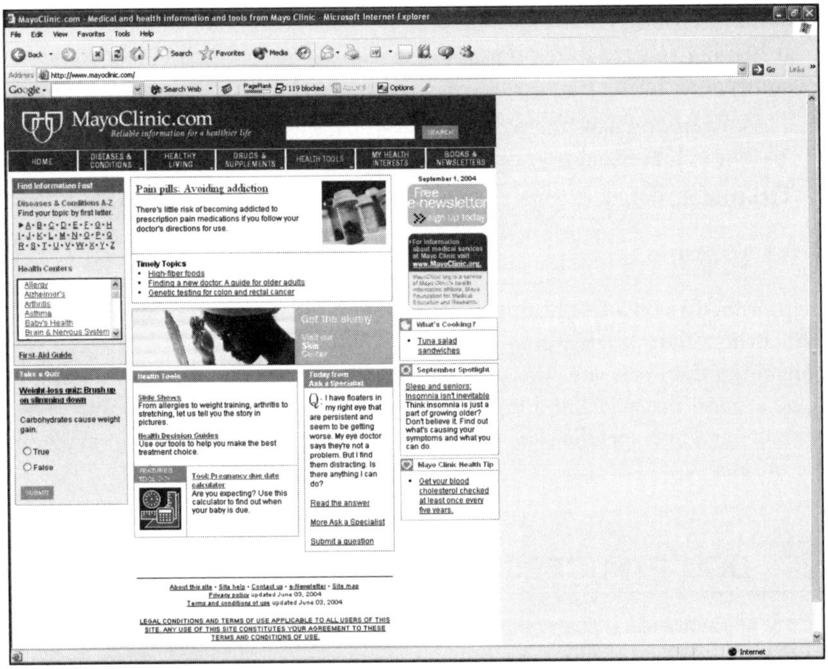

FIGURE 5.1 *MayoClinic.com home page*

The Diseases & Conditions category provides literally an A to Z guide to what ails you. Click on a topic, and you will get much more than a typical definition. For example, Figure 5.2 shows the Mayo Clinic's guide to back pain. The guide includes a short overview article, and then includes the following sections:

- Causes
- Complementary and alternative medicine
- Prevention
- Screening and diagnosis
- Self-care
- Treatment
- When to seek medical advice

The guide follows this up with further articles and tools, including a number of related slideshows. Finally, there is expert advice and a center for further information—in this case, the Pain Management Center. All this is presented in easily digestible bites of information, making it highly accessible. There are hundreds of topics in the Diseases & Conditions area, all treated in this excellent way.

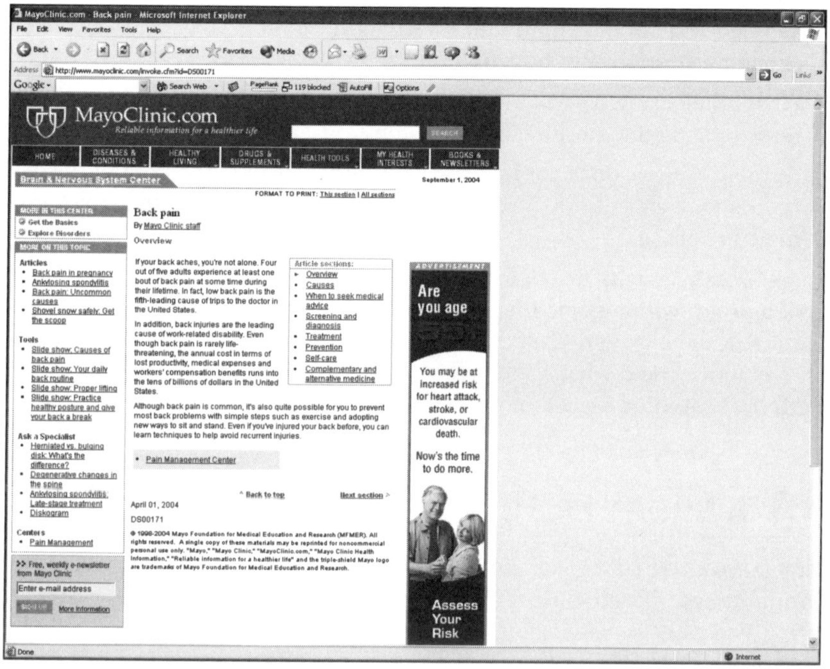

FIGURE 5.2 *Back pain is just one of hundreds of topics in MayoClinic.com's exhaustive Diseases & Conditions category.*

The Healthy Living category is broken up into subsections for different types of people, such as babies, children, men, women, pregnant women, and seniors. There are also areas that cover complementary and alternative medicine, fitness and sports medicine, food and nutrition, sleep, and working life. Each subsection includes a center feature, an area with basic articles, an area to explore the topic more deeply, and a take control section that provides tips, tools, and techniques to master the subject.

For example, in the Food & Nutrition Center, there are basic articles about portion sizes, nutrition guidelines, and a calorie calculator, as well as articles about disease prevention, weight control, and other topics (see Figure 5.3). And, there is a take-control area that provides shopping strategies, cookbooks, tips for making recipes more healthful, and meals and menus. There are also recipes, expert advice, and a poll on a topic of interest.

The Fitness & Sports Medicine Center is a typical, content-rich site that includes articles on a variety of subjects, tools such as a heart rate calculator, quizzes (this site is very big on quizzes), slideshows, tips, and expert advice (see Figure 5.4). One article takes a hatchet to many fitness myths and suggests the following tips:

- **Don't go for the burn.** Exercise shouldn't hurt. Soreness is okay, but if it hurts, stop.
- **Don't just do aerobic exercise.** Strength training and flexibility training, such as stretching, are also important.

- **Women will not bulk up if they do strength training.** In general, women don't have enough testosterone to bulk up.
- **Abdominal exercises will not flatten your stomach.** Crunches do strengthen those muscles and build posture, but they don't flatten your stomach.
- **Aerobic exercise does not increase your metabolism for the rest of the day.** However, it does for a short time. Strength training in conjunction with aerobic exercise is more beneficial.

The Drugs & Supplements area of MayoClinic.com is a great resource to prescription and non-prescription drugs, with a guide for nearly every drug sold. Each drug includes a description, brand names in the U.S. and Canada, and a discussion of how to use the medicine, including dosages, precautions, and what to do before using it (see Figure 5.5). There is also a discussion of side effects, broken up by common, less common, and rare side effects.

A SHORT HISTORY OF THE MAYO CLINIC

The Mayo Clinic's roots can be traced back to 1864, when the first Dr. Mayo, William Worrall Mayo, moved to Rochester, Minnesota, to examine recruits for the Union army. Twenty or so years later, his sons, Charles and William, joined his practice. They soon started recruiting other physicians with different specialties, hence establishing the first place where patients could go and get advice from doctors with varied backgrounds. This was the first instance of teamwork among doctors. It was also very popular; many patients, including a lot of well-known ones, came there.

Specialties that originated at the Mayo Clinic include orthopedics, neurology, thoracic surgery, dermatology, pediatrics, neurological surgery, and proctology, among others.

In 1907, the clinic opened its doors. Since then, many medical discoveries have been made. In 1920, for example, the Mayo Clinic developed a system for grading cancer numerically (stage 1, stage 2, and so on), a system that's still used today. In 1950, Mayo doctors Edward Kendall and Phillip Hench were awarded the Nobel Prize for medicine for their work on developing cortisone to treat arthritis. The clinic has also done pioneering work on heart disease, hip replacement, and psoriasis, among many other ailments.

Today, the Mayo Clinic has major locations in Jacksonville, Florida, and Scottsdale, Arizona, in addition to Rochester, and employs more than 40,000 physicians, scientists, and allied health workers. It has been a nonprofit organization since 1919 and is owned by the Mayo Foundation for Medical Education and Research.

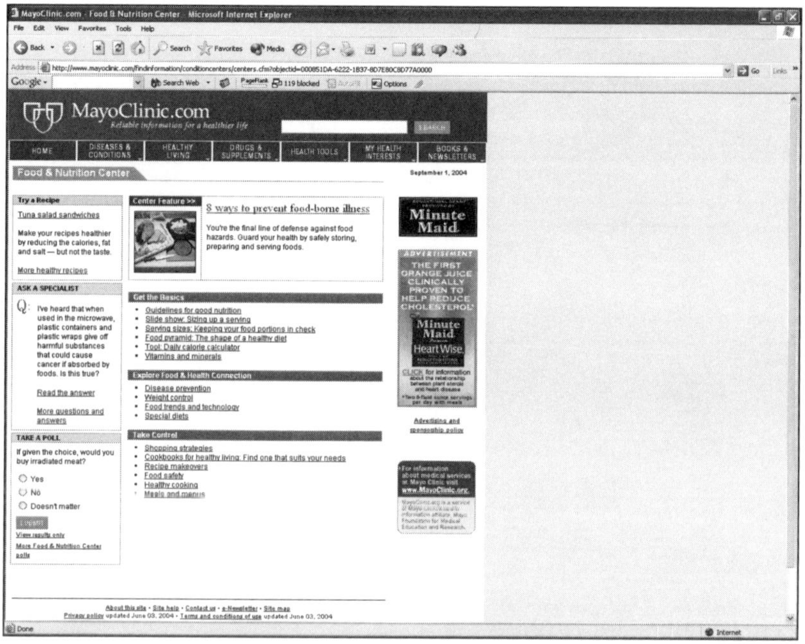

FIGURE 5.3 *MayoClinic.com's Food & Nutrition category features hundreds of articles and tools to aid in weight loss and nutrition.*

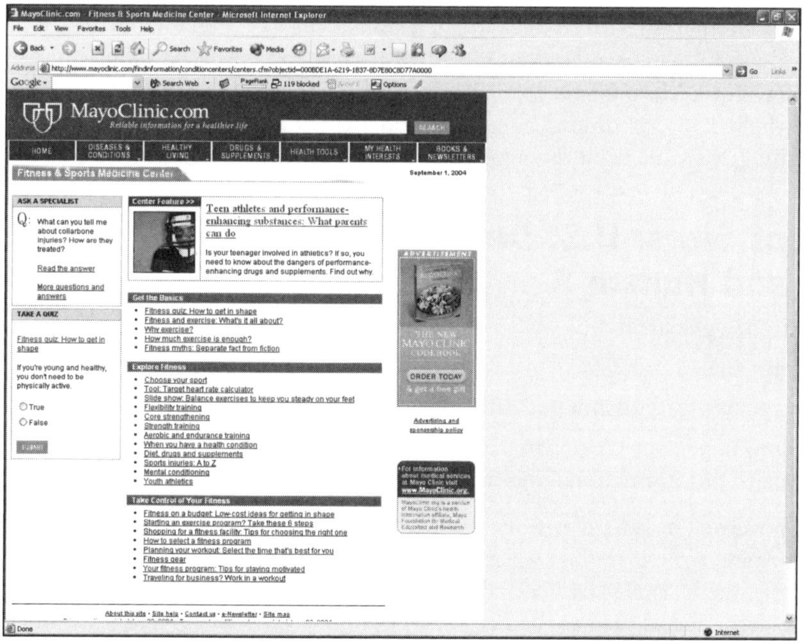

FIGURE 5.4 *The Fitness & Sports Medicine Center on MayoClinic.com*

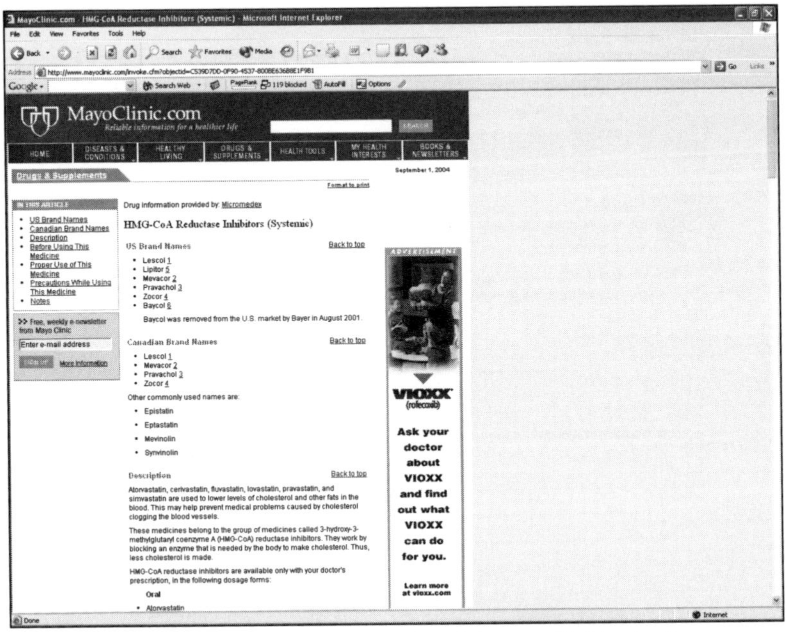

FIGURE 5.5 *Zocor is one of hundreds of medicines profiled in the Drugs & Supplements area on MayoClinic.com.*

Health Tools is a fun area that includes a lot of calculators, plus quizzes, slideshows, videos, and much more (see Figure 5.6). The most useful feature is the Decision Guides, which provide about 30 minutes of information on a given topic (see Figure 5.7). Decision Guides include treatment options, videos of a Mayo Clinic specialist discussing frequently asked questions, personal stories of people who've had a condition, things to consider, a dictionary, and links to related information. At this writing, there are eight different Decision Guides available on the site.

Government Sites: U.S. Department of Health and Human Services

http://www.smallstep.gov

http://health.nih.gov

http://www.niddk.nih.gov

Summary: Your tax dollars are at work in a great way via these sites, which provide a wealth of information about nutrition, health, and fitness.

The U.S. government is hard at work helping us get healthier. They have a variety of fine sites aimed at helping Americans lose weight, eat well, and live a healthier lifestyle. Many of the best sites are from the U.S. Department of Health and Human Services. They come from agencies within the department, such as the National Institutes of Health (NIH), National Institute of Diabetes and Digestive and Kidney Diseases (NIDDK), National Cancer Institute (NCI), and

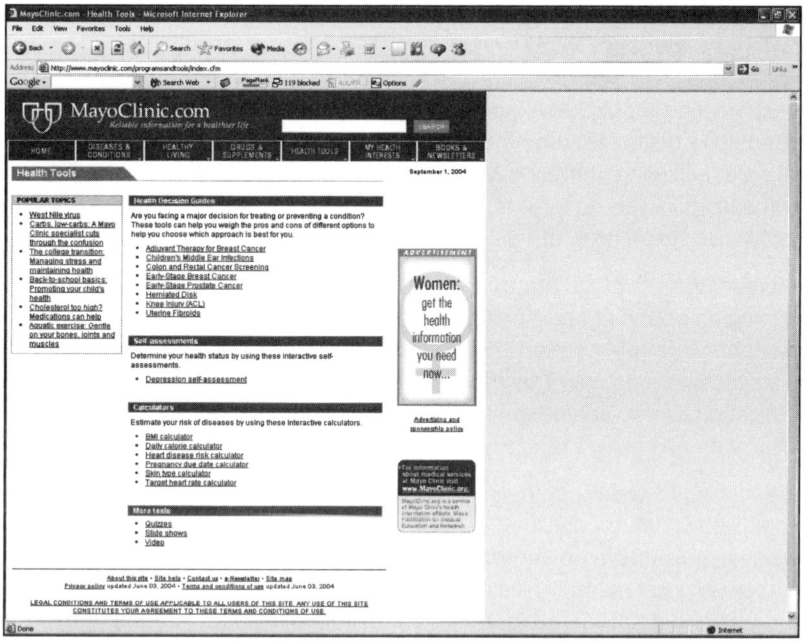

FIGURE 5.6 *The Health Tools category includes calculators, quizzes, slideshows, videos, and much more.*

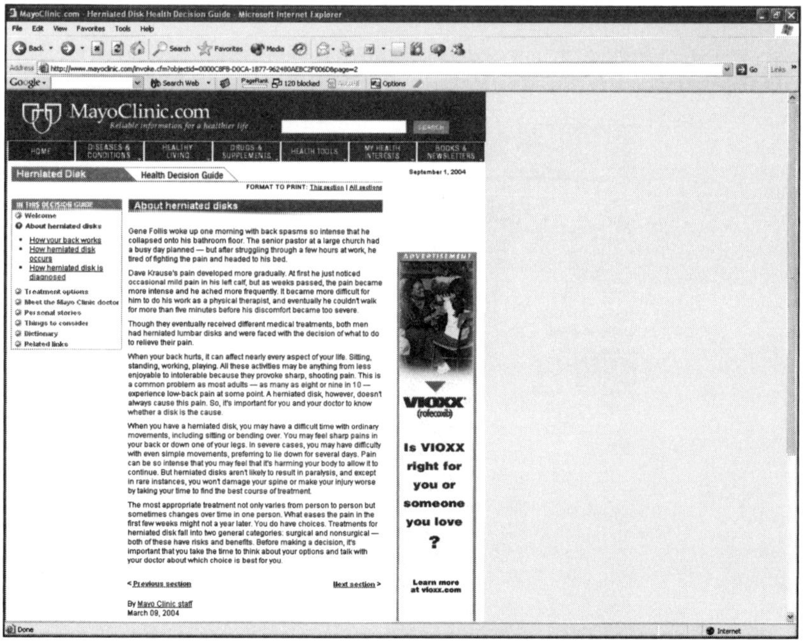

FIGURE 5.7 *Decision Guides provide about 30 minutes of information on each available condition.*

THE FOOD POLICE

Several years ago, Michael Jacobsen and his newsletter, *Nutrition Action Healthletter*, created quite a stir with their exposés about food areas that most Americans thought were safe, including various ethnic foods and movie theater popcorn. Jacobsen and his organization, the nonprofit Center for Science in the Public Interest (http://www.cspinet.org), are still at it.

The organization's goals are to act in people's best interests and provide objective information about diet and health. The organization claims that its efforts have led restaurants to introduce more healthful menu options, manufacturers to stop deceptive advertising, and major fast food chains to stop frying potatoes in beef fat. The organization is also behind much of the labeling that has gone on foods. Lately, the organization has been targeting trans-fats and promoting a trans-fat–free America.

The heart, so to speak, of their efforts, is *Nutrition Action Healthletter*, the widely read bimonthly newsletter published by CSPI (see Figure 5.8). The current issue of the newsletter is available on the Web site for free. Each newsletter is information-packed, with recipes, food ratings, articles, and more included. Food Porn is a great feature that skewers a brand-name food for infractions. Right Stuff is equal treatment for a food that CSPI praises.

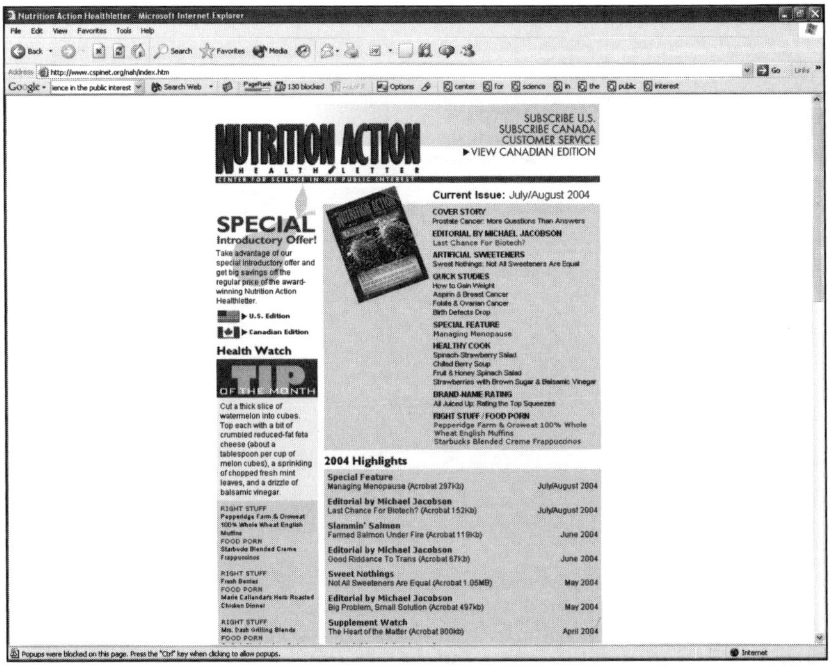

FIGURE 5.8 *Nutrition Action Healthletter is the centerpiece of CSPI's communications efforts.*

many others (see Figure 5.9). There are articles, dictionaries, quizzes, videos, pamphlets, charts, abstracts, and much more on these sites, which are well designed and well linked. There's also a site aimed specifically at weight loss, called smallstep.gov (see Figure 5.10).

The NIH, with its network of sites, is one of the most trafficked health-related areas on the Internet. As the government agency in charge of research, NIH provides a wealth of information about various diseases and health issues. Although it's fairly free of bells and whistles, NIH is a great resource to thousands of health-related articles. It includes separate sites for men, women, children, seniors, and minorities, as well as a general health and wellness section. There's also a health dictionary called MedlinePlus and links to other sites from departments within NIH, such as NIDDK and NCI. NIDDK provides at-a-glance, detailed data in a friendly manner. These data are actually online versions of the department's WIN publications. WIN stands for *Weight-control Information Network.* WIN provides a variety of publications, videos, abstracts, newsletters, and other information about controlling and losing weight (see Figure 5.11).

NOTE

For more information, contact WIN at the following address:

The Weight-control Information Network
1 WIN Way
Bethesda, MD 20892-3665
202-828-1025 or 1-877-946-4627
win@info.niddk.nih.gov

Although WIN provides a great deal of useful information, keep in mind that it's a government program, so it endorses other government programs. If you don't agree with a diet that is consistent with the USDA Food Guide Pyramid, you might not agree with WIN. However, here are some of the guidelines that it suggests for a healthy America:

- **Eat an appropriate amount of calories to help you lose between one-half and two pounds per week.** In other words, you should eat about 300 to 500 calories per day less than you need to maintain your weight.
- **Make sure that you are getting enough vitamins and minerals.** You might need to take vitamins, for example.
- **Diet should be high in carbohydrates.** Fifty-five percent of your carbs should come from complex carbohydrates, such as fruits, vegetables, and whole grains. They suggest that if you eat fewer than 130 grams of carbs each day, you'll suffer side effects, such as fatigue and nausea.
- **Diets should be low in fat.** No more than 30 percent of your calories per day should come from fat. At 1,500 calories, that's about 50 grams of fat. Remember, each gram of fat is about nine calories.

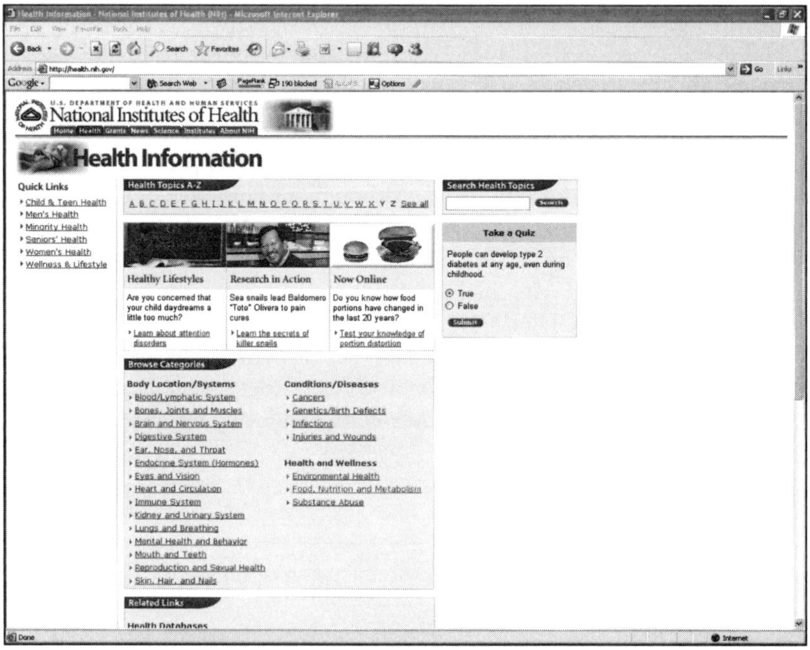

FIGURE 5.9 *The National Institutes of Health provide a great deal of useful information about health and fitness.*

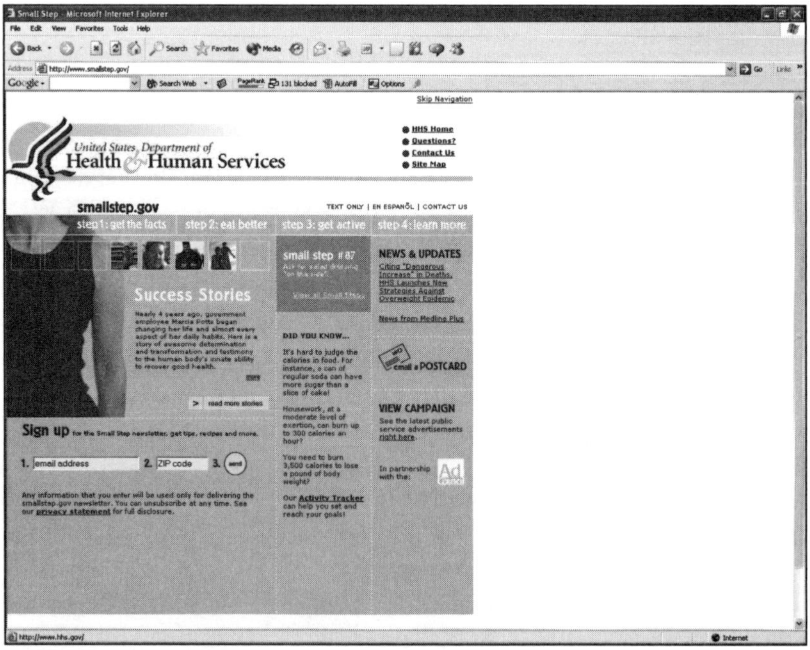

FIGURE 5.10 *Smallstep.gov is the Department of Health and Human Services' effort toward reducing obesity one small step at a time.*

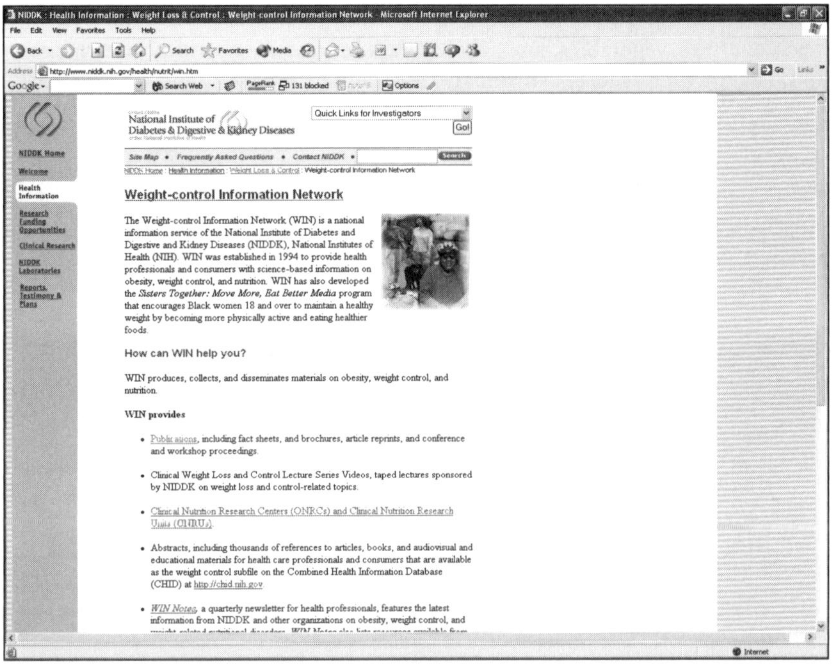

FIGURE 5.11 *WIN is at the heart of the NIDDK's effort at controlling weight through information and outreach efforts.*

In conjunction with WIN, the Department of Health and Human Services developed smallstep.gov. The organization realizes that it's not easy to develop a cure for obesity, but if everyone would take a series of small steps to move their own lives in the right direction, they would be able to fight obesity and lose weight. Among the 118 small steps included on the site are the following tips:

- Take the stairs instead of the elevator.
- Park a little farther from your office each day.
- Skip buffets.
- When eating in restaurants, ask your server to put half your entrée in a to-go bag before you are served.
- Take longer walks.
- Drink lots of water.
- Avoid food portions larger than your fist.
- Get a dog and walk it.
- Avoid labor-saving devices.
- Don't skip breakfast.

The site includes lots of other advice that can be boiled down into three main points: Eat healthy foods, such as fruits, vegetables, and whole-grain products; control portions; and get plenty of exercise. It also includes success stories and a variety of details about diet and exercise.

There are many links to other government agencies for more information, including a great deal of information from the Centers for Disease Control (CDC). One of the best is from the NCI, which is promoting its 5 A Day for Better Health program (http://5aday.gov; see Figure 5.12), intended to encourage Americans to get five servings of fruits and vegetables per day (nine servings per day for men). The National Cancer Institute also recommends at least 30 minutes of physical exercise per day as well.

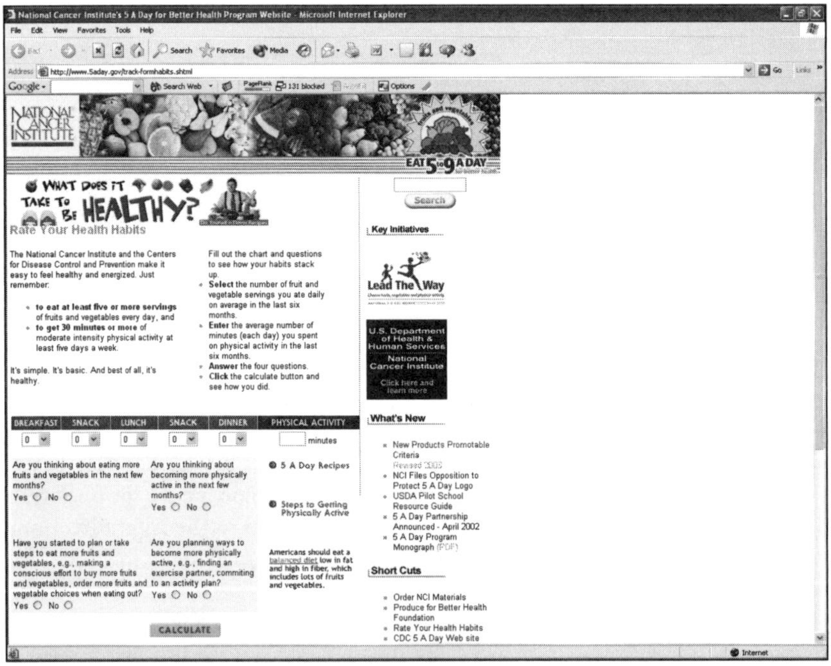

FIGURE 5.12 *The National Cancer Institute promotes its 5 to 9 per day program, encouraging Americans to eat more fruits and vegetables.*

WebMD

http://www.webmd.com

Summary: Lots of data here, both for medical professionals and non-professionals alike.

WebMD was formed to provide timely, credible medical information for consumers and physicians. With more than 20 million visitors each month and 575,000 physicians, WebMD is the number-one site on the Internet (see Figure 5.13). It provides health-related information for consumers and physicians through a number of programs. These include products for physicians

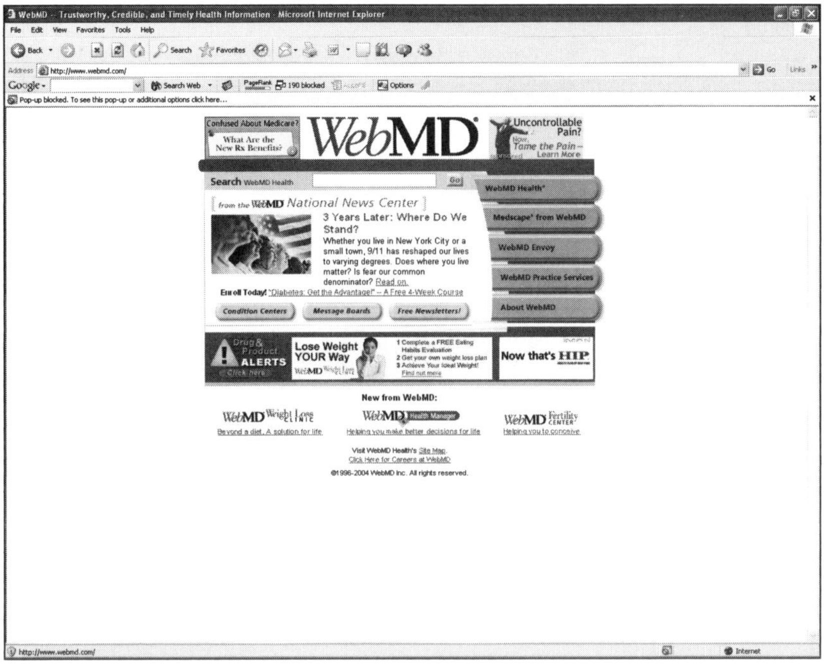

FIGURE 5.13 *WebMD is the number-one health-related site on the Internet.*

INSURANCE COMPANIES GET IN ON THE ACT

While consumer and government sites provide an abundance of information, don't forget your health insurance company. Many insurers, including Aetna, Blue Cross, Kaiser Permanente, Prudential, and others, have excellent sites with a great deal of health information. One of the best is InteliHealth from Aetna (see Figure 5.14).

Featuring data from the Harvard Medical School, InteliHealth provides news and information, health-related articles, expert advice, weight loss tools, medical and drug dictionaries, a health directory, message boards, and much more. It's free to everyone, not just Aetna subscribers, and the site takes great pains to assure visitors that it is independent and that content is created by Aetna editors and editors from the Harvard Medical School. Other health insurers are not as ambitious as Aetna, but they do offer resources with information for their customers. Kaiser Permanente, for example, offers HealthMedia, a site that provides basic information about living a healthy life. Several insurance companies don't have their own Web sites, preferring instead to provide information via WebMD. These providers let subscribers use the vast resources of WebMD for medical information and the WebMD interface to find health-plan–specific information, such as how to find a physician, request replacement ID cards, check the status of claims, change their address, and more.

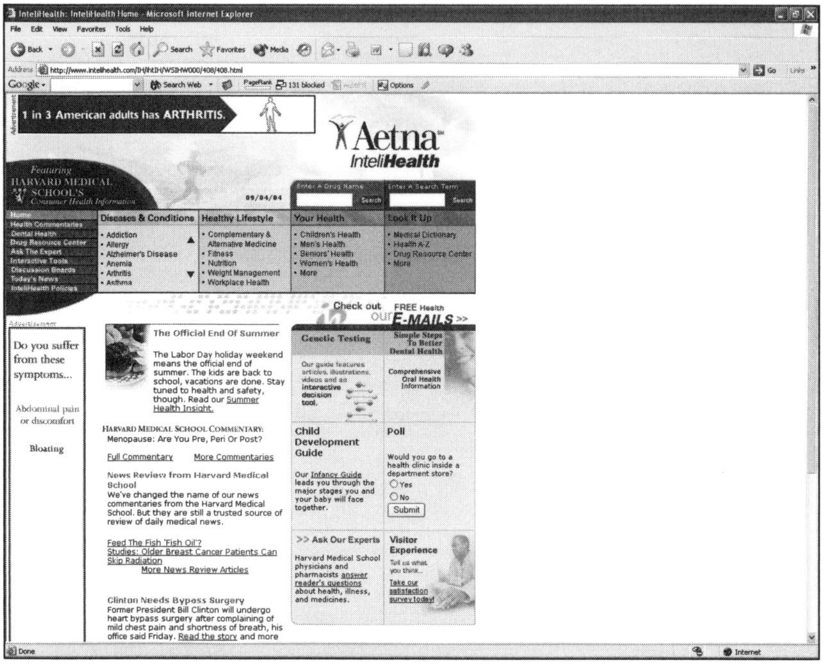

FIGURE 5.14 *Aetna's InteliHealth Site is one of the best from an insurance company and features data from the Harvard Medical School.*

(WebMD Practice Services and Medscape), healthcare companies (WebMD Envoy, as well as plan-specific sites, as mentioned in the preceding sidebar), and consumers (WebMD Health). We'll spend most of our time talking about WebMD Health (see Figure 5.15).

WebMD Health is a vast site covering nearly anything related to health. It includes news; quizzes; calculators; polls; expert advice; community services; symptom and disease information; message boards; a learning center; a drug and herb guide; women-, men-, and lifestyle-specific data; information about diet and nutrition; and much more. There are also subscription sites for weight loss and fertility, and an innovative product called Health Manager that provides personalized information and the ability to track medical history online.

Diseases & Conditions is one of the most used areas on WebMD (see Figure 5.16). It includes an exhaustive directory of diseases and conditions, including several links that are sponsored by advertisers. Clicking on a particular condition brings up an article about it, tips on how to deal with it, medical data from the Cleveland Clinic, a directory of clinical trials about your condition, quizzes and tools, and a section called We Knew You'd Want to Know, which covers tips and techniques for dealing with the condition.

Since being overweight is a condition, WebMD includes an excellent Weight Control Health Center (see Figure 5.17). There are articles, quizzes, tools, tips, facts from the Cleveland Clinic, and lots of data about a variety of obesity-related subjects.

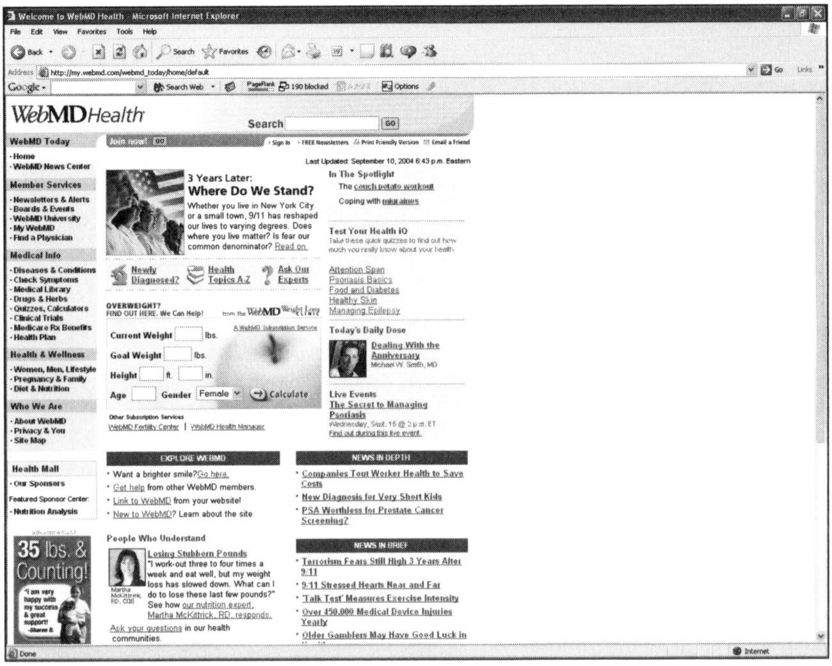

FIGURE 5.15 *WebMD Health*

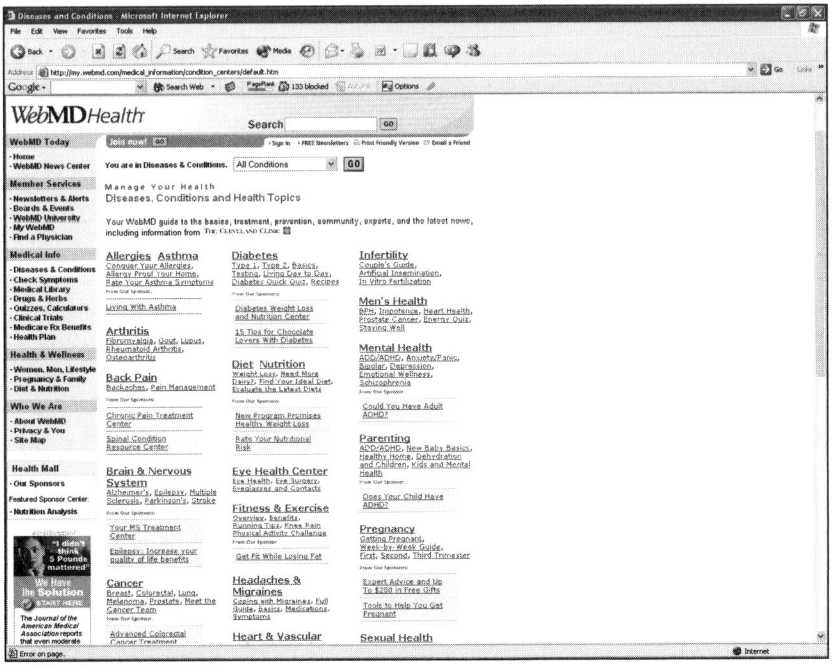

FIGURE 5.16 *Diseases & Conditions is an exhaustive database of information from WebMD.*

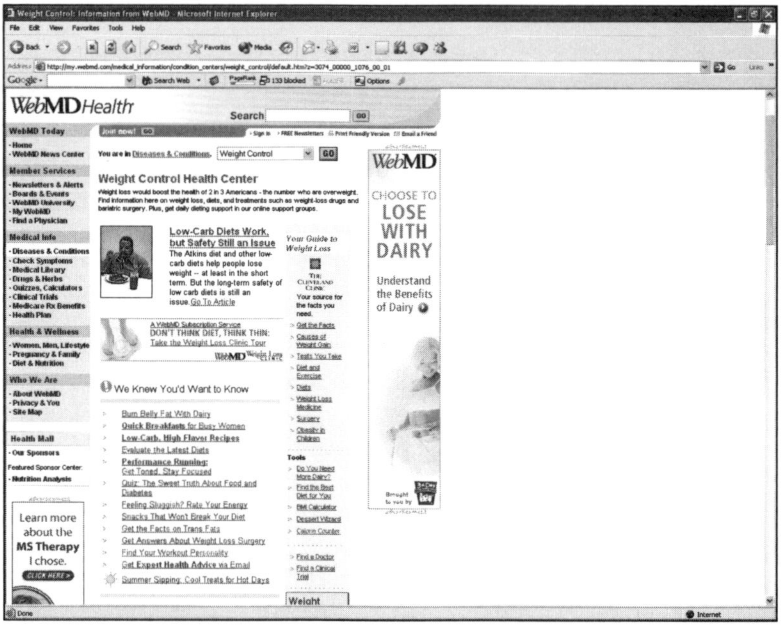

FIGURE 5.17 *The Weight Control Health Center on WebMD includes lots of articles, quizzes, tools, and other information.*

WebMD's Medical Library is without peer. It includes an interactive symptom checker (see Figure 5.18), an A–Z library of medical terms, a directory that describes nearly all medical tests, a drug and herb guide, and a listing of all clinical trials. You can also ask questions of the more than 30 medical experts on WebMD in a wide variety of areas, from weight loss to heart disease to female issues to attention deficit disorder.

The symptom checker features a number of yes or no questions that will lead you to a diagnosis. There is also an overview of the topic, health risks, home treatment, prevention, and a wide variety of related information that may lead you to determine what is ailing you (see Figure 5.19).

WebMD's more than 200 message boards are well traveled, with a variety of support groups on a number of topics (AIDS, aging, addiction, arthritis, cancer, cholesterol, dental health, infertility, men's issues, women's issues, and weight loss, among others) plus boards hosted by an expert (ADD/HD, cancer, diabetes, dieting, general health, sleep disorders) and some tips on topics such as skin care and others. There are also live events most weekdays at 2:00 pm Eastern time. These events are hosted by WebMD experts who cover a wide variety of topics from childhood obesity to parenthood to cancer and more. Archives of most live events are available long after the event has passed. Although most of WebMD is free, it also offers three subscription services for weight loss, health records, and infertility. The Weight Loss Clinic costs $99 for six months and $9.95 per month after that, or $60 for three months and $14.95 per month after that. It includes personalized meal plans, a food journal, community support from their message boards, news about weight loss, fitness tips, and recipe ideas, among other features (see Figure 5.20).

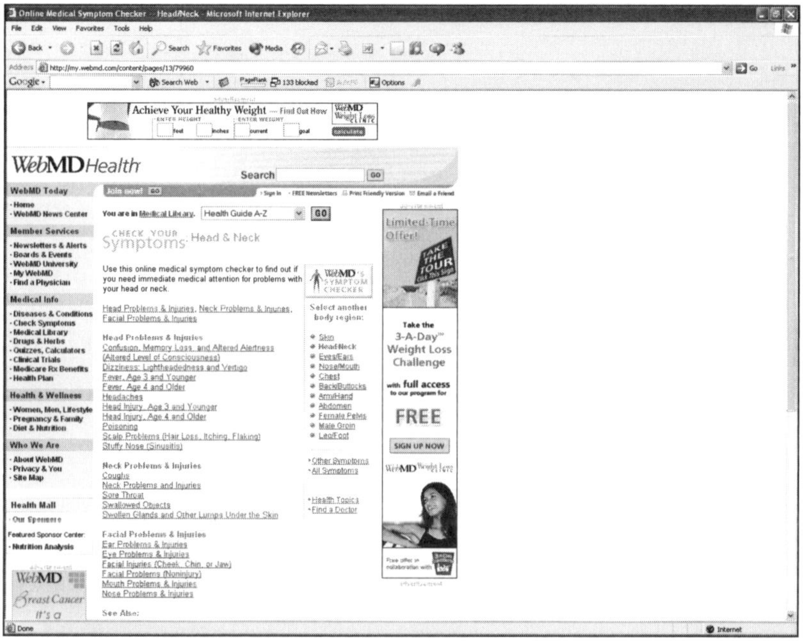

FIGURE 5.18 *WebMD's symptom checker provides data for literally hundreds of different injuries, diseases, and illnesses.*

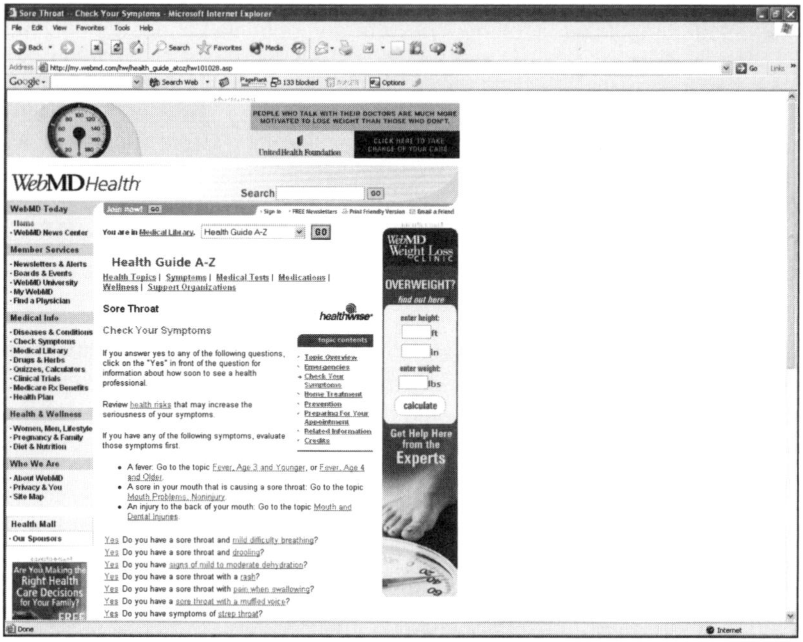

FIGURE 5.19 *WebMD's symptom checker helps you resolve common and uncommon maladies. In this case, there is lots of information about a sore throat.*

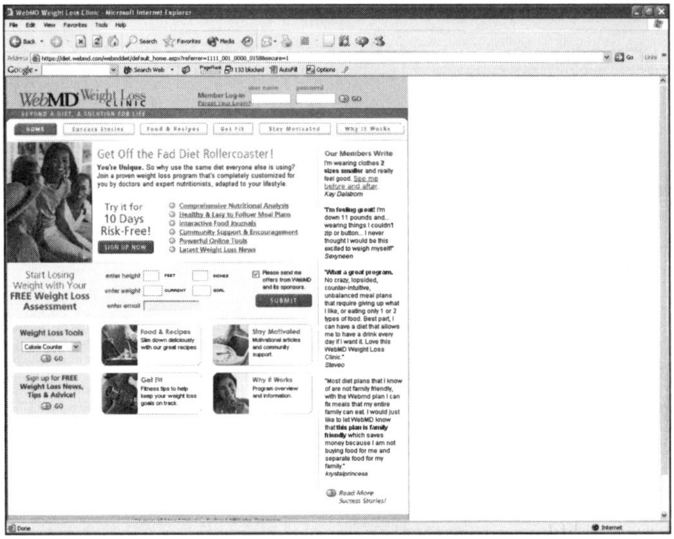

FIGURE 5.20 *The Weight Loss Clinic at WebMD provides meal plans, nutritional tools, and other information to help users lose weight.*

WEBMD AND CHILDHOOD OBESITY

WebMD articles are authoritative, with step-by-step instructions that are based on fact and sound medical reasoning. They are authoritative yet not condescending, informative but not preachy, and complete but not closed-minded. They read as if you have a doctor sitting in your living room.

For example, WebMD, in conjunction with the Cleveland Clinic, includes several articles about childhood obesity. There is an article that discusses what childhood obesity is, another that talks about prevention, another with tips for healthy eating, and an excellent article about how to help your child lose weight if he or she is already overweight. In short, this is nearly everything a parent needs, in bite-sized pieces, and provides enough guidance along the way.

One of the most interesting aspects of WebMD's recommendations about childhood obesity is that, in general, WebMD recommends that to prevent childhood obesity, you treat your child much as you would an adult who is trying to lose weight. Don't make them clean their plate, make sure that their diet is healthy, ensure that the child gets enough exercise, and don't bring home unhealthy snacks.

If a child is already overweight, WebMD recommends the same things it would for adults as well. Set goals in conjunction with the child, have him or her keep a food diary, ensure that the child is getting enough exercise, and help him or her with portion control. WebMD also recommends that you only enter your child in a weight-control program if his or her doctor recommends it.

LOSING WEIGHT WITH A LITTLE HELP FROM WEBMD

Thirty-three-year-old Sharon Ranch was searching online for information about croup in the fall of 2003; she was afraid that her one-year-old daughter, Elizabeth, might have it. She saw some information about the WebMD Weight Loss Clinic and decided then and there to do something about her weight. "I didn't want my daughter to grow up with a fat mom," she says. "I didn't want to transfer my body issues to her."

Ranch, who is 5'8", weighed 209 pounds in the fall of 2003 (see Figure 5.21). Her goal was to get to 169 pounds. At first, she tried to go it alone, by using the Journal feature on WebMD. After a few weeks, she realized that wasn't good enough; her old habits were still coming to light. So, she started to look for help. "I posted a note on the Friends Talking bulletin board, and the support and advice I got from the other members and moderators was incredible," she says.

Ranch had tried eDiets but found it too restrictive. "I just wasn't interested in what they prescribed," she says. She prefers WebMD's expert system technology that basically takes what you eat in a given week and helps you reduce the amount of food while still enjoying your own basic diet.

Practicing portion control, following the program, and exercising for 20 to 30 minutes per day three to four times per week, Ranch reached her goal in less than one year (see Figure 5.22). Now that she has gotten there, she's thinking about losing some more. The BMI for her height recommends 164, so she will strive for that.

Ranch expresses surprise and delight at her success. "I have never stuck with any program this far before," she says. Ranch attributes her "addiction" to the program to the message boards and the scheduled chats with experts, which she attends at least once per week. "If it wasn't for the community, I probably would have given up after my first stumble," she says. "But they boosted me back up into the saddle, and I'm happy to say I've done it."

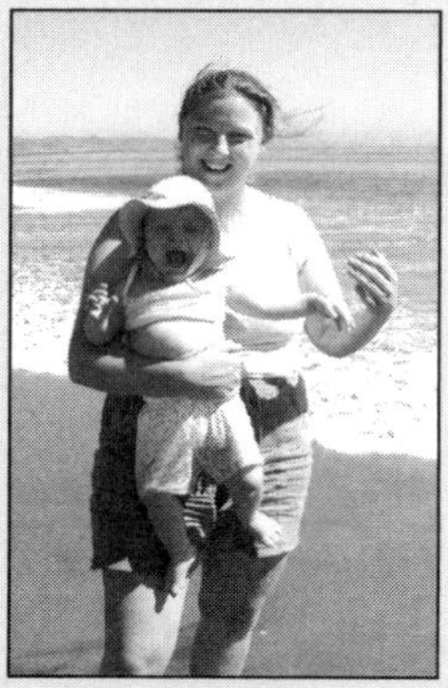

FIGURE 5.21 *Sharon Ranch and her daughter, Elizabeth, just before she started her weight-loss program.*

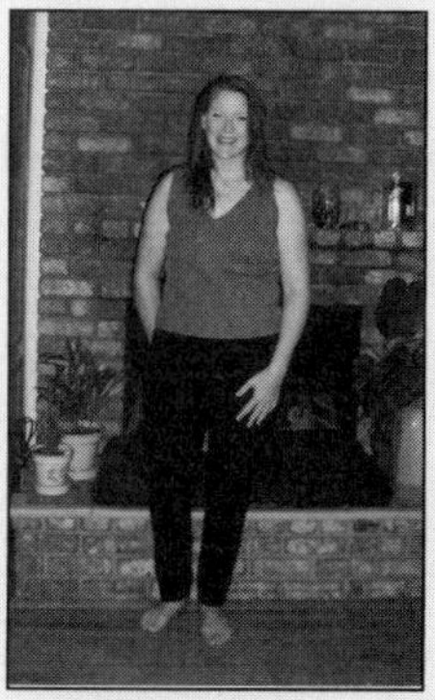

FIGURE 5.22 *Sharon Ranch one year later.*

HEALTH OUTSIDE THE U.S.

Excellent health-related information is not restricted to the U.S. There are a number of great sites that provide lots of interesting and varied content from other countries. One example is Canada's C-Health (http://chealth.canoe.ca), a service of Canoe (Canadian Online Explorer), the top news and information site in Canada. The site is heavy on articles from its news agency and major Canadian newspapers, and it also features information centers for a wide variety of issues, including men's, women's, seniors', and babies' health; sexual health; sleep health; diabetes; and other issues (see Figure 5.23). It also includes a drug information center, weight loss calculators, community support, dictionaries, quizzes, and other tools in a content-rich site tailored for Canadian readers. The Canadian government also offers a content-rich site called Health Canada, available in both English and French (http://www.hc-sc.gc.ca).

On the other side of the Atlantic is BBC Health (http://www.bbc.co.uk/health), a service of the British Broadcasting Company. BBC Health promotes the health-related programming offered by the BBC on TV, and it includes articles and expert advice about health issues, as well as special interest groups based on age group, gender, and other factors (see Figure 5.24). It also includes quizzes and guides to various illnesses, a weight loss center, and much more. Another popular U.K. site is NetDoctor (http://netdoctor.co.uk).

Down under, there's myDr (http://mydr.com.au), an Australia-specific site with special interest groups (called *Centres*), news and articles, and, of course, weight loss (see Figure 5.25). And the Australian government offers a popular site called HealthInsite (http://healthinsite.gov.au).

Of course, when you start talking about height and weight outside the U.S., some of the calculators and discussions change markedly because everyone else uses the metric system, in which one stone is equal to 14 pounds, and there are 28 grams in an ounce.

Gender- and Age-Specific Sites

While many of the health and wellness sites we've covered so far in this chapter include gender- and age-specific information, none of them cover these categories as well as those dedicated to the subject. This is somewhat like the difference between department stores and specialty stores. Department stores have departments for a variety of categories, but no department is as good as going to an entire store that specializes in the category in which you are most interested. In this section, we'll cover sites for men, women, and seniors. There are many great sites in this category; we've picked what in our opinion are the best ones. We picked one from each category, which wasn't an easy task.

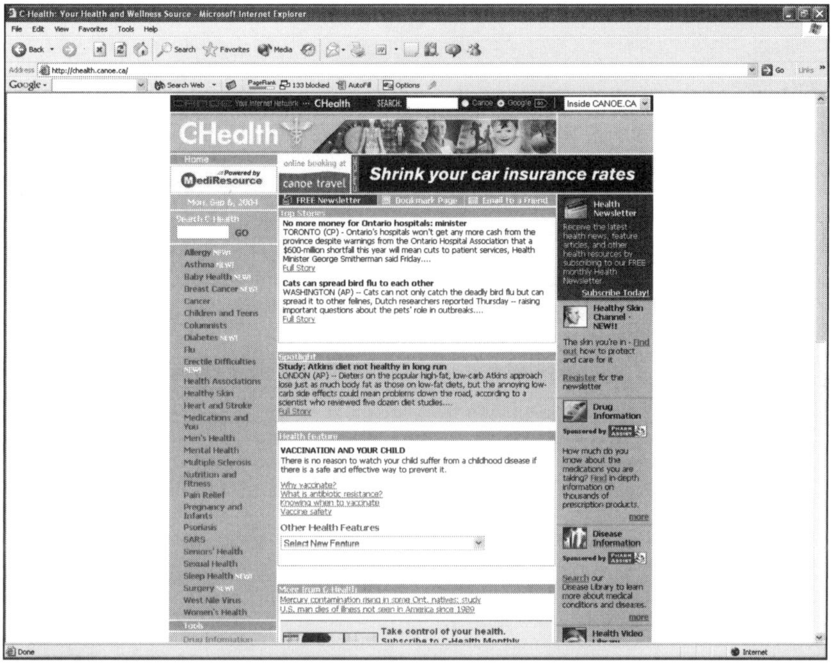

FIGURE 5.23 *C-Health is Canada's number one health site*

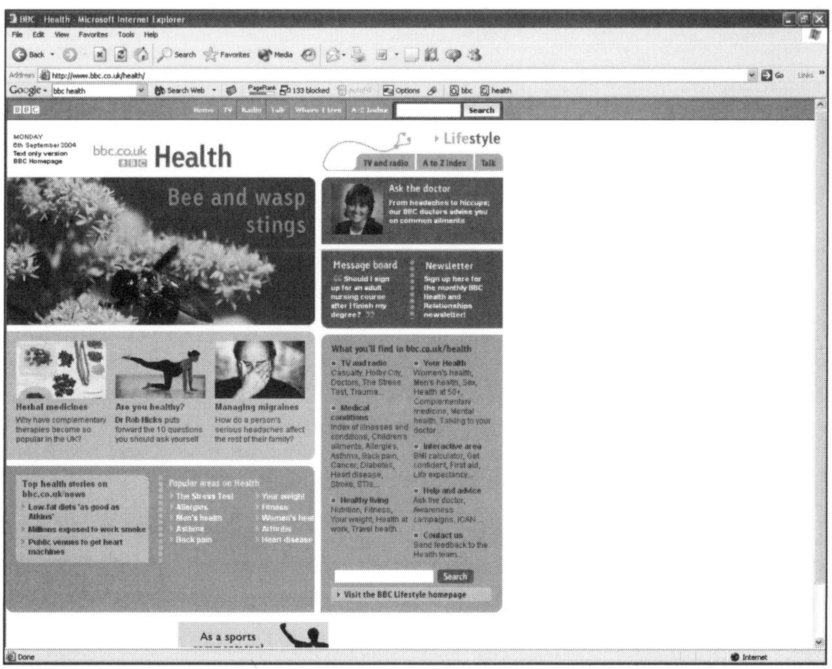

FIGURE 5.24 *The BBC offers BBC Health to British users.*

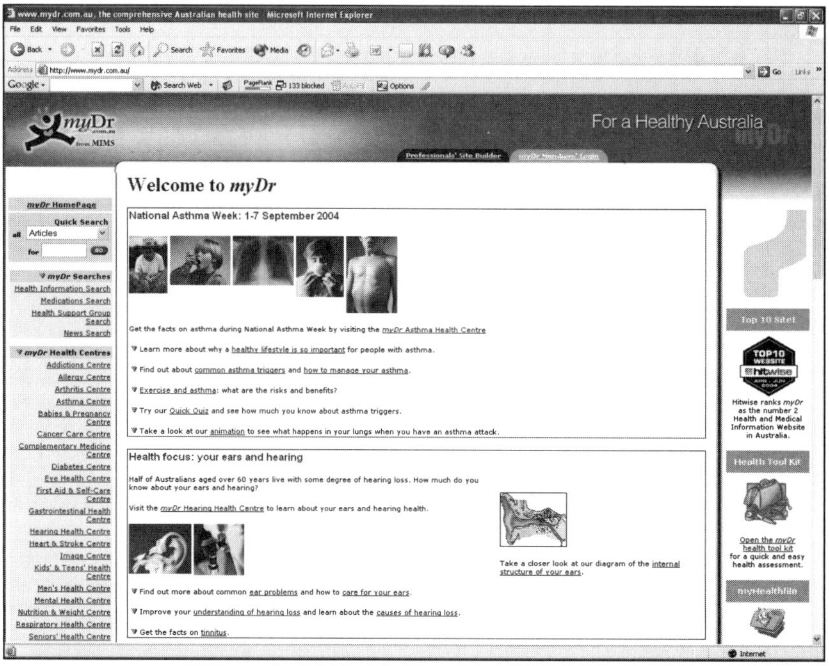

FIGURE 5.25 *From down under comes myDr, a health site aimed at Australian users.*

There are many differences in these types of sites. Women tend to be interested in body image, health, nutrition, and family issues. They make most of the decisions about what families eat and the activities in which they participate. As a result, women's health sites include lots of family information, cooking tips, and relationship issues. These sites also focus on subjects of particular interest to women, and because women tend to communicate more, the sites tend to have much stronger communities than men's sites.

On the other hand, if a man's site has cooking tips, they're likely about grilling, the macho cooking trend of the moment. Plus, while women will follow meal plans and diet plans, men generally would much rather lose weight through fitness and exercise, with some discipline thrown in for good measure. Most men would rather make their own meal choices and cut calories in their own way. In general, they don't want to have someone else tell them what to eat via a meal plan. That's why the folks at eDiets introduced eFitness; they wanted a site for men. While eDiets is not aimed at women, most of the members who follow meal plans at eDiets are women. Men tend to join eFitness.

Seniors, on the other hand, are more interested in simply feeling better day to day. They generally are worried about their health, insurance, drug plans, Alzheimer's disease, protecting themselves, and avoiding major injuries and illnesses. Seniors are interested in leading active, healthy lives.

iVillage

http://www.ivillage.com

Summary: It's not called "The Internet for Women" for nothing. The number-one women's site on the Internet is chock full of female-oriented information about diet, fitness, weight loss, and health.

It's no wonder that iVillage is the number-one community Web site for women (see Figure 5.26). With more than 370 million page views per month from more than 17 million unique visitors, iVillage gets a lot of attention.

More than 1,400 message boards; topics rich with content that women want to know about; lots of information about health, fitness, diet, exercise, weight loss, and more—and all of it aimed at women. iVillage is that and more. It has sister sites (of course, no brothers), including women.com, all the female-related magazine Web sites for the Hearst Corporation (*Country Living*, *Cosmopolitan*, *Good Housekeeping*, *House Beautiful*, *Marie Claire*, *Redbook*, and *Town and Country*), and so much more. And by the way, there's lots of good information here for everyone, not just women. Although the articles are slanted toward women, iVillage strikes me somewhat like that old campaign for Secret deodorant, which was "strong enough for a man, but made for a woman." iVillage content is useful enough for everyone, but made for women.

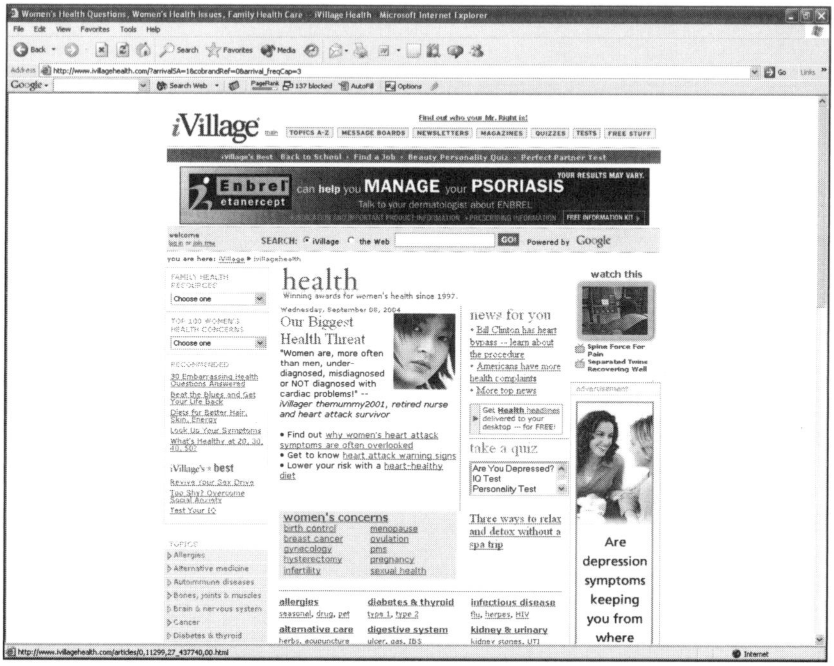

FIGURE 5.26 *The Health site at iVillage.com is fun, informative, and a great women's resource.*

All areas of iVillage are organized in a similar fashion, with news, articles, videos, quizzes, tips, issues particularly suited to women, and a Best of iVillage section that features the most popular articles. There's an A–Z health dictionary, message boards on many subjects, chats, expert advice, and more. All topics are written for women. For example, in the section on cholesterol, iVillage admonishes women who think high cholesterol is only a problem for middle-aged men and elderly men and women. And in the weight management section, iVillage provides some great facts particularly oriented toward females. (For example, dividing a woman's waist measurement by her hip measurement can help determine her risk of diabetes and heart disease. If her waist measurement divided by her hip measurement is greater than 0.8, she is at greater risk of developing those diseases because that ratio means that she has a high amount of visceral fat, which is associated with those diseases.) Developed in conjunction with the National Women's Health Resource Center, each health topic includes an overview, diagnosis and treatment information, prevention, facts, questions to ask, and tips, as well as a test to see how much you know about a subject (see Figure 5.27).

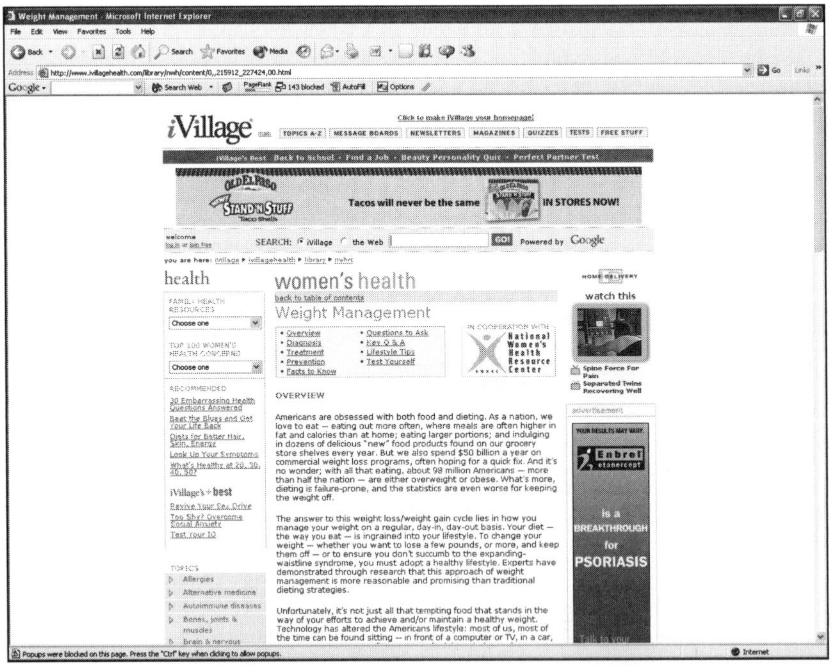

FIGURE 5.27 *A typical topic on women's health at iVillage.com*

In the Diet & Fitness area, iVillage provides a lot of great information aimed at helping women achieve a healthy weight (see Figure 5.28). Taking content developed from all of the Hearst magazines in addition to their own content, iVillage provides information that is every bit as good as any of the other weight loss sites we've covered. The Diet & Fitness area is broken down into nine main categories. Each category has essential information about the topic, articles, newsletters, message boards, expert advice, quizzes, tools, and a community challenge to help you lose weight. The categories include:

- **Diet Plans.** This is a nice area that compares diet plans, offers diet tips, and much more.
- **Eating Habits.** This area helps you deal with cravings, healthy eating plans, and portion control, as well as helping you create new habits.
- **Safety & Health.** This is an excellent source that evaluates the safety of some of the "lose weight quick" programs, such as surgery, fad diets, and drugs. This category contains lots of hints and tips.
- **Workouts.** This area helps users decide which cardio workouts are for them. It discusses all cardio workouts, including aerobics, biking, jumping rope, martial arts, running, spinning, sports, and more. This area also includes a fitness video finder, with reviews, previews, and user feedback.
- **Diet Blocks.** This area helps women deal with issues that invariably come up during dieting, including staying motivated, dealing with emotional issues, and getting past plateaus.
- **Nutrition.** This area contains lots of data about essential nutrients, carbs, fats, proteins, and much more. It also includes recommendations for particularly nutritious foods. (Did you know that soy contains phytoestrogens to help relieve hot flashes during menopause for women?)

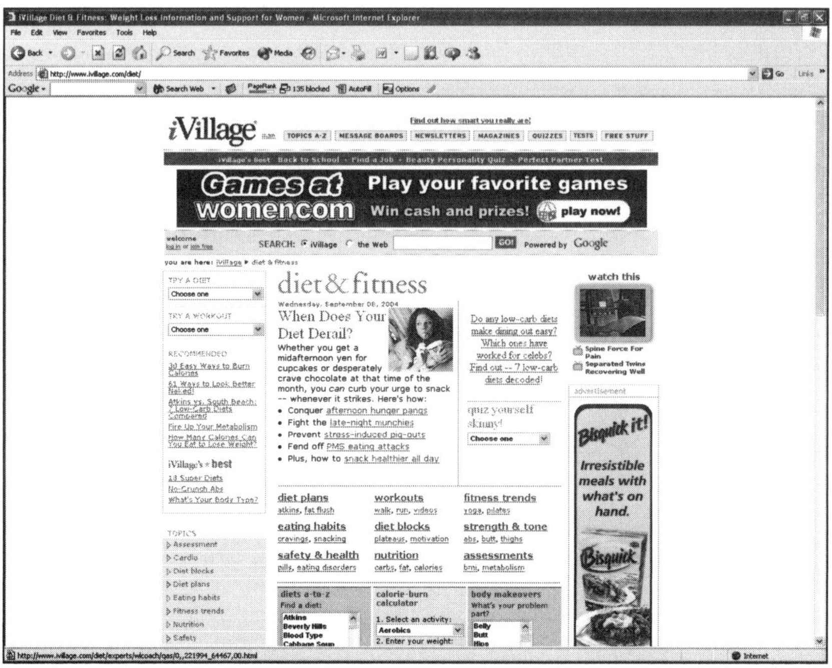

FIGURE 5.28 *The Diet & Fitness area on women's health at iVillage.com*

- **Fitness Trends.** This area discusses essential fitness gear, meditation, Pilates, yoga, and other popular trends and workout programs.
- **Strength & Tone.** This area discusses the essential exercises you should do to tone and strengthen various parts of your body. It includes a lot of good information about getting started in weight training, among other topics.
- **Assessment Tools.** This area presents quizzes, calculators, and tips to help you assess your overall body health. It includes a BMI calculator, a health calculator, heart rate thresholds, bone density information, tips for improving your metabolism, and much more.

Each section is heavy on tips, "secrets," and tricks, such as how to lose 10 pounds, 101 tricks to avoid overeating, or 10 easy ways to eat healthier. Many of these articles come from the pages of the Hearst magazines featured on iVillage; others come from iVillage editorial staffers or experts. Here are some tips for saving calories:

- Have a flavored bagel without cream cheese or butter.
- Use fat-free instead of regular salad dressing.
- Eat an English muffin instead of a donut.
- Eat tortilla chips with salsa instead of guacamole.
- Remove the skin from a chicken breast after cooking it.
- Use light mayo instead of regular mayo when making tuna, chicken, or pasta salad.
- Leave the bottom crust of a piece of pie on your plate.
- Use nonstick spray instead of oil when cooking.
- Order a small order of fries instead of a large one.
- Have virgin drinks instead of the same drinks with alcohol.

The Food area on iVillage.com is more of the same, with lots of tips for cooking, entertaining, nutrition (the same area as on Diet & Fitness), and healthy eating, plus a large recipe database and an area for baking and desserts (see Figure 5.29). Although the Food area is filled with useful information, be cautious. Not all of the recipes are healthy, and many don't include nutritional information. However, if you use the recipe finder, you can narrow down essential recipes and find the ones that are nutritionally sound. A special diets option in the recipe finder lets you choose low-fat, low-salt, heart-smart, low-calorie, and vegetarian entrées, among others.

Men's Health

http://www.menshealth.com

Summary: The popular magazine has much to offer online. A content-rich site provides much more information than the magazine offers alone, while keeping the edgy nature of the publication alive.

The *Men's Health* magazine and Web site have the same slogan: "Tons of useful stuff." It's an appealing slogan because Men's Health provides just that. There is a plethora of information

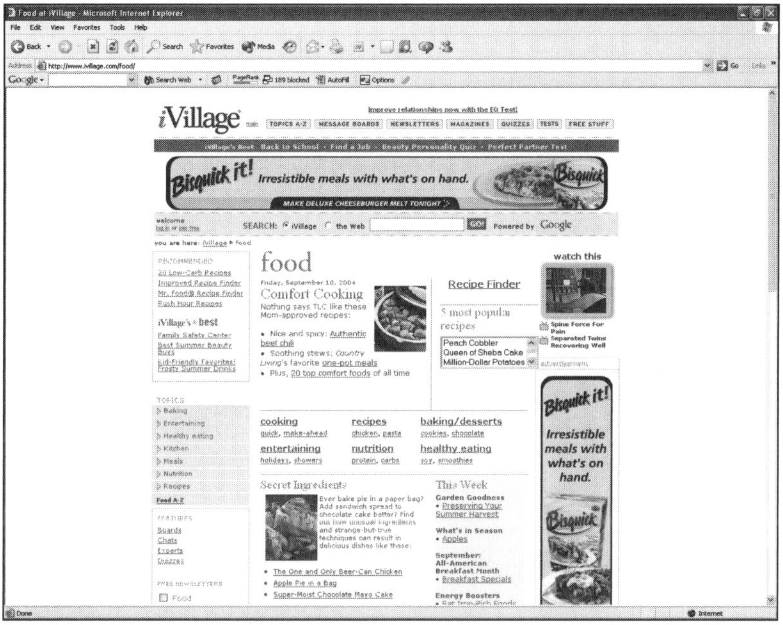

FIGURE 5.29 *iVillage Food section*

HEALTH AND FITNESS FOR KIDS

Men, women, and seniors have an abundance of sites devoted to their health, but kids aren't left out in the cold. Kidsnutrition.org is a service of the USDA about kids, intended for parents. It's produced by the Children's Nutrition Research Center at the Baylor College of Medicine.

Kidsnutrition.org includes a children's BMI calculator, which is slightly different than a BMI calculator for adults. An energy calculator intended to show parents the importance of making sure their kids get enough exercise also adds value. The site also includes articles about diet, exercise, and childhood obesity, plus links to other nutrition sites.

Plus, the Nemours Foundation, a nonprofit organization dedicated to the well being of children, offers KidsHealth (http://kidshealth.org), a Web site that helps kids, parents, and teens with health issues (see Figure 5.30). For younger children, KidsHealth explores such topics as dealing with feelings, safety, children's health problems, a kid-friendly glossary of medical terms, health games, information about what different kinds of doctors do, and more. There are also recipes for kids, including kids with diabetes, cystic fibrosis, and other conditions. The teen site has some of the same content as the kids site, but it also includes information about teens' changing bodies and much more information about diets and diet safety. The parent section features advice for talking to your child's pediatrician, general health issues, child development, and parenting. All these sites are also available in Spanish.

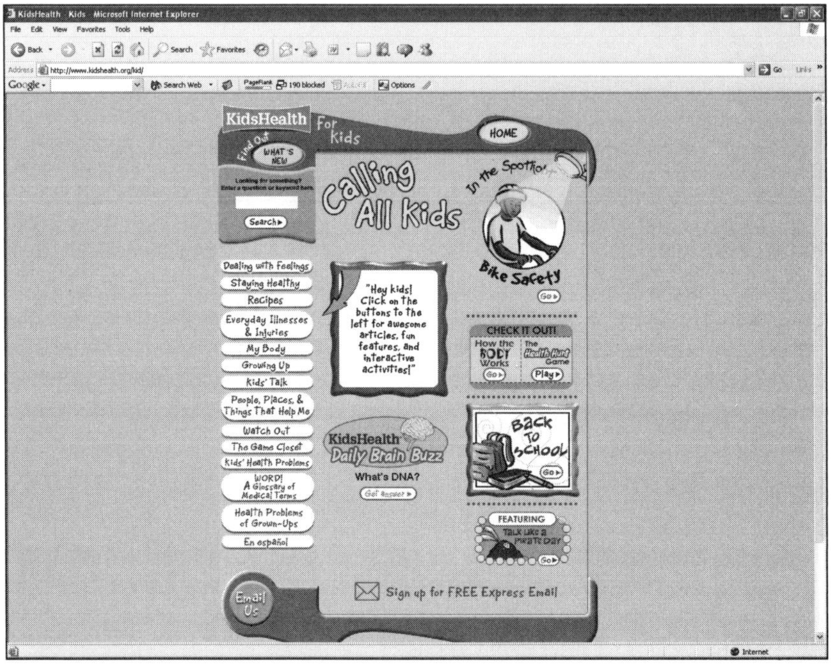

FIGURE 5.30 *KidsHealth offers separate home pages for parents, kids, and teens. This is the kids home page.*

about style, gadgets, and sex, plus the topics that we're covering, including weight loss, nutrition, and health (see Figure 5.31). The Web site combines content from the magazine and adds community features and original online content to create even more useful stuff. There are daily tips on a variety of subjects, surveys, contests, and a subscription site for folks who want to lose weight.

The Fitness section includes videos to help you do exercises right, articles about fitness, quizzes, a fairly active forum about fitness (of course, they call it the "best fitness message board on the Web"), and a subscription site that provides personal training information, including animated demos and a personal training regimen (see Figure 5.32). There's also a message board promoting the Abs Diet, a book written by a *Men's Health* editor, as well as a six-week challenge for men to try the diet themselves and sculpt their abs and improve their sex life (always a good selling tool on this Web site).

The Health center includes a great Conditions center that provides at-a-glance information about a condition (called a "Crash Course"), and then follows that up with tools, articles, and information that help men "Fight Back" against the condition (see Figure 5.33). For example, the section on cholesterol includes a quick guide to the statin drugs that help lower cholesterol, plus weight control, diet, and exercise tips and a guide to good and bad fats and the foods that they are in. (In short, eat more salmon, nuts, olive oil, and avocados; eat fewer processed snack foods, fried foods, and whole milk.)

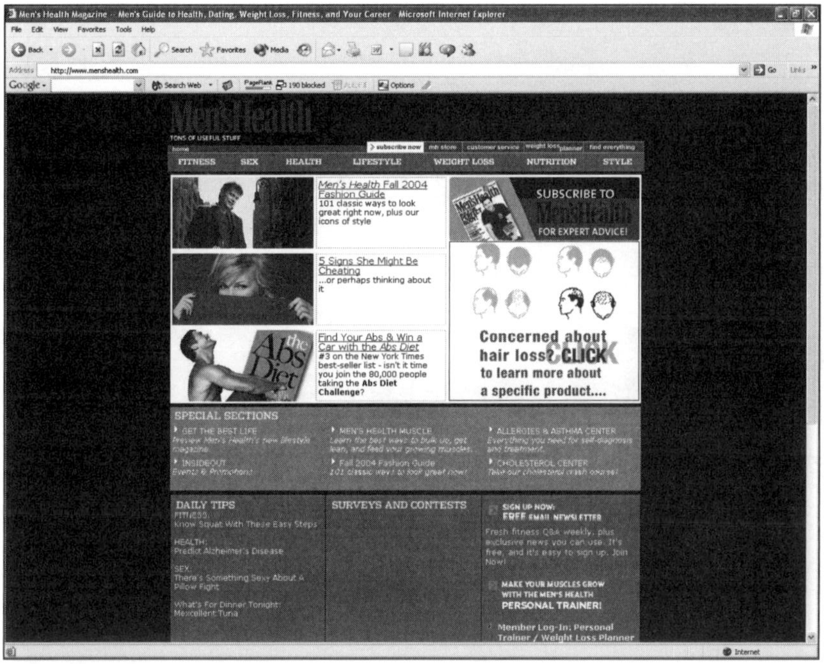

FIGURE 5.31 *Men's Health*

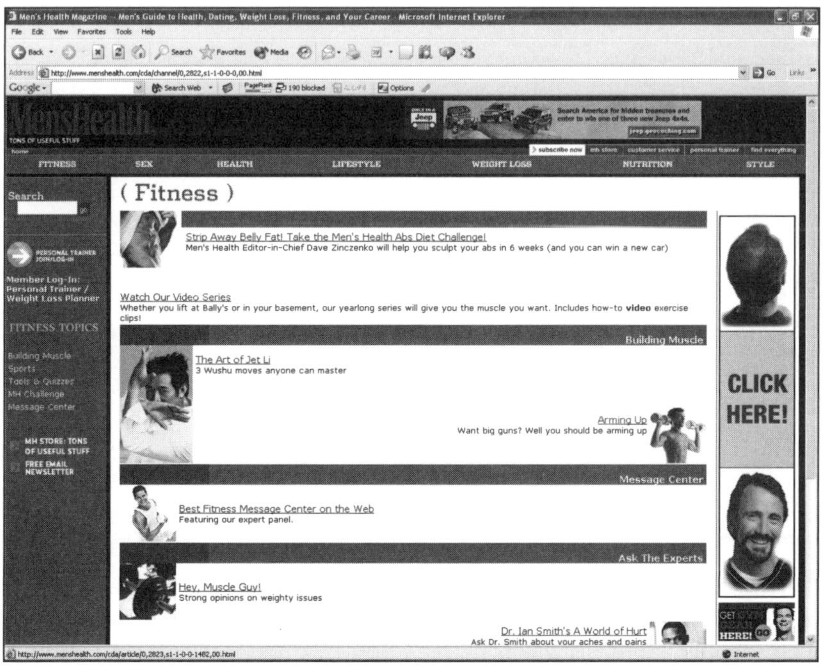

FIGURE 5.32 *Men's Health Fitness center*

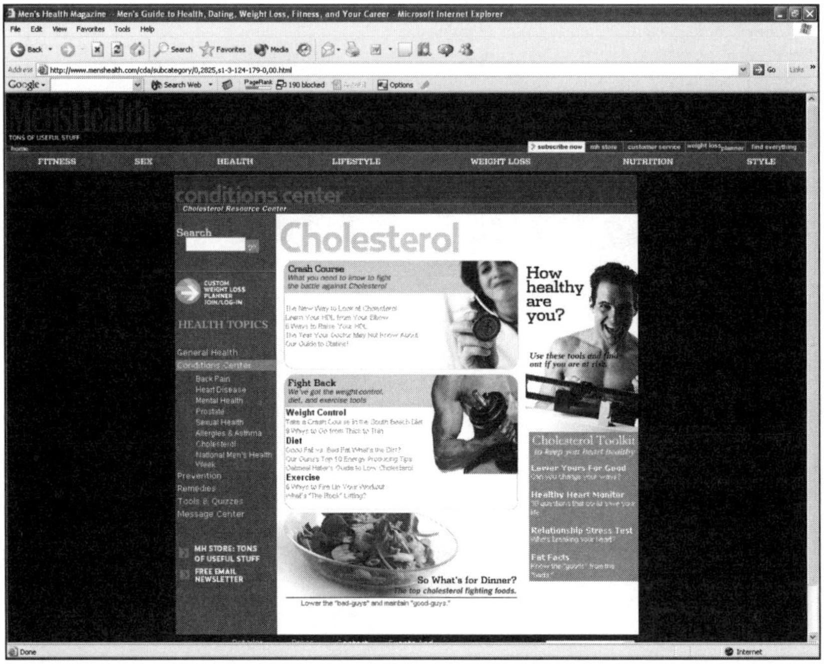

FIGURE 5.33 *The Men's Health Conditions centers, such as this one on cholesterol, include lots of tips for preventing and fighting back against illnesses and conditions.*

MensHealth.com is light on recipes and food-related information, but it does include grilling tips! And the recipes that are on the site (a few hundred) include nutritional information. And, as a member of the family of Rodale publications, there's good information on the South Beach diet on the site.

AARP

http://www.aarp.org

Summary: With millions of members, AARP is a great place for those who are over 50 to get the information they need.

In 1958, Dr. Ethel Percy Andrus, a retired high school principal, founded the American Association of Retired Persons (AARP) as an offshoot of the National Retired Teachers Association, which he founded in 1947. AARP's mission is to enhance our quality of life as we age. Open to anyone 50 or older, AARP has more than 25 million members in the U.S. and another 40,000 worldwide. Its Web site is dedicated to the same principles as the organization itself.

AARP's Health and Wellness center features articles about health care, prescription drugs, Alzheimer's disease, exercise, and more (see Figure 5.34). Sections are devoted to prevention, nutrition, insurance, stress management, prescription drugs, and exercise. Its Eating Well area (see Figure 5.35) includes weight loss tips and advice specifically for those over 50.

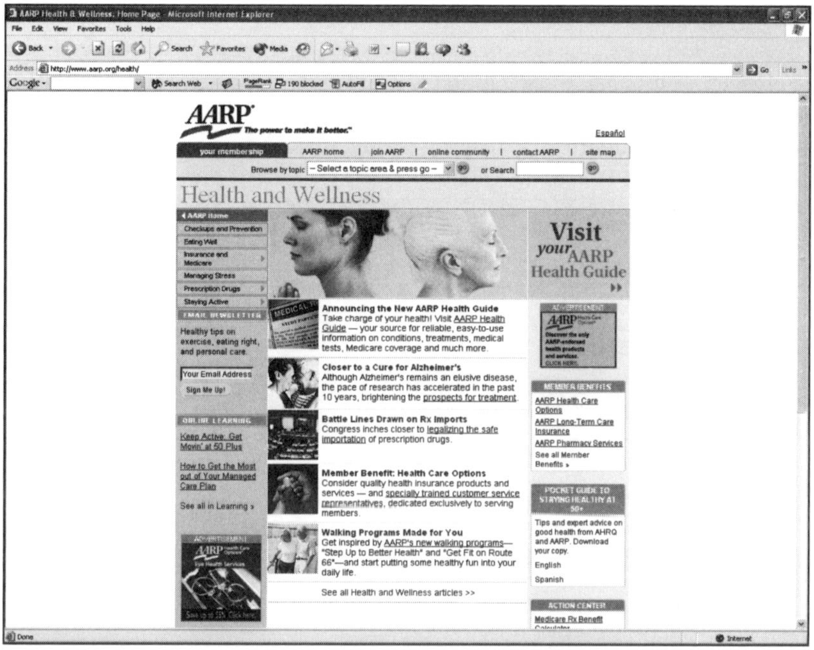
AARP Health & Wellness: Home Page - Microsoft Internet Explorer
AARP
The power to make it better.
Español
your membership
AARP home | join AARP | online community | contact AARP | site map
Health and Wellness
Visit your AARP Health Guide
Announcing the New AARP Health Guide
Take charge of your health! Visit AARP Health Guide — your source for reliable, easy-to-use information on conditions, treatments, medical tests, Medicare coverage and much more.
Closer to a Cure for Alzheimer's
Although Alzheimer's remains an elusive disease, the pace of research has accelerated in the past 10 years, brightening the prospects for treatment.
Battle Lines Drawn on Rx Imports
Congress inches closer to legalizing the safe importation of prescription drugs.
Member Benefit: Health Care Options
Consider quality health insurance products and services — and specially trained customer service representatives, dedicated exclusively to serving members.
Walking Programs Made for You
Get inspired by AARP's new walking programs—"Step Up to Better Health" and "Get Fit on Route 66"—and start putting some healthy fun into your daily life.
See all Health and Wellness articles >>

FIGURE 5.34 *AARP Health and Wellness center*

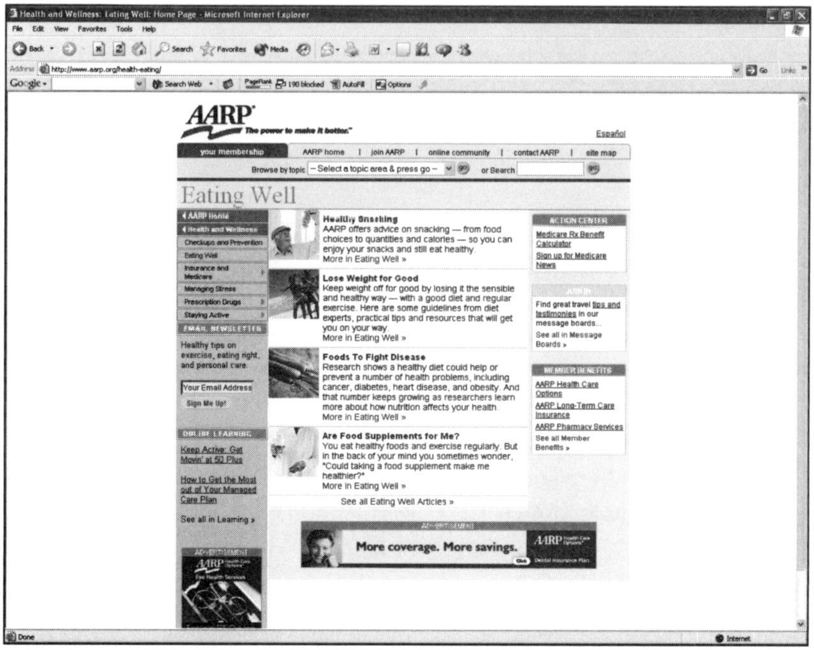

FIGURE 5.35 *The AARP Eating Well center features tips and advice for healthy eating and weight loss.*

Perhaps even more helpful is the AARP Health Guide (see Figure 5.36). It includes an A–Z guide to health tailored specifically for those over 50, tips on healthy living, a guide to medications, a glossary of medical tests, a guide to Medicare, and more than 1,000 support groups for various topics. These are powered by Healthwise, Inc.'s medical knowledgebase. Healthwise is a nonprofit organization aimed at helping people make better health decisions.

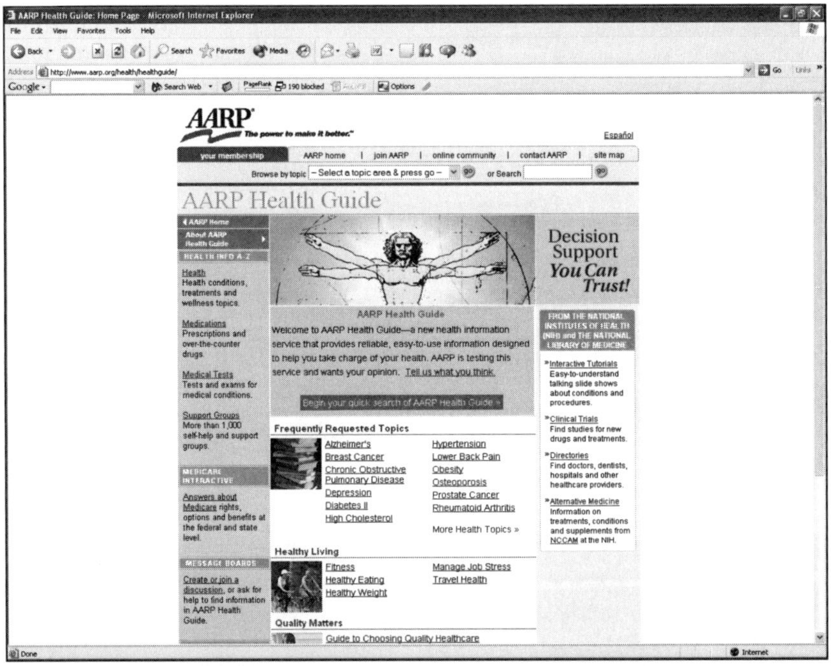

FIGURE 5.36 *AARP Health Guide*

The AARP Health Guide also offers much of the content on the National Institutes of Health sites mentioned earlier in this chapter, including the MedlinePlus directory. It features interactive tutorials and slideshows, listings of clinical trials, healthcare-provider directories, and information on alternative medicine sources. AARP also offers a variety of health tips for seniors, including videos and case histories. Their fitness for seniors area offers lots of safety information, demonstration animations of the correct ways to do exercises, and quizzes to test your knowledge. Some tips from the AARP and NIH include the following:

- **You're never too old to start exercising.** Older adults can hurt themselves more by not exercising than by exercising. However…
- …**Safety first.** Check with your doctor before beginning any exercise program. Also, consult your doctor if you have any symptoms after exercise, including chest pains, severe shortness of breath, an irregular or fluttery heartbeat, or any new symptom that you've never experienced.

- **Start slowly.** As little as five minutes per day helps, particularly if you haven't exercised in a while.
- **Workouts.** NIH recommends four types of exercises for older adults—strength (moderate weight lifting), balance (leg raises), stretching, and endurance (cardio exercises, such as aerobics, running, or walking).
- **Chart your progress.** This will help keep you motivated.

Summary

In this chapter, we looked at the various health and wellness sites on the Internet, including general, government, and international sites, and sites for men, women, children, and seniors. All of these will help keep you healthy. Many will help you lose weight and improve your fitness. And even more important, each site is a place where you can go and feel like you belong. Many of these sites are great places for you specifically because you believe that they are for you. I like the Men's Health site, for example, because I feel like many of the articles are written for me. And I'm sure I'll like the AARP site when I get to that age, too!

In Chapter 6, "Fun Fitness Gadgets," we're going to move away from the computer and discuss devices and gadgets that will help you improve your fitness while you're having fun. Many of these work in conjunction with your computer, which provides a level of power that no generation has ever had before. After using one of these devices, you'll know more about your fitness habits then you might want to!

Chapter 6

Fun Fitness Gadgets

"Never eat more than you can lift."

—Miss Piggy

It's easier to lose weight when you're having fun. For me, gadgets are fun. I have more fun with gadgets and get more motivation out of the right ones, so I lose weight without even thinking about it. Add competitiveness to fun, and I'm on my way.

In this chapter, we'll look at the best fitness gadgets that work with your computer and some that work on their own, and we'll talk about the technologies behind them. We'll examine pedometers, calorie calculators, heart rate monitors, GPS devices, and more. The field of fitness technology is constantly changing, and we'll tell you how to keep up with the changes.

Pedometers

A pedometer can help you lose more weight than the foods that you eat. Pedometers count your steps, and some track the distance you go, the speed at which you walk or run, and the calories you burn. Used along with a fitness tracking spreadsheet or other journal, a pedometer can get you motivated to keep moving.

You wear a pedometer along your waistline, usually along your dominant leg. Pedometers are built to clip there; some also include a safety strap so that you don't lose them. In general, pedometers have pendulums inside that move along with your hip; they record a step when the pendulum swings past a magnetic field each time you move. Electronic pedometers count a step when your foot hits the ground.

Most pedometers have a built-in display that tells you the basic statistics of how many steps you took. For a pedometer to know how far you walked, it needs to know your stride length, which you can easily measure by taking 10 steps, measuring how far that is, and dividing by 10. For calories burned, the pedometer needs to know your gender, age, and weight.

Like a food diary keeps track of what you eat, pedometers keep track of the amount of activity in which you engage. After getting a pedometer, I parked my car farther from the office each day, walked a little more each evening, exercised more, and tried to take as many steps as possible each day. As a result, I lost weight without even trying. Experts say that you should aim for at least 10,000 steps per day for optimal fitness (the average American averages approximately 6,000 steps per day). For weight loss, I recommend at least 15,000 steps per day. One mile equals approximately 2,000 steps. To be useful, a pedometer must be accurate. Otherwise, it either overestimates or underestimates your steps, which won't provide you with the information you need to ensure that you're exercising enough. This problem is similar to a food diary that underestimates the number of calories you're eating.

Pedometers are great for walking or running, using a treadmill or an elliptical trainer, or engaging in a sport, such as baseball, soccer, or football. But you can't wear one while swimming, and they are close to useless for biking. Other devices do a much better job of measuring these types of activities, and we'll cover those devices later in this chapter.

The price of pedometers varies widely. McDonald's is giving away pedometers with their new Go Active! adult Happy Meals. You can also buy one for as little as $10. I recommend spending a little more than that and getting a pedometer that calculates your distance and speed during workouts, as well as counting steps. Some of the best pedometers come from vendors such as DIGI-WALKER, OMRON, and SportBrain. But there are others from Freestyle, Sportline, and Walk4Life that are also very good quality.

The really cool pedometers, of course, are those that work with your computer. To date, the only pedometer in this category is from SportBrain. However, there are many step-counting software programs that will provide you with the ability to keep a record of your steps no matter what pedometer you use.

DIGI-WALKER

http://www.new-lifestyles.com

Summary: A variety of reasonably priced pedometers, all providing accurate readings.

DIGI-WALKERs have been around for several years, and the company has grown dramatically along with the rise in popularity of pedometers. The company offers several different pedometer models, which vary in price primarily due to the features offered.

The units have been very well reviewed and are considered to be very accurate. I wore an NL-2000 for about a year and was impressed with its features and accuracy (see Figure 6.1). Table 6.1 shows the various models, features, and prices for DIGI-WALKER products.

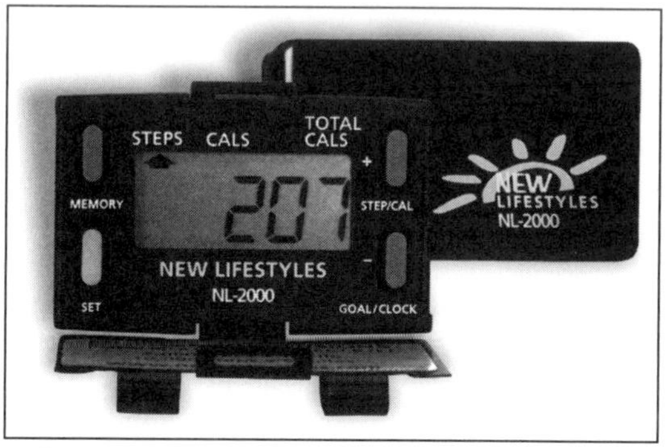

FIGURE 6.1 *NEW-LIFESTYLES calls the NL-2000 an "Activity Monitor" because it does more than just count steps.*

The NL-2000, of course, is the most advanced DIGI-WALKER. It includes a built-in accelerometer to measure actual calories burned. You input your age, gender, height, and weight, and the DIGI-WALKER determines your BMR. From there, it measures activity calories burned, adds that to your BMR, and tells you how many calories you burn each day. The NL-2000 also measures the distance you traveled. It includes a metal clip for added security. However, one of the problems with that is it takes some getting used to in order to get it on and off your belt.

A nice feature is the NL-2000's seven-day memory and clock, so that you can scroll through the last seven days to see how many steps you took, how far you went, and how many calories you burned.

Table 6.1 DIGI-WALKER Models and Prices

Model	Features	Price
Skeletone	Steps only	$14.95 (security strap $5)
SW-200	Steps only	$21.95 (security strap $5)
SW-401	Steps and distance	$24.95 (security strap $5)
SW-651	Steps, distance, stopwatch, and clock	$29.95 (security strap $5)
SW-701	Steps, distance, and calories	$29.95 (security strap $5)
NL-2000	Steps, activity calories, total calories, seven-day memory, and clock	$54.95 (security strap included)

OMRON

http://www.omron.com

Summary: A medical devices company branches out into fitness products and scores big.

When SportBrain went out of business temporarily in the summer of 2001, many suddenly addicted pedometer users were in a quandary—if they couldn't use their SportBrains, what then? Word got around about a pedometer from OMRON, a medical devices company, that was accurate, inexpensive, and feature packed. The OMRON HJ-104 was a nonimpressive looking device with a seven-day memory and a simple way to set your stride length—count your steps, see how many the pedometer says you went, and adjust the sensitivity accordingly (you can also set your stride length the normal way). Within days, you couldn't find an HJ-104 anywhere, as the unexpected demand of tens of thousands of SportBrain users needing a pedometer overwhelmed the supply. At less than $20, the HJ-104 remains one of the best pedometers on the market. Another model, the HJ-105, appears to be identical to the HJ-104.

OMRON recently introduced a new device, the HJ-112, which is nicer looking and adds more features to the mix (see Figure 6.2). It also includes two acceleration sensors to more accurately measure steps. OMRON claims that a user can even put the pedometer in his or her pocket or purse and still get an accurate step count. The HJ-112 counts both steps and aerobic steps, so it tracks workouts of 10 minutes or more in which you take at least 60 steps per minute. It also counts calories and distance and, like the HJ-104, it has a seven-day memory. The list price for the HJ-112 is $40, but we've seen it for as little as $24.99.

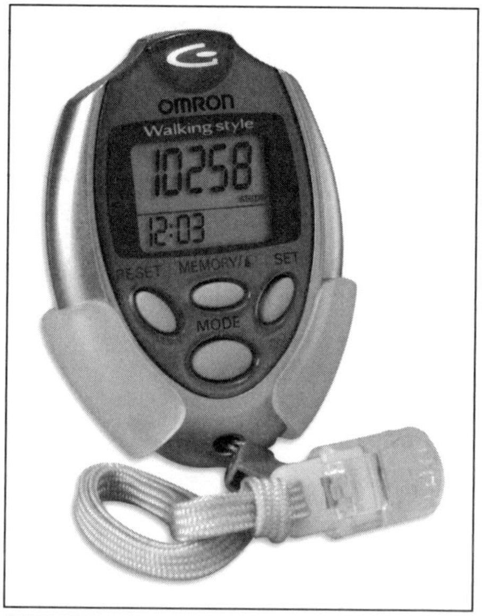

FIGURE 6.2 *The Omron HJ-112 is one of the most impressive pedometers on the market.*

SportBrain

http://www.sportbrain.com

Summary: Very interesting, computer-related technology, but pricey.

I've been using a SportBrain on and off for nearly four years. I got one in February, 2001, as a gift, and I used it religiously until the company exploded in a ball of high-flying, dot-bomb dust in July, 2001. Sixteen months later, the company returned to life in a much less ambitious form, and I've been using my SportBrain ever since.

When it first came out in 2000, SportBrain revolutionized the pedometer market; it brought tens of thousands of people to a market who never would have gotten there. I was one of them. As a technology geek, I love new gadgets, and SportBrain was an old gadget in new clothing—a Web-enabled pedometer that offered community to its new fangled content.

SportBrain measures distance, calories burned, steps taken, and "Sportivities" (any activity that takes 10 minutes or more). You also get to see how you're doing in relation to others if you join a club on the SportBrain Web site. I like this because it keeps me motivated. While I was writing this book, I joined the 500,000 steps per month club on SportBrain's Web site and promptly registered my three best months ever, all in a row, with each month breaking the previous month's record. Until I joined the club, I'd only had one month of more than 500,000 steps. Now I have four, and my record is now up to 540,000 steps in a month. Does this help me keep my weight down? You bet!

SportBrain calculates your stride length based on your height and weight. You can reset this by using a treadmill, but I've found SportBrain to be very accurate when measured with my elliptical trainer, so I use the automatic stride length.

The original SportBrain, which is the one that I use, doesn't even have a digital step counter to read how many steps I take. Instead, it uses a SportPort device that's plugged into the phone line. You plug the SportBrain into the SportPort, and it calls SportBrain and uploads your data so you can view it on your own homepage. The new SportBrain iStep connects to your PC via the USB port and uploads your data directly through the Internet. The iStep also includes a digital readout so you can see your progress in this way (see Figure 6.3).

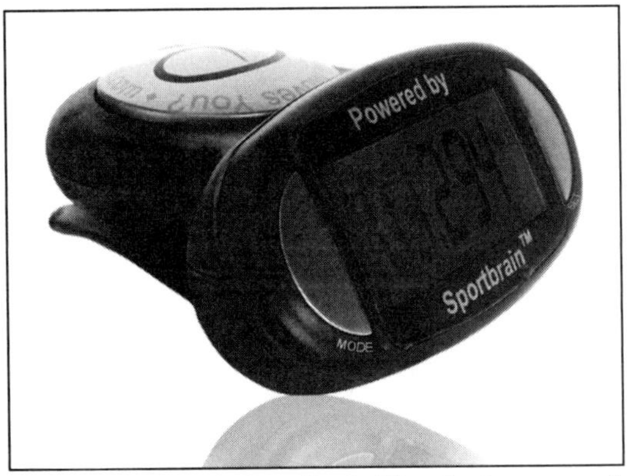

FIGURE 6.3 *The SportBrain iStep is the company's first offering since coming back from being a dot-com bust.*

Whichever device you use, your homepage tells you how many steps you took, how fast you went, how many calories you burned, and how you compare to others in your age group. It also has charts and graphs illustrating your progress (see Figure 6.4).

SportBrain features periodic rewards programs for its members where they can qualify to win little things, such as towels and cups, for averaging 10,000 steps per day over a 30-day period, for example, or bigger things, such as iPods, for averaging 20,000 steps per day over that same period. SportBrain gives away a limited number of items in each rewards period, which is generally every three months or so.

SportBrain is not cheap. If you have an older model, which sells for $99, you have to pay a monthly membership fee to access the SportBrain Web site. You can pay $12.95 per month, $29.95 per quarter, or $99 per year to access this site. However, given that SportBrain has recently cut way back on its community features, this has become less and less attractive. The company now offers a Silver membership, which is free to its iStep customers. These customers can't qualify for rewards or join clubs, but they do get access to the last two weeks' worth of their data. So, if they use a spreadsheet to track their steps, they are fine. And, since the new iStep costs as little as $34.99 at other Web sites, it's worth a look.

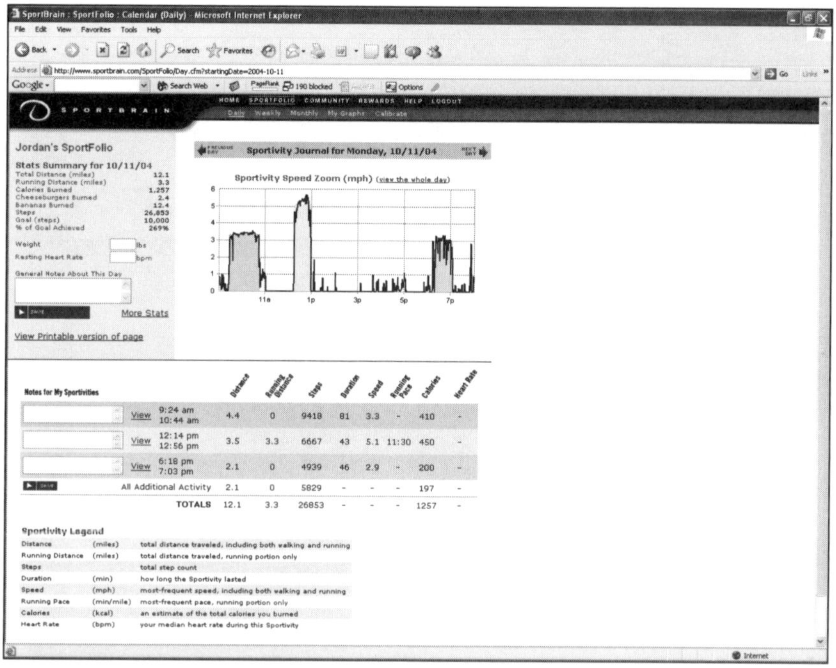

FIGURE 6.4 *A typical SportBrain homepage*

FRIENDS OF SPORTBRAIN

When SportBrain went down in a cloud of dust in July, 2001, many members flocked to Thom and Alley Kirby's Friends of SportBrain site (http://bearykirby.com/sb; see Figure 6.5). Thom and Alley were former employees of the original SportBrain, and they quickly formed the best place to commiserate with other SportBrain addicts. Their site features forums on a wide range of topics, including areas for general discussion, a place to discuss what's happening at SportBrain, forums for fitness and training, reviews of the latest gadgets, and more. Although traffic has died down considerably since SportBrain came back to life in late 2002, the Web site still provides some of the best information anywhere about SportBrain and other fitness products.

Sportline

http://www.sportline.com

Summary: The market leader in pedometers boasts the best distribution and has a few impressive models along the way.

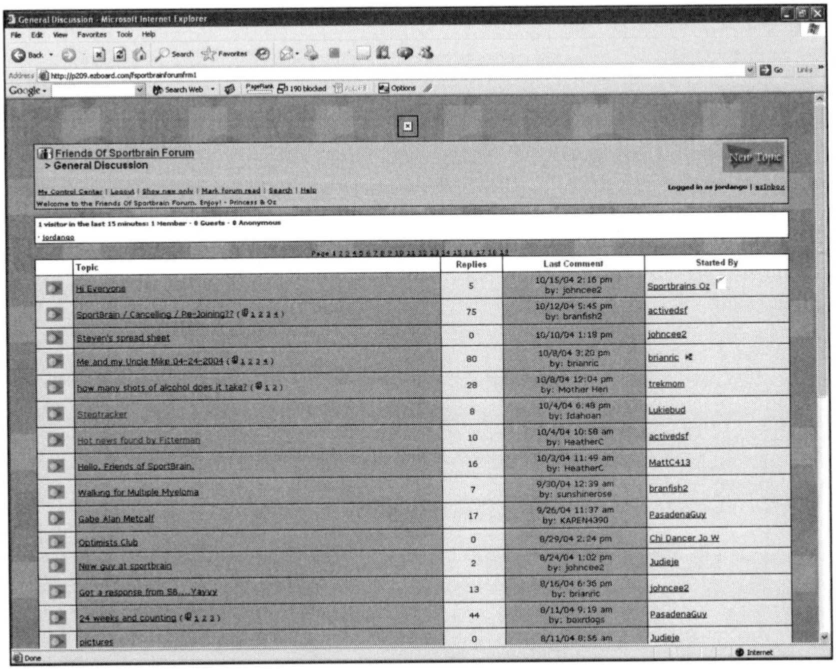

FIGURE 6.5 *The Friends of SportBrain Forum provides information about SportBrain as well as other fitness equipment.*

When you go into a sporting goods store and see pedometers, Sportlines are invariably available. Sportline arguably has the best distribution in the business, if not the best pedometers. Their pedometers are reasonably priced and well reviewed, and they are a good choice for anyone looking for a pedometer.

The company's best reviewed pedometer is the Fitness Pedometer 360, which features a seven-day memory and clock and measures your distance (in 1/100 mile increments), steps (including steps per minute and miles per hour), calories, speed, and time spent exercising (see Figure 6.6). A scan feature automatically cycles through all of the pedometer's functions, showing you how you've done at a glance. Its retail price is $39.95.

Sportline offers many other pedometers; a partial list is provided in Table 6.2.

Because of its distribution capabilities and the number of people who sell its pedometers, the retail price and the actual street price could vary considerably. For example, the lowest price we've seen for the Sportline 360 is $18.76 at Wal-Mart.

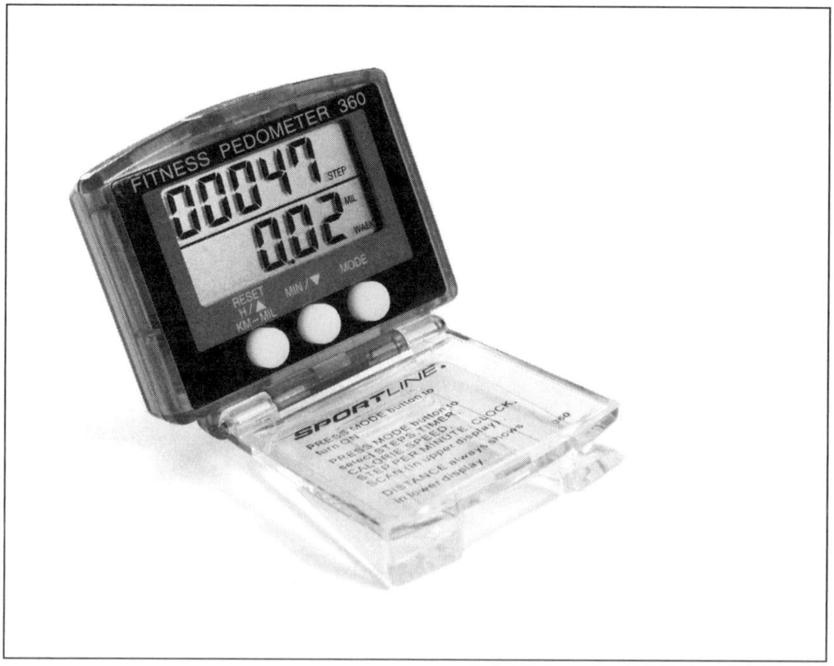

FIGURE 6.6 *Sportline's Fitness Pedometer 360 features a seven-day memory and much more.*

Table 6.2 Sportline Models and Prices

Model	Features	Price
330	Steps only	$12.95
343	Talks—tells you time, distance, steps	$29.95
345	Time, distance, steps, calories	$29.95
346	Nightlight, steps, distance	$29.95
347	Time, distance, steps, stopwatch, exercise splits	$29.95
349	Time, steps, distance, workout results	$34.95
360	Seven-day memory, clock, steps, distance, calories, speed, time spent exercising, scan feature	$39.95
355	Time, distance, steps, workout data, pulse monitor	$44.95

Heart Rate Monitors

Pedometers are just the tip of the iceberg when it comes to fitness gadgets and motivational tools. The next step up the ladder to fitness awareness comes in the form of heart rate monitors. While a pedometer can show you how far you've gone and how much you exercised, a heart rate monitor can show you how *well* you exercised. Monitoring your heart rate is the best way to tell just how much you've exerted yourself during a workout.

When you are exercising, your heart moves blood from your lungs, where it picks up oxygen, to your muscles, where it burns the oxygen as fuel, and sends it back to your lungs again. The harder you exercise, the more fuel your body needs and the harder your heart has to work to get oxygen to your muscles. The harder your heart works, the faster it beats. This is where a heart rate monitor comes in.

You need to get your heart rate (beats per minute) to a certain threshold to ensure that you are working hard enough and getting more fit. If your heart rate is too low, you're not working hard enough and your body won't benefit as much. If your heart rate is too high, you might be damaging your body. By exercising too intensively, you're putting your heart at risk and increasing the chances of injury. A heart rate monitor can literally tell you when your exercise is at the right point. Keeping your heart rate in this so-called *target zone* is key to burning fat and getting into shape.

Figuring out your target zone is not that difficult. It is typically 60 to 80% of your maximum heart rate. First, figure out your maximum heart rate, which is typically 220 minus your age. (This is a general measurement; more extensive tests are available at your doctor.) Multiply that number by .60 to get the bottom end of the target zone and by .80 to get the top end. Table 6.3 does this for you in a few age groups.

LISTEN TO YOUR BODY, NOT JUST YOUR HEART RATE MONITOR

When some people first use a heart rate monitor, they go by the readings on the watch to tell them how tired they are or how much they're exerting themselves. This is a mistake. Always listen to your body when you're working out. If you are tired, dizzy, or not feeling well in general, it doesn't matter what your heart rate is. Stop exercising at any point if you don't feel well.

Think of exercising as a continuum. Your resting heart rate is your heart rate when you aren't exercising. This is typically 60 to 80 beats per minute for the average person, and as low as 30 beats per minute for a very fit athlete. As you start exercising, you gradually get to 50% or so of your maximum. You burn body fat as you enter the target zone, at 60 to 70% of your maximum heart rate. You build aerobic endurance but you don't necessarily burn body fat at 70 to 80%. Professional athletes, who don't care about burning body fat, generally stay in the 80 to 90% or even higher zone. The key is to stay in the zone that you desire for as long as you can, at least 20 minutes per session for effective exercise.

Table 6.3 Target Heart Zone

Age	Maximum Rate	Target Zone
20	200	120–160
25	195	117–156
30	190	114–152
35	185	111–148
40	180	108–144
45	175	105–140
50	170	102–136
55	165	99–132
60	160	96–128
65	155	93–124
70	150	90–120
80	140	84–112

Intensity is different for everyone, by the way. Someone who is not in very good shape and is walking three miles per hour might be struggling and have a very high heart rate, while another person might hardly be working out at all. It's all a matter of fitness. As your fitness improves, you can go faster, jump higher, and exercise longer at the same heart rate than you did at slower performances in the past.

Heart rate monitors keep you motivated to do more and provide you with a benchmark from which to judge the effectiveness of your workouts. They teach you to exercise at your own ideal pace, they maximize your workout so you exercise as efficiently as possible, and they effectively serve as a training partner, providing you with real-time feedback on your workout. Also, unlike pedometers, many heart rate monitors are waterproof, so you can use them while swimming, and most will accurately measure your workout during cycling.

In general, you use a heart rate monitor by wearing a strap across your chest that wirelessly sends signals to a watch on your wrist. This strap is essentially performing a continual electrocardiogram, monitoring your heart rate. Some monitors track this data for later upload to your computer. Others just tell you your heart rate so you can monitor it during your workout. Some models use earphones instead of a watch to literally tell you your heart rate. And a few heart rate monitors forego the chest strap completely, effectively serving as glorified pulse monitors. Because these devices don't use a chest strap, they can't continually monitor your heart rate. However, many people don't like wearing a chest strap while exercising. It can be uncomfortable and it takes some getting used to.

Many heart rate monitors double as a wristwatch. However, since they were designed by exercise and medical device companies, some of these watches are not exactly attractive. This is changing, however, as many manufacturers are emphasizing fashion in their devices.

You can get a heart rate monitor for as little as $50, or you can splurge and get a feature-packed device for several hundred dollars. It all depends on how many features you want. Basic models simply give you your heart rate. Others can sound an alarm when you are in the zone, above the zone, or below the zone; monitor the length of your workout; offer stopwatch features, workout splits, and lap times; and offer calories burned and the ability to upload your workout to your PC, among other features. Before buying a heart rate monitor, check it out to be sure you like how it works. The following sections detail a few of the leading manufacturers of heart rate monitors.

EXERCISING EFFECTIVELY

Fitness professionals offer the following tips for exercising effectively and reducing the risk of injury during exercise:

- First, warm up for at least five to 10 minutes before beginning an exercise session. Stretch, do some calisthenics, and start your exercise slowly.
- Then, stay in your target zone for as long as you can, at least 20 minutes. This helps you build your endurance over time.
- Finally, cool down. Spend at least five minutes gradually slowing down and moving at a slower pace before stopping your exercise.

As always, check with your doctor before beginning any exercise program.

Cardiosport

http://www.cardiosport.com

Summary: A nice variety of excellent heart rate monitors.

Cardiosport is a UK company with excellent distribution in the US. They feature several excellent heart rate monitors at affordable prices that provide accurate readings without a lot of features. For example, the Cardiosport Go provides the time of day and your heart rate. It allows you to set your target zones with an alarm function that tells you when you've reached your zone. And, it includes an exercise session timer and tells you how well you did on your last workout. It offers an excellent value for $69.

The GraphX, at $159, which features a color display (one of the few color displays on the market), displays heart rate in numerical as well as percentage terms (as a percent of your own maximum), shows how long you've been exercising, and includes a stopwatch.

Cardiosport's high end is appropriately named the Ultima, a $300 heart rate monitor that records up to 80 hours of training and up to six sessions at a time, which you can then upload to your PC for analysis later. Used in conjunction with the included software, it can tell you your average heart rate per lap, your actual heart rate per session, and your time in, above, and below your target zone.

Street prices for Cardiosport heart rate monitors are much lower then I've mentioned here. For example, we saw the GraphX for as low as $89.

MIO

http://www.miowatch.com

Summary: Heart rate monitors with no chest strap required.

The great thing about the MIO heart rate monitor watch is that it doesn't require a chest strap (see Figure 6.7). The bad thing about the MIO is that it doesn't have a chest strap. This feature is good because no one really likes to wear a chest strap while exercising (or at any other time, for that matter). It's bad because there's no way to truly analyze your workout. Also, because you're not wearing a chest strap, the MIO can't tell you whether you're in your target zone. It can only tell you your heart rate when you put two of your fingers on the watch and press down. Believe me, this is distracting, and it sometimes doesn't work right.

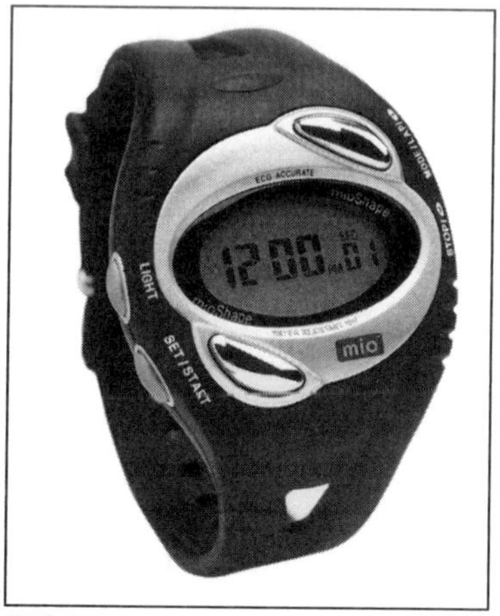

FIGURE 6.7 *The MioSHAPE SELECT heart rate monitor watch does not require a chest strap.*

The MIO heart rate monitor watch features a stopwatch for exercising, and will track your heart rate and relationships to the target zones, including percentages. It also tracks calories burned in a workout and can track calories eaten throughout the day. To get your heart rate, put your thumb and index finger on the MioSensors on top of the watch for a few seconds. The MIO takes your pulse and displays your heart rate.

The folks at MIO call it a "lifestyle monitor" because it tracks your heart rate during workouts, as well as calories burned. Then, throughout the day, you can enter how many calories you've eaten, and MIO tells you how well you're doing from that standpoint. You subtract calories burned from calories eaten to help you determine whether you're on track for the day from a diet and exercise standpoint.

Once you tell the MIO that you've started a workout, it automatically calculates your expected heart rate in between the times that you get your heart rate. So, if you get your heart rate after five minutes and then again after 15, MIO will calculate what it expected your heart rate to be in those intervening minutes and determine how many calories you've burned in your workout as a result. They claim that this is accurate, and they have a research study to prove this online. However, their study says that MIO was able to get a heart rate 79% of the time (because of the difficulty of using the sensors), while a heart rate monitor with chest strap was successful 100% of the time. In any case, using a MIO watch will give you fairly accurate results and without the hassle of a chest strap. MIO offers several variations of the watch, all with similar features, ranging in price from $89.95 to $149.95.

Nike

http://www.nike.com

Summary: Nike offers stylish alternatives in the heart rate monitor market.

Nike offers both low-end and very high-end heart rate monitors, all very stylish. For $99, you can get the Imara, which is designed for women and features a calorie counter, programmable heart rate zones, a data mode that offers exercise time, and a two time-zone watch. It displays heart rate in both beats per minute and as a percentage of maximum.

Step up a bit to $299 for the Triax Elite HRM or the $359 Triax Elite HRM/SDM, both intended for serious athletes (see Figure 6.8). Both devices are feature-packed and provide heart rate zones and numerous features. Both include software so you can upload your workouts to your PC. The SDM includes a pod that clips to your shoe and measures speed and distance features so that it not only monitors your heart rate, but it also tells you how far you went and how fast you went. The watch displays your performance in real time as well, so you can turn it up a notch during a workout. This is a pretty serious product that works on both PCs and Macs. You connect it to your computer through a USB dock that's about the size of a hockey puck. These devices sync with your computer, downloading workout data from the watch to the computer and uploading workout plans and watch settings to the watch. Either device is great for training purposes, but they are both probably more than the average person needs.

Polar

http://www.polarusa.com

Summary: The market leader in heart rate monitors offers a device for every budget and need.

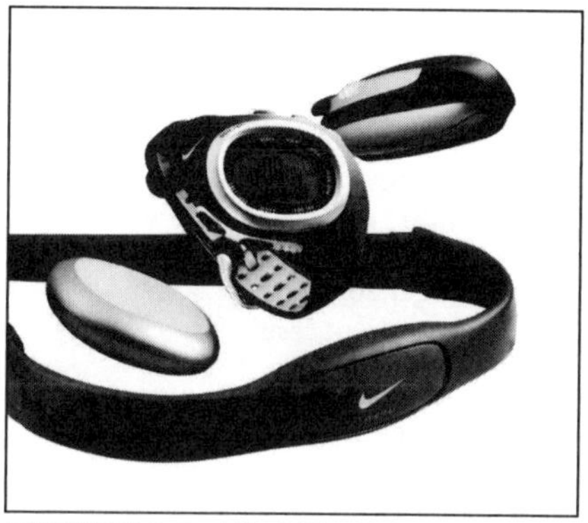

FIGURE 6.8 *The Nike Triax series features pricey heart rate monitors that do much more than just monitor your heart rate.*

Whatever you want in a heart rate monitor, the odds are, Polar offers it. With models starting at $59.99 and going up to $399.99, you can get nearly anything you want in a Polar heart rate monitor. And it's no wonder; Polar has been making heart rate monitors since 1977, when they invented the first wireless heart rate monitor. Now, Polar offers more than 20 models, optimized for cycling, swimming, running, or mountain climbing. Plus, many watches include barometric readers, altimeters, compasses, and other devices (see Figure 6.9). Table 6.4 shows a selected list of various Polar models.

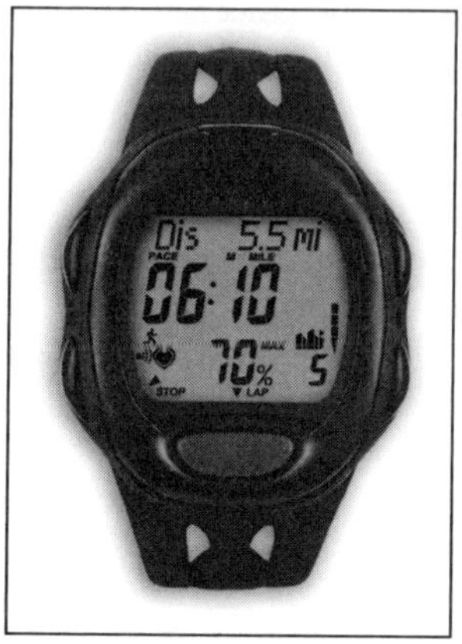

FIGURE 6.9 *The Polar S625X provides all the features that anyone could dream of in a heart rate monitor.*

Table 6.4 Polar Heart Rate Monitors

Model	Recommended For	Features	Price
F1	Beginners	Heart rate, exercise time, and average heart rate	$59.99
A3	Cardiac rehab	Heart rate, target zone tracker, time in zone, workout results	$89.99
A5	Walking	Same as A3 but with calorie tracking and built-in walk test as well	$109.99
S120	Running	Exercise features, target zones, uploads to PC	$119.99
S150	Triathlon	Same as S120, but with cycling features including bike mount	$149.99
M32	Weight management	Counts calories and fat, and automatically determines target zone each day	$149
M61/F92Ti	Weight management	Same as M32, but with a fitness level feature; F92Ti is titanium and more stylish	$179/$249.99
S210	Running	Stores five workouts, includes PC uploading, fitness test, calories	$199.99
S520	Triathlon	Adds cycling features and other bells and whistles to the S210	$259.99
S625X	Triathlon	Provides continuous running speed and distance, optimizer recovery test	
S720i	Triathlon	Adds altitude and terrain data for cyclists	$309.99
AXN300	Mountain climbing	Includes slope counter, vertical speed feature, and a barometer	$199
AXN500	Mountain climbing	Same as AXN 300 but with compass, a stainless steel design, and a more comfortable strap	$299
AXN700	Mountain climbing	Adds the heart rate test and a titanium design to the AXN 500	$399

The street prices for these units vary widely from the retail prices in Table 6.4. For example, we've seen the Polar S720i for as little as $250, the A5 for as low as $89, and other Polar heart rate monitors for approximately 20% off the list price.

As you can see, Polar offers a dizzying variety of heart rate monitors. And, they offer a dizzying variety of software as well. Most of their heart rate monitors upload data to PCs and download data from PCs as well. And Polar's Personal Training Software lets users manage their progress along the way (see Figure 6.10).

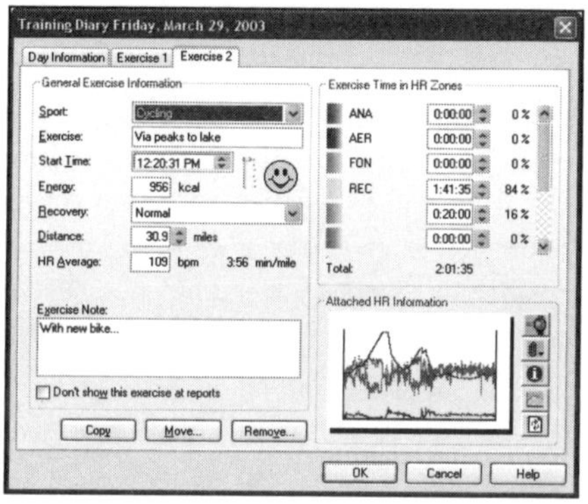

FIGURE 6.10 *Polar Personal Training software*

Reebok

http://www.reebok.com

Summary: Reebok offers stylish, inexpensive, high-quality heart rate monitors.

While Nike is spending much of its time developing high-end exercise monitors, Reebok is tackling the low end, offering four heart rate monitors, all around $100 or less. Their top of the line is the Reebok Fit Trainer Heart Rate Monitor, which features a target zone alarm; exercise timer; and time in, above, and below your target heart rate in a stylish watch that you can wear when you're not working out. The Fit Trainer sells for $89.99. Reebok also offers a more basic unit, the Personal Trainer, for $59.99. It's not as attractive as the Fit Trainer and it doesn't feature the exercise timer or zone alarm. The $79.99 Strapless Heart Rate Monitor is Reebok's answer to the MIO. It features a timer, pacer mode, and touch sensors to take your heart rate up to 42 times during a workout.

Other Cool Gadgets

Some devices just don't fit in with the others mentioned in this chapter. They're not really heart rate monitors—or maybe they are, but they're more than that. Some track calories burned or body composition, or include GPS positioning to tell you precisely how much you've worked out. They always let you upload your data to your computer or a Web page, and they're generally pretty expensive. But they are also fun, useful, and motivating.

HOW TO KEEP EXERCISE GOING

Ever look in the paper and see all those exercise bikes, treadmills, weight sets, and other products for sale? Those are the remnants of someone's failed exercise plan. How can you make sure that you don't wind up in that boat someday? It's fairly easy. Just follow the steps below:

1. **Pick a time of the day to exercise and do it regularly.** Most experts say that people who exercise in the morning are more likely to stick with it than people who exercise in the evening. This makes sense, because it's easier to develop excuses in the evening, and the day can sometimes get away from you when you're at work. However, if you're not a morning person, just pick a time, whether it's noon instead of lunch, just after work, or after the kids go to bed. Then stick with it.
2. **Vary your workouts.** Know why those exercise bikes wind up on the trash heap? They're BORING. You can't do those every day; you'll get deathly tired of them and give up exercise altogether. Instead, vary your workouts and do something different each day. Walk, bike, run, swim, play a sport, use an exercise machine, do weights. Walk in different neighborhoods, swim in a variety of pools. Don't get too set in your ways. The best way to exercise is to make it seem like you're not doing it.
3. **Love those chemicals.** You really *can* become addicted to exercise because the body releases chemicals that can make you feel really good—commonly called an "exercise high." Try to get high on exercise as much as possible without overdoing it.
4. **Get a gadget or two.** A pedometer, heart rate monitor, or other device can motivate you to keep going, even when you're bored. And a TiVo in your workout room lets you watch something that you're interested in while exercising, passing the time so that you don't even notice the calories you're burning. An iPod is also good, but if you're exercising outdoors, make sure you don't wear the iPod on the street! It's not safe.

Fitness Expert

http://www.fitnessexpert.com

Summary: Interesting products that measure your body composition and calories burned.

Fitness Expert, formerly Stay Healthy, Inc., offers two very interesting products—the Body Analyzer and the Calorie Tracker. The Body Analyzer will tell you your hydration level, lean muscle mass, and body fat percentage, all within two-percent accuracy of a water immersion test, and much more accurately than a typical body-fat scale, according to company president John Collins (see Figure 6.11). I was happy with that fact because the Body Analyzer showed my body-fat level at a full six percentage points less than my body-fat scale showed.

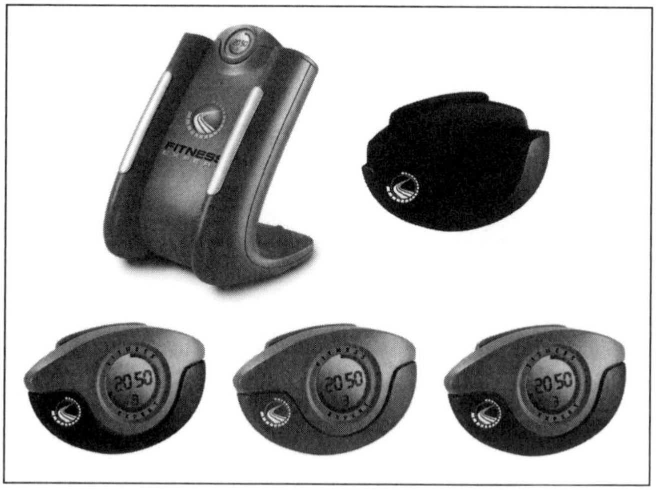

FIGURE 6.11 *The Fitness Expert Body Analyzer*

The Body Analyzer essentially takes a bio impedance reading of your body by sending a low-level electrical charge through it. You place one hand on each side of the device, keep your elbows straight, and wait a few seconds. A painless charge is sent through your body, and data is stored in the device. You then upload the data over the Web to Fitness Expert's medical devices, where it is analyzed and provided to you on your own Web page. "All of the expensive devices are on the Internet site," Collins explains.

You wear Calorie Tracker on your waist. It's a pager-like device that counts calories you've burned, including those burned outside of typical exercise. I wore the Calorie Tracker for several weeks and worked out regularly, and I found that I was burning between 2,700 and 3,300 calories per day, depending on how much I worked out.

The Calorie Tracker detects motion and converts that motion into calories burned. You have to enter your own personal information, including height, weight, gender, and age, and then Calorie Tracker does the rest. Calorie Tracker uses ergometric technology that includes three accelerometers to deliver what Collins claims is extremely accurate calorie burning information. Each accelerometer tracks a separate movement—forward and backward, side to side, and up and down. As with the Body Analyzer, Calorie Tracker uploads this data to the Web, where it is analyzed and results are provided (see Figure 6.12). Body Analyzer and Calorie Tracker retail for $350. Access to the Web site is $9.99 per month.

FitSense

http://www.fitsense.com

Summary: The FS-1 provides speedometer, heart rate monitor, and PC upload capabilities.

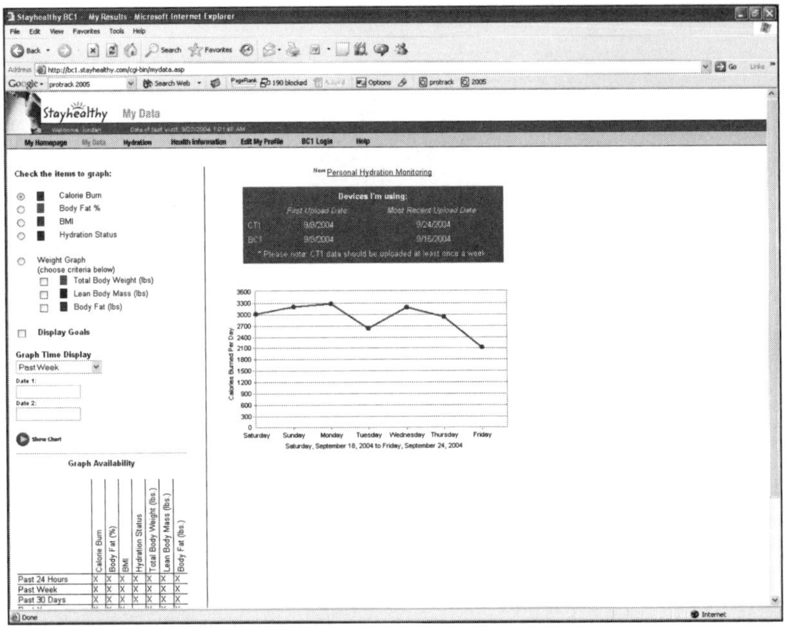

FIGURE 6.12 *The Fitness Expert software*

In many ways, the FitSense FS-1 is similar to the Nike Triax Elite. It measures heart rate, speed, and distance, and uploads it to your PC. The FS-1 includes a full-featured heart rate monitor and adds a speedometer and a PC upload capability to measure speed, pace, distance, heart rate, calories burned, splits, and target zone alerts (see Figure 6.13).

In its most basic form, the FS-1 is a speedometer. It's a watch with a foot pod that tells you your speed and distance, and it retails for $124.99. The FS-1 + Heart Monitor is a $174.99 product that adds a chest strap to the device. And the FS-1 + Heart Monitor + NetLink adds a USB adapter and software so you can track all of your workouts online (see Figure 6.14). It retails for $224.99.

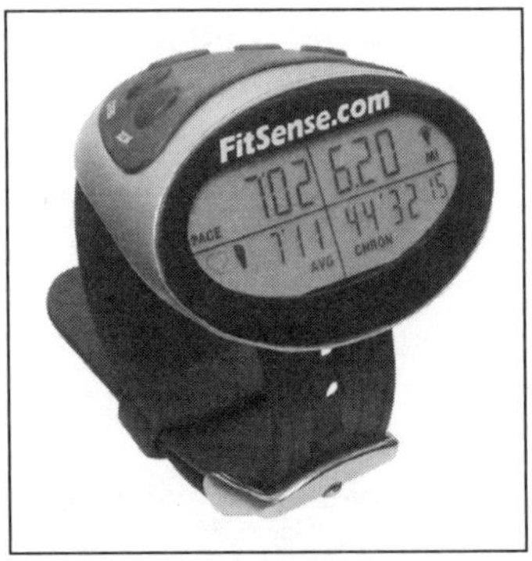

FIGURE 6.13 *FitSense FS-1*

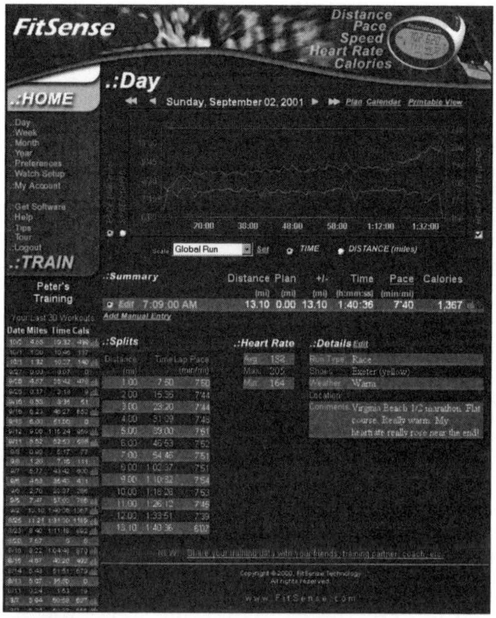

FIGURE 6.14 *The FitSense FS-1 software works via the NetLink connection to the Web.*

NetLink and FitSense create your own personal Web page, where you can access your workout data and results. For more robust training software that works on your PC without you having to connect to the Internet, the company offers a third-party product that is compatible with FitSense, called CrossTrak. It's an additional $39.99.

Garmin

http://www.garmin.com

Summary: The Garmin Forerunner series provides sophisticated GPS technology to help you track your outdoor workouts.

The Garmin Forerunner 101 and 201 are GPS devices that provide speed and distance data for runners, hikers, and bikers. Don't use one of these things inside, because the device will think you're standing still. It includes software that uploads your workouts to your computer, a three-level split-screen display, and a unique design that includes the GPS and watch in the same body. The large display looks funny on your wrist and takes some getting used to. The only differences between the devices is that the 101 is a little bigger, works on AAA batteries, and doesn't interface with your PC, while the 201 uses rechargeable lithium-ion batteries and does interface with your PC (see Figure 6.15). The Forerunner 101 retails for $114.27, while the Forerunner 201 retails for $160.70.

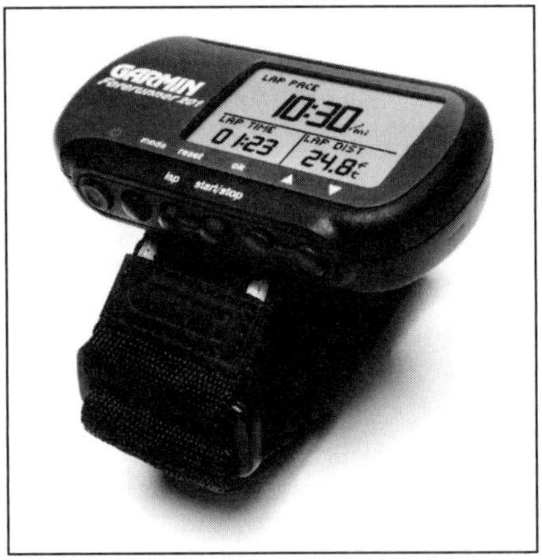

FIGURE 6.15 *The Garmin Forerunner 201*

The device stores up to 100 locations and displays training time, elevation, calories burned, pace, and distance. It also includes a stopwatch and a lap timer; you can store up to two years of lap data. Because it's a GPS, the Garmin Forerunner graphically shows you where you are at any given time, including longitude and latitude information. Plus, if you come across an interesting place on your running path, the Forerunner lets you mark the location for future reference.

A unique feature of the Forerunner is the Virtual Partner. You set your goals for the workout in terms of distance and pace, and your "virtual buddy" is displayed onscreen, running at that pace. Your character is shown either ahead of or behind your virtual partner, depending on your performance. This is an extremely motivating feature. A pace whistle alerts you when you are traveling either faster or slower than your desired pace, and a distance whistle tells you when you've reached the specified distance in your workout. The Forerunner also includes a built-in timer that pauses when you stop running, giving you an accurate picture of your workout.

The Forerunner connects to your PC, enabling you to upload your workout data from the Forerunner to your PC and the Forerunner's Logbook software. Logbook includes a detailed workout history that lets you view workout statistics broken down by day or week.

Pam

http://www.pam.com

Summary: A unique device that features accelerometer technology to provide you with feedback about your workouts.

The $147 Pam Activity Monitor is a unique device that gives you points based on how much energy you expend in a day (see Figure 6.16). Your wear it on your waist like a pedometer, and it measures your movements and provides you with a readout of your activity level.

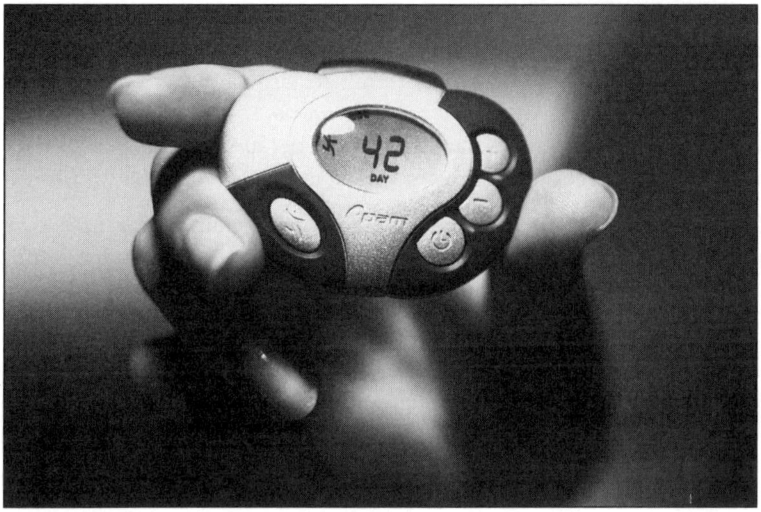

FIGURE 6.16 *The Pam Activity Monitor*

After connecting to your PC via Pam's docking station, your personal Pam Web site shows your actual activity for the day, converting your score into calories burned, steps taken, and how you're doing from a personal fitness standpoint. It will tell you how much time you've spent working out in a given day, either low impact (the Health Zone) or high impact (the Sport Zone). You get 30 days' worth of data on the Web site at a time, more if you join the Pam Fitness Society, which is free with your Pam purchase for the first two years, and $99 per year thereafter.

Similar to the Fitness Expert Calorie Tracker, Pam uses accelerometer technology to measure your movements. It tracks the full motion and force of your hips and torso as you work out each day. After uploading to the Internet, Pam takes the data that you've uploaded and uses your age, weight, height, and gender to determine just how many calories you burned. The accelerometer determines the steps you've taken.

Timex

http://www.timex.com

Summary: The Timex Bodylink works on a different level than other exercise devices.

The Timex Bodylink System features nearly everything you'd need in a workout device, including a fashionable watch, a heart rate monitor, a GPS system, and data uplink to your PC and the Internet. It includes the Timex Ironman Triathlon Bodylink Performance Monitor, which is a watch that provides real-time workout data, the Timex Digital Heart Rate Sensor (the chest strap), and the Timex Speed + Distance Sensor (the GPS).

The Performance Monitor includes a three-line display that lets you view heart rate, speed, pace, and distance simultaneously; a 100-hour chronograph with lap and split times; and a 100-lap memory with recall of average and maximum speed, average and maximum pace, average heart rate, and time in the target zone, as well as lap and split times for your workout. You can set alerts to tell you if you are outside any predetermined targets (heart rate, pace, speed, or distance). Plus, an odometer tracks your distance for a workout or a group of workouts, which is helpful if you want to run a certain distance per week because the watch will tell you how far you've run this week at a glance. You can swim with this watch; it is water resistant to 50 meters.

Data Recorder software uploads your workout information to your PC for further analysis, using Timex Trainer Software, which generates graphs, workout logs, and summary information.

The Bodylink is not an inexpensive product. The heart rate sensor alone is $125; the GPS without the heart rate sensor is $250; and the Bodylink system without the data recorder is $300 (with the data recorder, it's $375). Street prices can be much lower than this, though. We've seen the entire Bodylink System with Data Recorder for as low as $255.

The Future

The world of fitness technology is changing pretty quickly. PCs get more powerful, the Internet and broadband connections are becoming ubiquitous, and technology keeps improving. Heart rate monitors, for example, have become much more powerful, attractive, and feature-filled in the last few years. Heart rate straps used to be very uncomfortable and PC uploads were nonexistent, but as PCs become partners to these devices, they have gotten much more interesting. Expect to see more powerful gadgets at lower prices over the next few years.

One of the most interesting fitness gadget rumors we heard this summer is that a major shoe manufacturer is going to come out with Bluetooth-enabled sneakers that transfer workout data from the sneakers to an MP3 player that you wear while running or walking. You then upload that data to your computer. This is something that would have sounded like science fiction a few years ago, but it is plausible today.

Summary

Fitness gadgets keep you motivated and moving. You'll exercise more if you wear one. And most are small enough that no one will notice that you're wearing one (or they'll think it's a pager). They're comfortable enough that you'll forget it's on, and they're powerful enough that you'll be grateful you're wearing it and wonder how you got along without it in the past.

Pedometers represent the low end of the fitness gadget world. You can get a good one for less than $30 and a great one for less than $50. Heart rate monitors provide much more information and cost more, but you can get a good heart rate monitor for less than $100, and a bells-and-whistles one for less than $300. You can also buy fitness gadgets that monitor the calories you burn, where you are, how fast you're going, and how you're doing in relation to your goals. You can spend as little as $100 for one of these gadgets, or you can spend up to $350 or more.

When you're beginning your workout routine, you'll be fine with a pedometer. Use a spreadsheet and track your steps on your PC to measure your progress. As you progress in your fitness, you might want to buy something more powerful, such as a heart rate monitor, but that's up to you.

In the next chapter, we'll show you how to spend less money for the gadgets mentioned in this chapter, as well as other products.

Chapter 7

Shop Naked

"The waist is a terrible thing to mind."

—Tom Wilson (in the *Ziggy* comic strip)

Okay, so maybe don't shop naked until you've minded your waist. But this chapter explores the many places at which you can shop however you're dressed and at whatever time you want, without burning any calories—online. There are many options for online shopping. You can buy food, cooking utensils, and fitness gadgets online, and you can learn a lot and save a lot of money in the process.

In this chapter, we'll examine the best sites for buying health- and fitness-related products. As usual, we're covering the best. If a site is not up to our standards, you won't see it here. We'll show you how to get the best deals and provide tips and advice for shopping safely and wisely.

CHECK THE WHOLE PRICE

When shopping, either online or off, most of us look at offered price and neglect to consider everything. When evaluating the pricing of items, make sure to check the whole price, including shipping and sales tax. Some sites even sneak in an extra "order fee" that essentially pays for the free shipping that they're allegedly offering.

Superstores

With apologies to Arlo Guthrie, you can get anything you want at many of the superstores on the Web. And this isn't limited to health and fitness products in any way. The stores in this list offer everything from books to electronics to lawn furniture. These so-called superstore sites boast large departments and a variety of choices. They are also very good places to buy health- and fitness-related equipment.

Amazon.com

http://www.amazon.com

Summary: Amazon offers a plethora of health and fitness products, including books, gadgets, utensils, and even food and drugs.

Amazon.com has come a long way from its days as "Earth's Biggest Bookstore." It still holds that title, but it also holds much more, as founder and CEO Jeff Bezos ventures to offer a selection of products as "wide as the Amazon." Its growing list of stores is shown in Figure 7.1.

Health and fitness aficionados will not be disappointed by a trip to Amazon's wide range of specialty stores. Besides the thousands of health- and fitness-related books it offers, Amazon has a Kitchen & Housewares store, a Health & Personal Care store, an Electronics store, and a Medical Equipment & Supplies area to satisfy any gadget freak (see Figures 7.2 and 7.3). Plus, Amazon's Outlet store offers used and reconditioned products at a significant discount. Because some of these "stores" are managed by third parties, you don't always get Amazon's free shipping offer on orders of $25 or more. For example, at the Vitamin Shoppe in the Health & Personal Care store, shipping is free after you spend $40 or more.

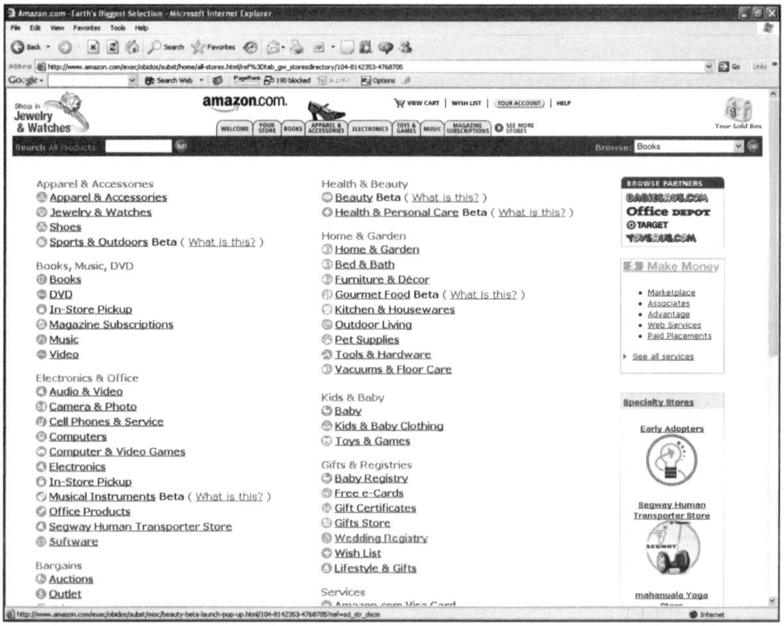

FIGURE 7.1 *Amazon.com's growing list of stores*

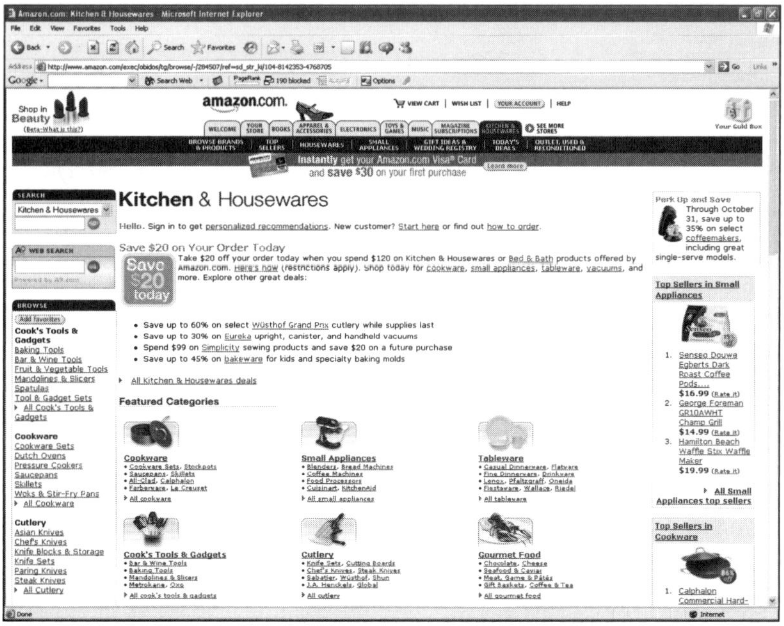
Amazon.com: Kitchen & Housewares - Microsoft Internet Explorer
amazon.com.
Shop in Beauty
Kitchen & Housewares
Hello. Sign in to get personalized recommendations. New customer? Start here or find out how to order.
Save $20 on Your Order Today
Save $20 today
Take $20 off your order today when you spend $120 on Kitchen & Housewares or Bed & Bath products offered by Amazon.com. Here's how (restrictions apply). Shop today for cookware, small appliances, tableware, vacuums, and more. Explore other great deals:
Save up to 60% on select Wüsthof Grand Prix cutlery while supplies last
Save up to 30% on Eureka upright, canister, and handheld vacuums
Spend $99 on Simplicity sewing products and save $20 on a future purchase
Save up to 45% on bakeware for kids and specialty baking molds
All Kitchen & Housewares deals
Featured Categories
Cookware
Small Appliances
Tableware
Cook's Tools & Gadgets
Cutlery
Gourmet Food
Top Sellers in Small Appliances
Top Sellers in Cookware

FIGURE 7.2 *Amazon.com's Kitchen & Housewares store offers lots of cooking utensils, pots and pans, and even gourmet foods.*

To make things easy, Amazon uses the same structure for every page. If it can, it strives to make recommendations to you based on your previous purchases and/or searches. It offers specials on the home page as well as featured sellers, a list of bestsellers, and links to related stores. You can browse by section, just as you would in an offline store, and you can buy multiple items from separate stores using the same shopping cart.

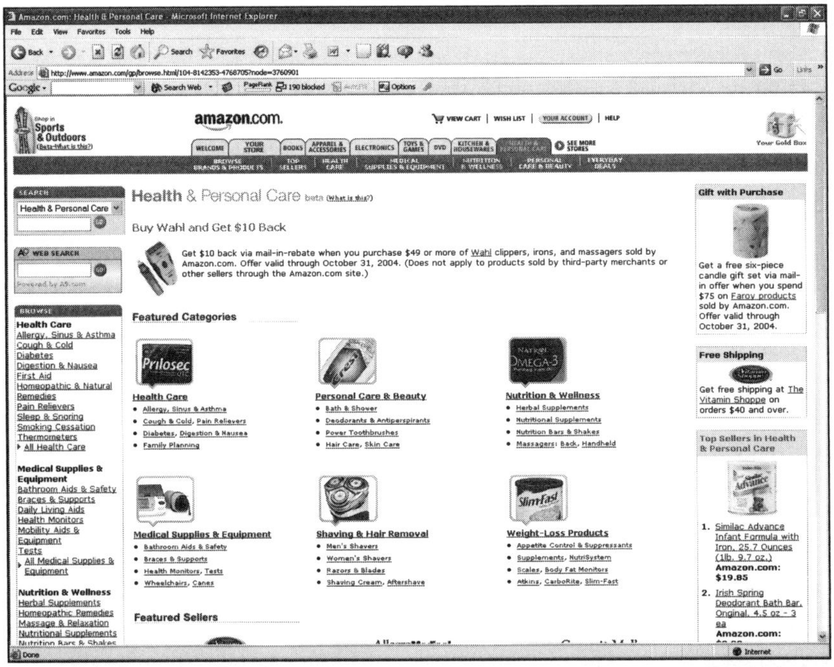

FIGURE 7.3 *Amazon.com's Health & Personal Care Store is one of its newest offerings*

In general, Amazon discounts books by about 30% (although that varies). Its other discounts vary as well, so shop wisely. We found that their prices for health gadgets, such as body fat monitors and pedometers, were competitive but not great. But their selection was good, with offerings from many different vendors, although they were scattered throughout the site (see Figure 7.4). Amazon also sells other gadgets, such as heart rate monitors and body monitors.

One fun new feature on Amazon is their Gourmet Food store (see Figure 7.5). While many of the offerings are not the healthiest, being able to get foods from Dean & Deluca, Godiva, Harry and David, Legal Sea Foods, and literally hundreds of others all in one place is very convenient. And among the numerous vendors are a variety that specialize in low-carb and low-calorie foods, so you can shop there guilt free.

Amazon also offers an Outlet store, where reconditioned and closeout products are available. We found some great bargains there, but you have to shop carefully. Many of these products are offered by third parties. Check those third parties out before buying anything from them.

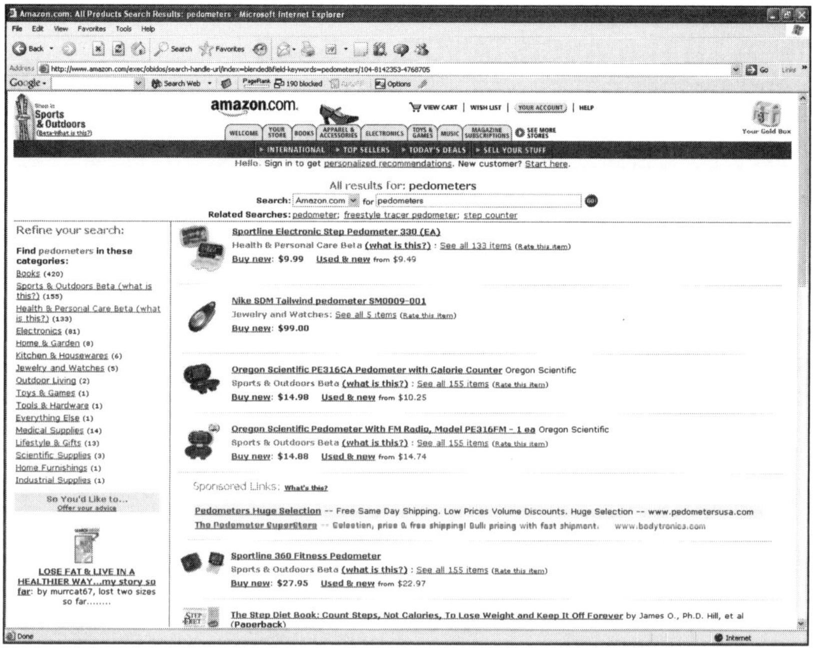

FIGURE 7.4 *Searching for pedometers brings up a lot in many different locations.*

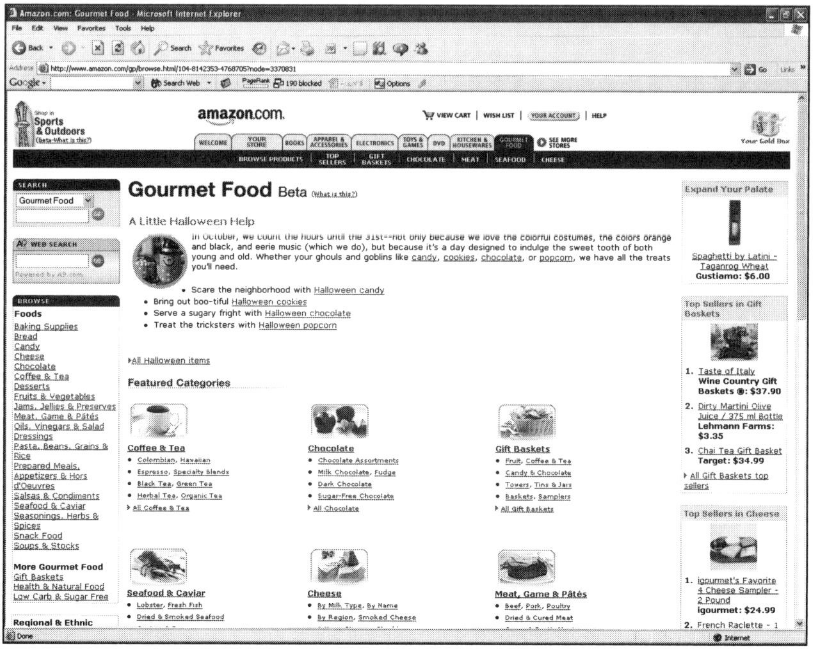

FIGURE 7.5 *Amazon's new Gourmet Food store was created in conjunction with a variety of gourmet foods vendors.*

A LITTLE ASSISTANCE, PLEASE

The Internet provides a great way to shop. And bots, or robots, offer help in finding the best price. To use a bot, go to one of the many shopping sites online, such as ActivShopper (http://www.activshopper.com), BizRate (http://www.bizrate.com), bottomdollar.com (http://www.bottomdollar.com), Google's Froogle (http://froogle.google.com), mySimon (http://www.mysimon.com), NexTag (http://www.nextag.com), PriceGrabber.com (http://www.pricegrabber.com), Shopping.com (http://www.shopping.com), and StreetPrices.com (http://www.streetprices.com); see Figure 7.6. These sites offer a way to compare prices quickly across sites. Many searches will provide a results box along with the price that the vendor offers, and reviews of the vendor by users as well as the site in some cases. One issue with these sites is that some ask vendors to pay to be included in the search and especially to receive a vendor rating, so you might have to go to several sites to find the lowest price because all sites don't include all vendors. And even then, if a discount site that you know about isn't listed, you might have to check there also. But with persistence, you can find the lowest price online from a vendor you trust.

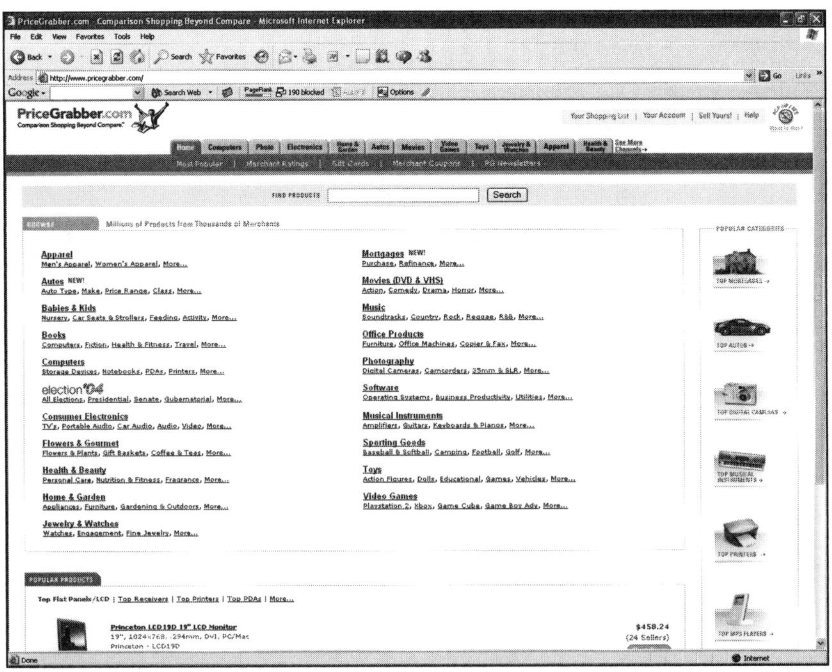

FIGURE 7.6 *PriceGrabber.com is one of the many shopping comparison sites on the Internet.*

Costco.com

http://www.costco.com

Summary: Shop early and often at this superstore. They provide great deals, if you move fast.

I'm the kind of customer that Costco doesn't like. I hate long lines, I don't like to bag my own groceries, and I can't figure out why I'd need a bottle of ketchup that can barely fit in my car. I've never been of fan of warehouse membership clubs, such as Costco. Costco.com, however, is another story.

Costco.com offers a wide variety of products at the same or better prices than its stores (see Figure 7.7). You don't have to be a member (membership fees start at $45) to shop at Costco; you simply pay 5% more than their listed prices if you're not. If you're not a regular shopper at a physical Costco, you'd have to spend $900 online in a year to justify the cost of membership. Even 5% over their listed prices is a good deal for infrequent shoppers.

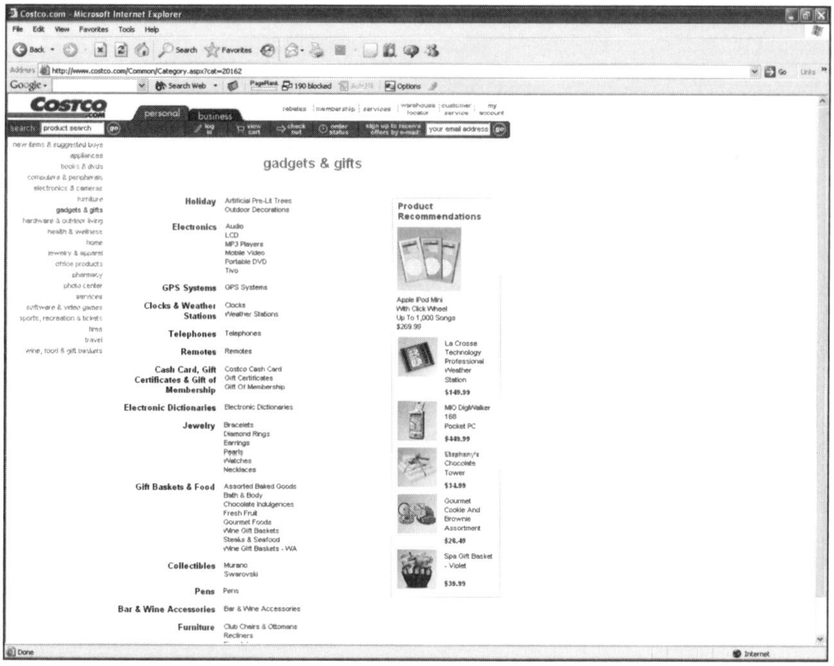

FIGURE 7.7 *Costco.com takes their great prices online, but without the long lines and searches for parking spots.*

Think of Costco.com as being several miles wide, but only an inch or so deep. They offer a large number of types of products, but only a few selections in each category, if that. When we shopped, their selection of health bars was limited to one vendor's products. But this changes often, so just like at the physical warehouse membership clubs, you have to shop often to find the best products. However, you can subscribe to one of Costco.com's many online newsletters and get an update of what's available.

Costco.com offers a wide variety of health and fitness products, including books, gadgets, health and wellness products, food, and a pharmacy that offers some of the best prices anywhere and is an excellent drug reference.

Costco is well known for its book section. Because of Costco's aggressive pricing, many books sell more copies at Costco than anywhere else. Costco's online bookstore doesn't offer a wide selection, but there are many choices and a wider variety than what you'd find in the store. The Costco Book Club offers a monthly selection that includes discussion questions and an interview with the book's author. Costco.com's nonfiction section always offers a few cookbooks and diet books for sale, typically at more than 40% off of the list price.

Costco.com's Health & Wellness section offers a variety of products, all at substantial discounts (see Figure 7.8). For example, they offered the OMRON HJ-112 pedometer for $24.99. We couldn't find it anywhere else for less than $28, and most places were well over $33.

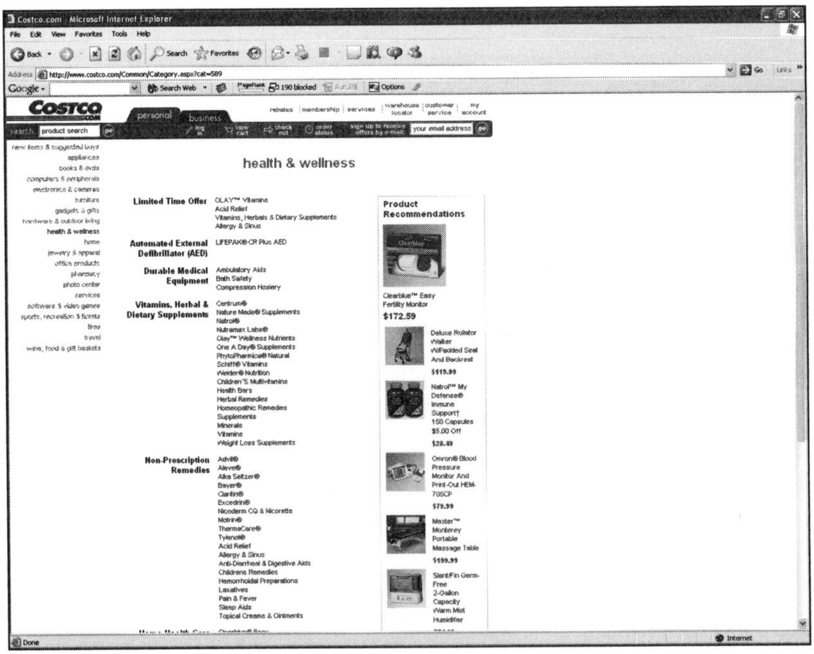

FIGURE 7.8 *Costco.com's Health & Wellness section features vitamins, non-prescription drugs, and health gadgets.*

In its warehouse clubs, Costco provides a wide selection of foods and quite often offers high-quality bakery items, meats, and other delicacies. This is not so online. Their food items are heavy on wines (which can only be shipped to a limited number of states), gift baskets, and some foods, but those are primarily for gifts also (see Figure 7.9).

Costco.com's pharmacy is one of the best on the Internet. It provides low-cost prescriptions and lots of information about them. You can manage your prescriptions online, store health information in a password-protected area, research medications, and consider natural medications as well.

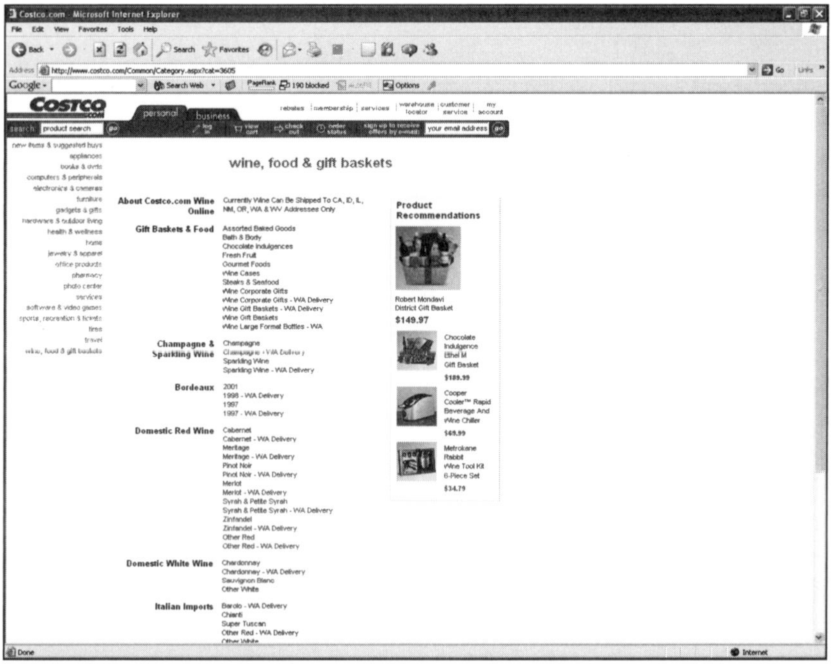

FIGURE 7.9 *Costco.com includes wine, gift baskets, and some food items.*

Drugstore.com

http://www.drugstore.com

Summary: Beautiful Web site, very well designed, good selection of fitness products. Their regular prices, however, are higher than most.

Drugstore.com is one of the best-designed sites on the Internet. It's well thought out, seems to anticipate your next move, shows you where you've been, and is a great place to shop. This makes sense, because Drugstore.com's roots come from Amazon.com. Amazon still owns about one-sixth of the stock in Drugstore.com and helped the company be the only health and beauty online store to survive the dot-bomb bust of 2000 and 2001.

As a result, Drugstore.com has built a niche in health and beauty, aligning with other retailers such as General Nutrition Centers, offering beauty aids at Beauty.com, working with Rite Aid on pharmacy orders, and working with VisionDirect for contact lens orders.

COUPONS SAVE THE DAY

I always get frustrated when I'm shopping at a site and the shopping cart includes a space for a certificate or coupon and I don't have one. It's like there's a secret club out there and I'm not a member. Luckily, there are a variety of sites to help you with that. Some vendors on eBay actually sell discount coupons, which are useful if you're buying a computer or a car. Other sites, such as DealCatcher (http://www.dealcatcher.com), dealcoupon.com (http://dealcoupon.com), DealofDay (http://www.dealofday.com), FatWallet (http://www.fatwallet.com), and ValueConsumer.com (http://www.valueconsumer.com) offer coupons and often much more (see Figure 7.10). Some sites will let you set up alerts, so if one of your favorite vendors offers a coupon, you'll get an e-mail informing you about it. Some also feature deals and special sales in addition to coupons, so they're a great place to go to get the latest bargains. In many cases, these sites are also selling their own discount programs, so evaluate those carefully. But often, they're just trying to get you the best deals.

With these partners and others, Drugstore.com sells a variety of fitness products, foods, pharmaceuticals, health and beauty aids, and other products. Its Fitness store features pedometers, heart monitors, blood-pressure monitors, and other devices, while its Vitamins & Diet store features vitamins, health foods, books, scales, and body-fat monitors (see Figure 7.11).

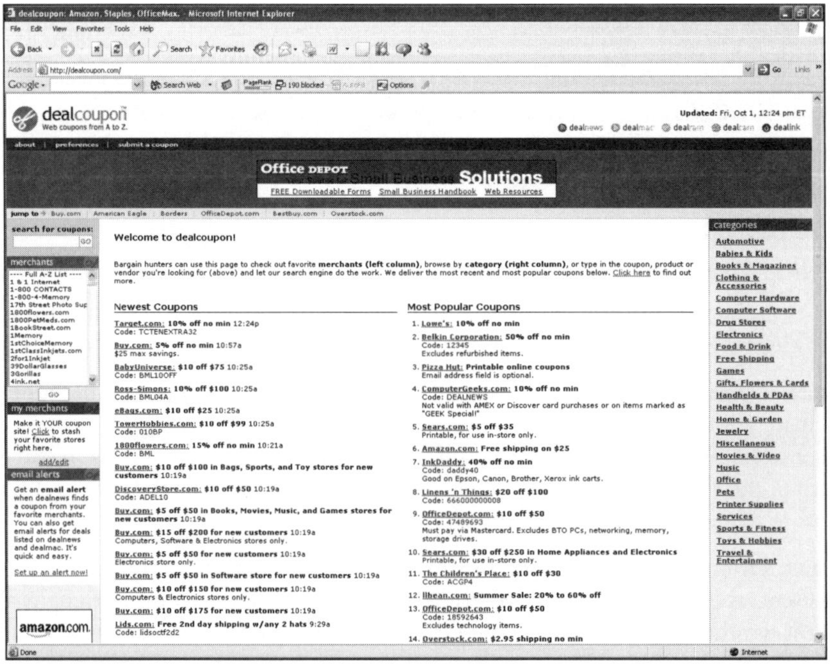

FIGURE 7.10 *dealcoupon.com offers coupons for nearly any type of online purchase.*

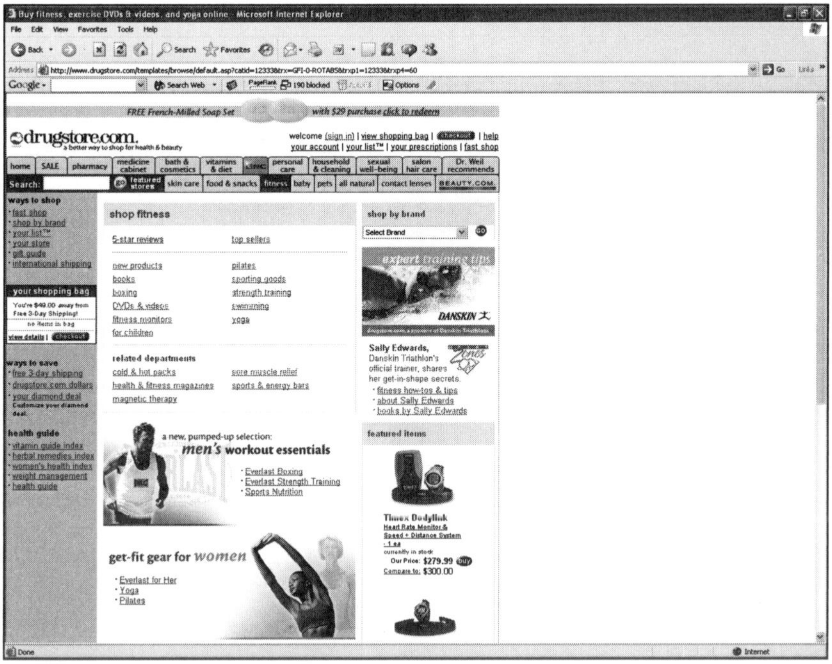

FIGURE 7.11 *The Drugstore.com Fitness store*

Their selection is good, but Drugstore.com's normal prices are somewhat higher than other locations on the Web. However, there are a number of sales and clearance items that provide excellent values, plus the company aggressively offers coupons for free shipping and other incentives to drive sales.

eCOST.com and Overstock.com

http://www.ecost.com

http://www.overstock.com

Summary: Both sites specialize in clearance items and aggressive pricing.

Think of Overstock.com as a large clearance center (see Figure 7.12). There's nothing new here; there are just lots of items to choose from. On the health and fitness side, they offer pedometers, heart monitors, and other health devices, plus a variety of books. When we visited, they had many health and fitness books and videos for 40 to 50% off of list price, heart monitors for as much as 70% off, and yoga equipment for 50% off. Because they are selling items on closeout, you have to visit often and shop carefully to find the product you want. Some products might seem like a great deal, but after looking more closely, sometimes they aren't because they're old models that have been replaced by better ones. Still, Overstock.com is a great source and should always be considered when you're looking for health and fitness equipment.

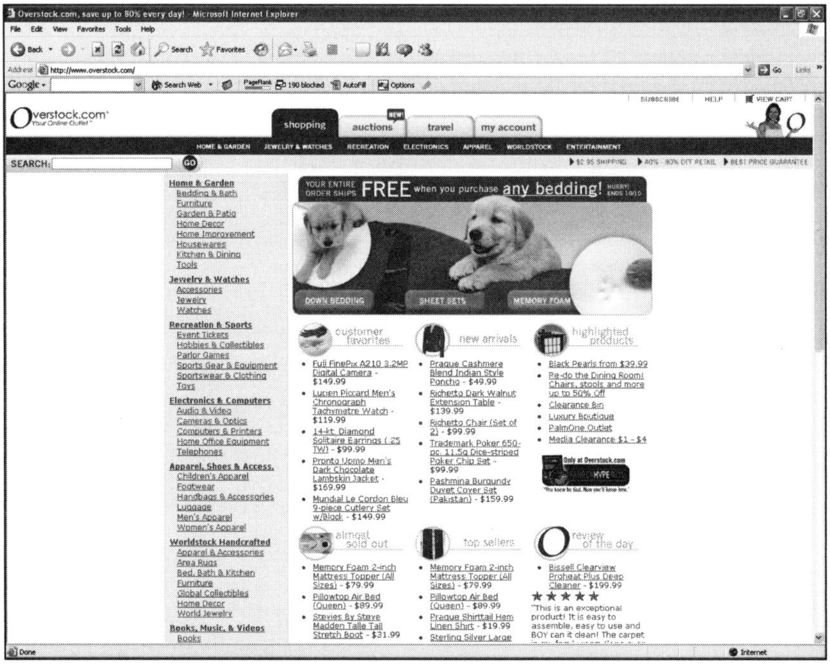

FIGURE 7.12 *Overstock.com offers thousands of items at clearance prices.*

On the surface, eCOST.com seems very similar to Overstock.com, and in many ways, it is (see Figure 7.13). Both sites offer aggressive discounting on a wide variety of items. eCOST.com seems to offer more products, but their pricing is somewhat sneaky. They show the price onscreen, but then mention that there's a "shopping cart special." In reality, this means that you don't see the actual discount price until you put the item in your shopping cart. Amazon.com does this also, because it tends to pique shoppers' curiosity, but eCOST.com does it a lot more often.

Items on clearance at eCOST.com are shown with the quantity and time remaining before they are gone, seemingly forever (see Figure 7.14). These are the truly hot buys on the site; there are often some tremendous buys on this site. I bought a pair of Sennheiser headphones for my iPod that were fully half the price of anywhere else. You just have to visit the clearance center early and often.

Both Overstock.com and eCOST.com sell products that are not necessarily old or out of date. They could also be a stock of refurbished products that came back for repair, or they could be products that the manufacturer simply ordered too many of. It happens, and you benefit. You just have to look for the products.

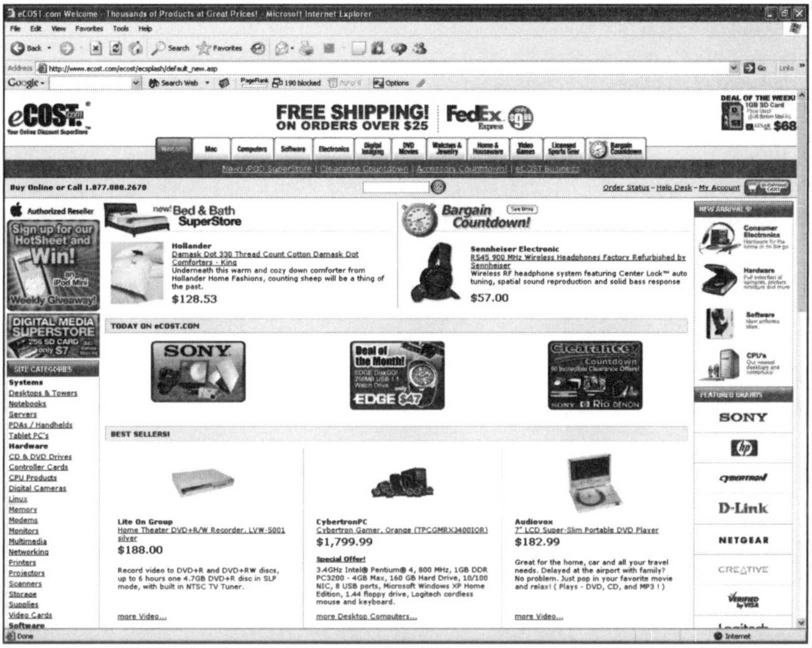

FIGURE 7.13 *eCOST.com features a wide variety of health and fitness equipment plus cookware and other devices.*

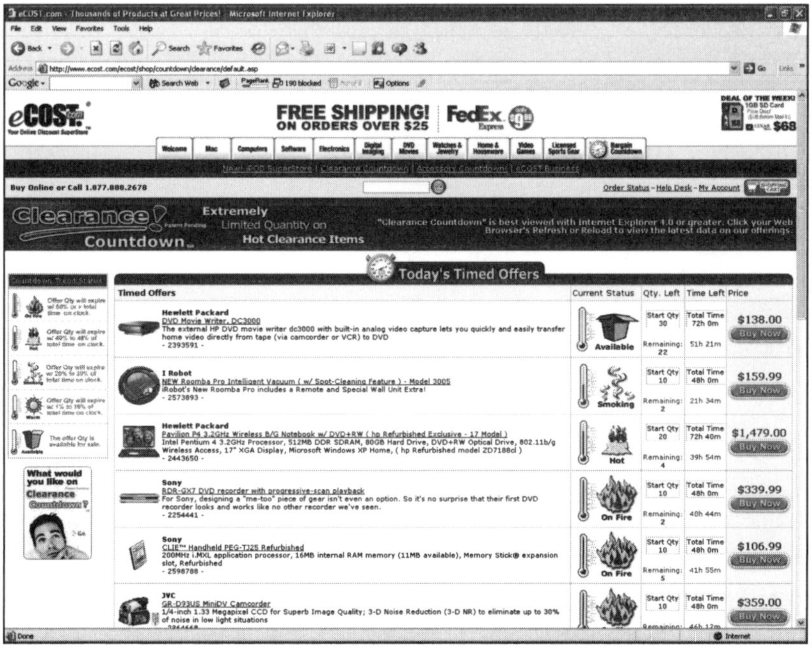

FIGURE 7.14 *Clearance items on eCOST.com get special treatment, with numbers of units remaining and time remaining shown onscreen.*

Walmart.com

http://www.walmart.com

Summary: They provide a surprising array of health and fitness products at excellent prices.

When it comes to health and fitness, most of us don't think about Wal-Mart. Lawn furniture, yes. Tires, sure. But health and fitness? Well, actually you should. Walmart.com has some of the best prices around on health- and fitness-related equipment (see Figure 7.15). They don't sell much in the way of food or drug products online, but they do offer an excellent selection of books, pedometers, heart monitors, exercise equipment, and a nice pharmacy with drug lookup information, a specialty health center for diabetes sufferers, and discount prices.

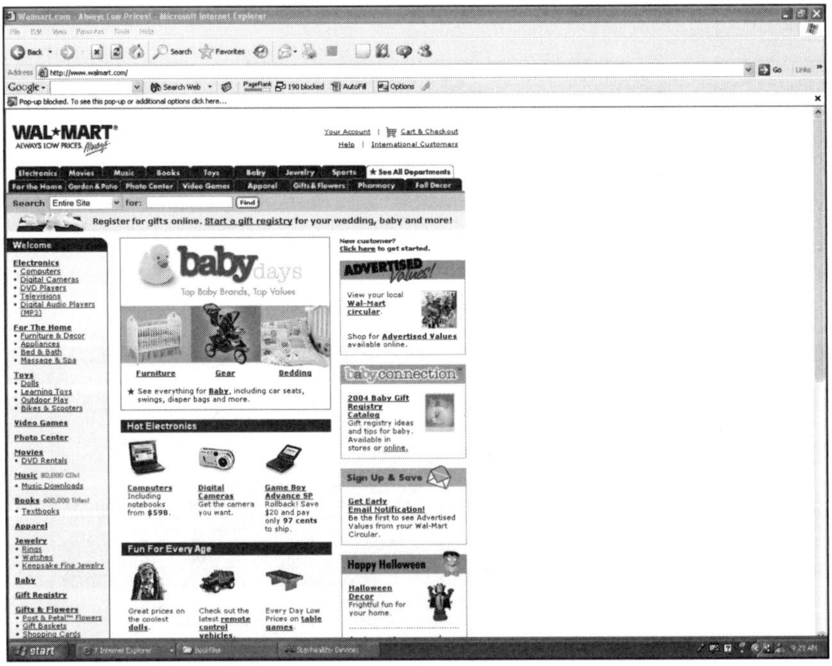

FIGURE 7.15 *Walmart.com features the same great prices online that they offer in stores around the country.*

Walmart.com also offers their famous Rollback feature to highlight prices that have dropped. In general, their pricing is among the lowest on the Internet, much lower than most. They don't have the same free shipping options that some sites, such as Amazon, offer, so you have to consider that when making a decision.

Their fitness equipment is the biggest surprise; Walmart.com features a virtual superstore of treadmills, elliptical trainers, weight sets, pedometers, and heart monitors at excellent prices (see Figure 7.16). Shipping can get pricey on some large pieces of fitness equipment, so Walmart.com often offers discounted shipping prices on these big-ticket items.

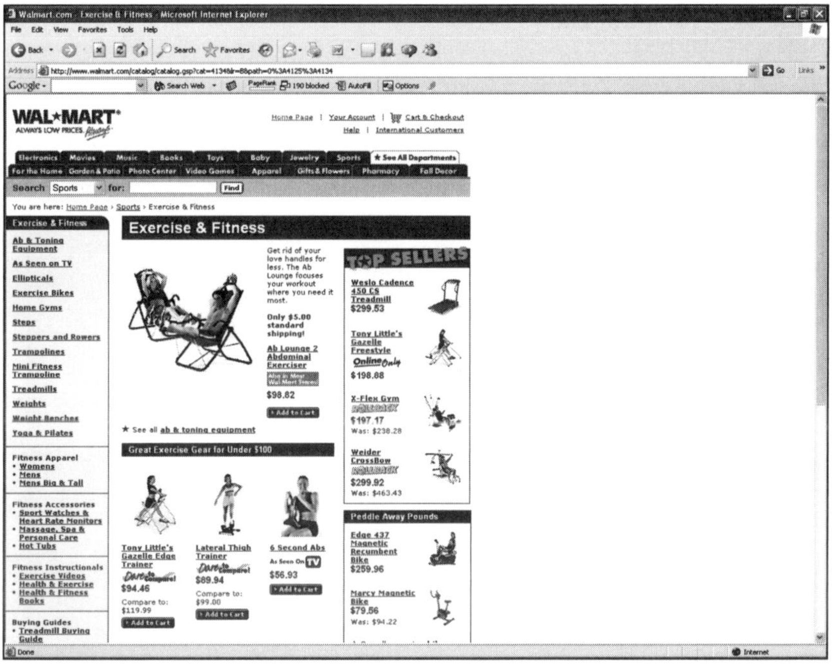

FIGURE 7.16 *Walmart.com offers a wide array of fitness equipment at excellent prices.*

Specialty Stores

While superstores are nice, specialty stores are often a better option when buying online. You'll almost always get a better selection, better expert advice, and sometimes better pricing at a specialty store than at a superstore. What follows are some of the better health, fitness, and food specialty stores on the Internet, with an eye toward those that actively work to get you the best deals and service in a particular area.

Bodytronics

http://www.bodytronics.com

Summary: Excellent selection of health and exercise equipment, particularly pedometers, heart monitors, and other devices.

Bodytronics focuses on health and fitness gadgets, offering a wide variety of pedometers, heart monitors, blood pressure monitors, stopwatches, GPS devices, body fat monitors, scales, books, and first aid kits, all at excellent prices (see Figure 7.17). Bodytronics includes an outlet center, but, at least when we visited, it was pretty weak, with only a few products available and at prices that weren't very good at all.

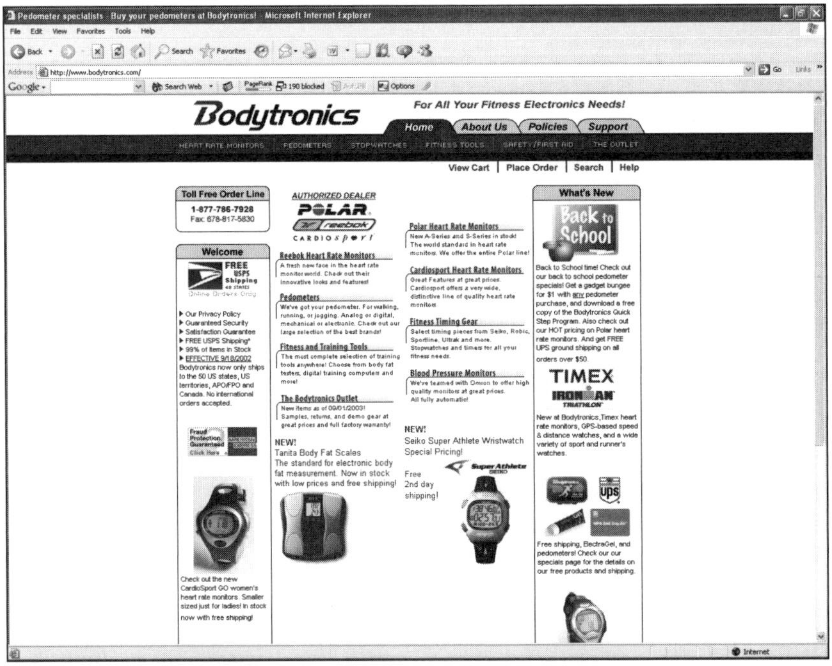

FIGURE 7.17 *Bodytronics specializes in health and fitness equipment.*

Most major manufacturers are represented on the site, including Garmin, OMRON, Polar, Reebok, Seiko, SportBrain, Sportline, Tanita, and Timex. Some of the products are sold under the Bodytronics name, including the SportBrain iStep, available on Bodytronics.com for half the price that SportBrain sells it for. Bodytronics does a good job of offering a lot of products at competitive prices.

Bodytronics could be better designed. It provides some good information, but you have to dig for it in many cases. For example, one nice feature of the site, although under-promoted, is that Bodytronics offers free shipping on many products, free ElectraGel to make heart monitors work better, and a free pedometer with certain purchases.

Epicurious Shop

http://www.epicurious.com/shop

Summary: One of the best stores anywhere for cooking, food, and related products.

As we showed you in Chapter 4, Epicurious is one of the best cooking-related sites on the Internet. A venture of Condé Nast and its *Bon Appetit and Gourmet* magazines, Epicurious features great information about food and cooking. Its shop is decidedly gourmet, with cookware, food products, travel offerings, wine, and other products, all aimed at the top of the market (see Figure 7.18). Epicurious doesn't do this alone; they have partners such as iGourmet, Jessica's Biscuit ecookbook, RedEnvelope, illy Caffè, LobsterAnywhere, and the California Wine Club, among others.

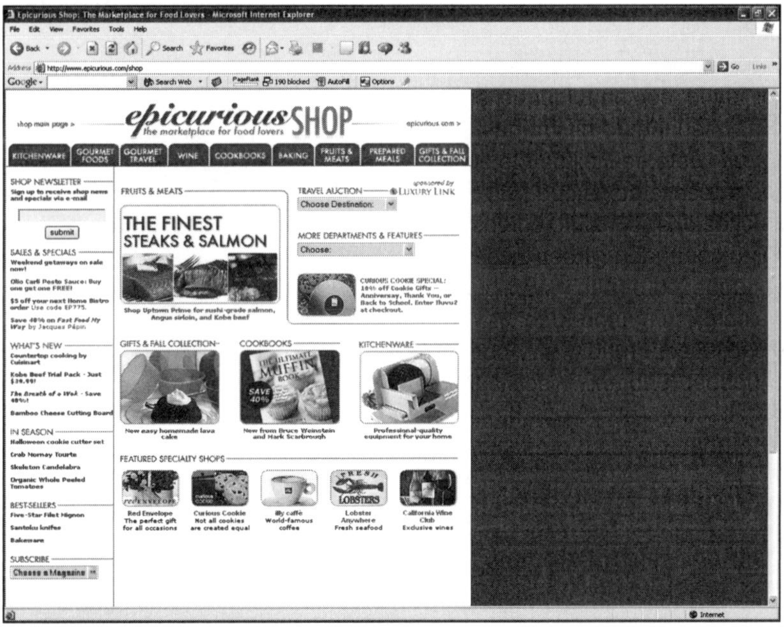

FIGURE 7.18 *The Shop at Epicurious.com features everything related to cooking and food.*

Epicurious Shop's pricing is not particularly aggressive, but there are some bargains in the clearance center (see Figure 7.19). We visited in early fall, when the shop featured summer items on clearance. There were a few items at substantial discounts (more than 50% off) and others at 10 to 15% off.

You have to look hard for healthy choices at Epicurious.com, but they do exist. Some can be found at Home Bistro, which is in the Prepared Meals section. Home Bistro specializes in high-quality prepared meals sent to you. They offer a wide variety of low-carb meals designed for those on Atkins or other low-carb diets. Other healthy choices include regular and organic fruit clubs, which send healthy fruits to your door, low-fat gourmet cheeses, and lots of cookware choices to help you prepare your foods just right.

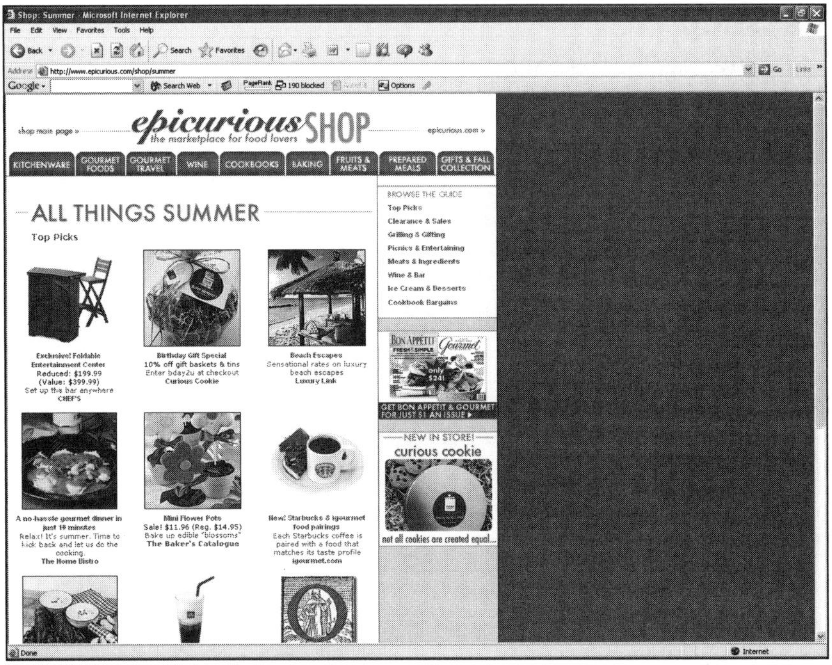

FIGURE 7.19 *The Epicurious Shop's clearance center*

Foot Locker

http://www.footlocker.com

Summary: Way more than just shoes.

When you think of Foot Locker, you think of shoes. Of course, you get lots of those at Foot Locker's online store, but you also get sports gear, fan gear, fitness equipment, and gadgets (see Figure 7.20). Foot Locker's online store features shoes from vendors such as Adidas, AND 1, ASICS, Converse, Dada, New Balance, Nike, Puma, Reebok, and Timberland for nearly any sport or training activity. Their search feature makes it easy to find shoes in your size for your needs. Plus, Foot Locker offers an innovative sales product called Wheel of Deals, which lets you pick products based on deals you select, such as all products under $30 (see Figure 7.21).

Foot Locker's sports gear includes jerseys, hats, and uniforms from all major teams in all major professional and college sports, plus the Olympics. The NFL Shop is also included at Foot Locker's online store, as are branded stores from vendors including Converse and Timberland. There aren't a lot of gadgets, only a few, but the heart monitors offered are useful and stylish.

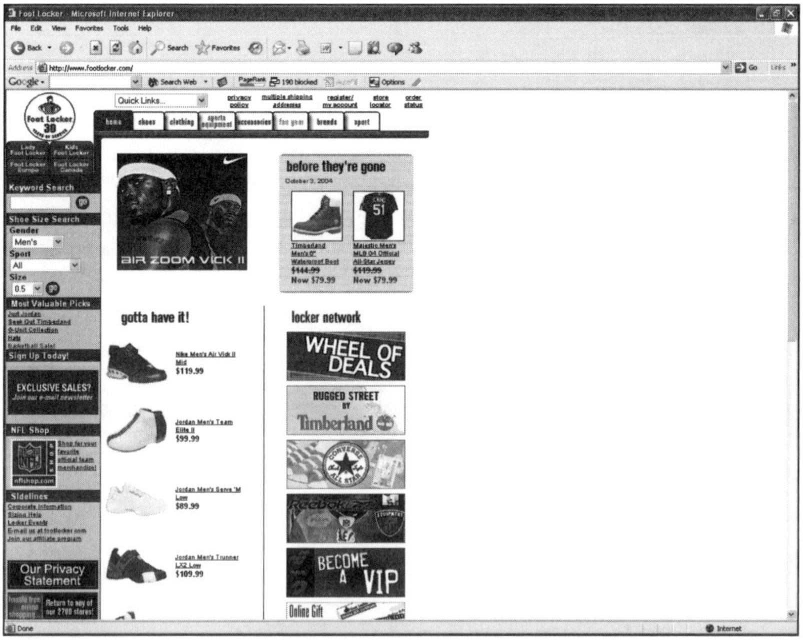

FIGURE 7.20 *Foot Locker features a great selection of athletic shoes, sports gear, and fitness equipment at competitive prices.*

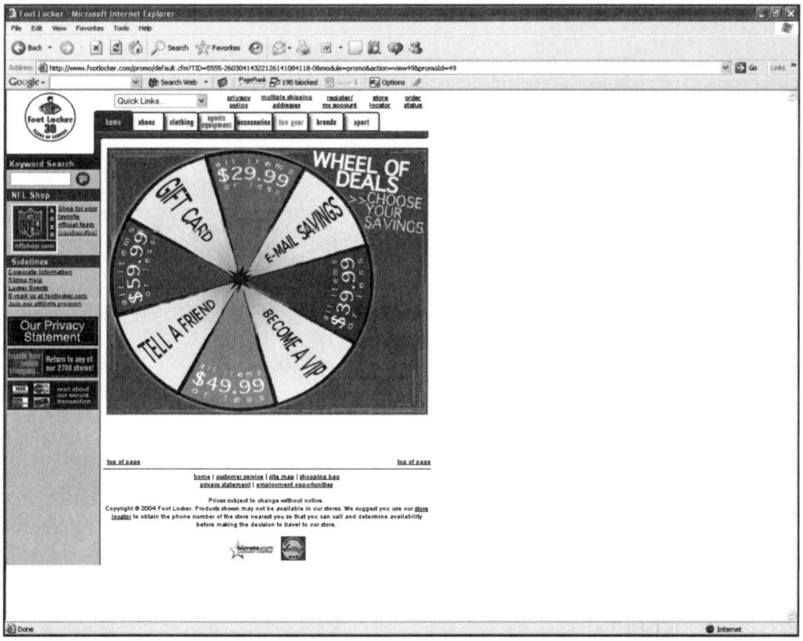

FIGURE 7.21 *Foot Locker's Wheel of Deals features low-priced products based on specs that you choose.*

Heart Monitors

http://www.heartmonitors.com

Summary: Lots of good information, plus a wide selection of heart monitors.

To borrow an old phrase, with a name like Heart Monitors, this site better specialize in heart monitors. And it does. Heart Monitors offers heart monitors from all the major vendors, including Cateye, Cardiosport, FitSense, Impulse, MIO, Polar, Polar Horse (heart monitors for horses), Reebok, and Timex (see Figure 7.22). Plus, the site includes a wealth of information about heart monitors, why they're important, and how to get the most out of using one. You can also find a heart monitor based on the features that are most important to you. The site recommends specific models for you based on your experience and exercise level.

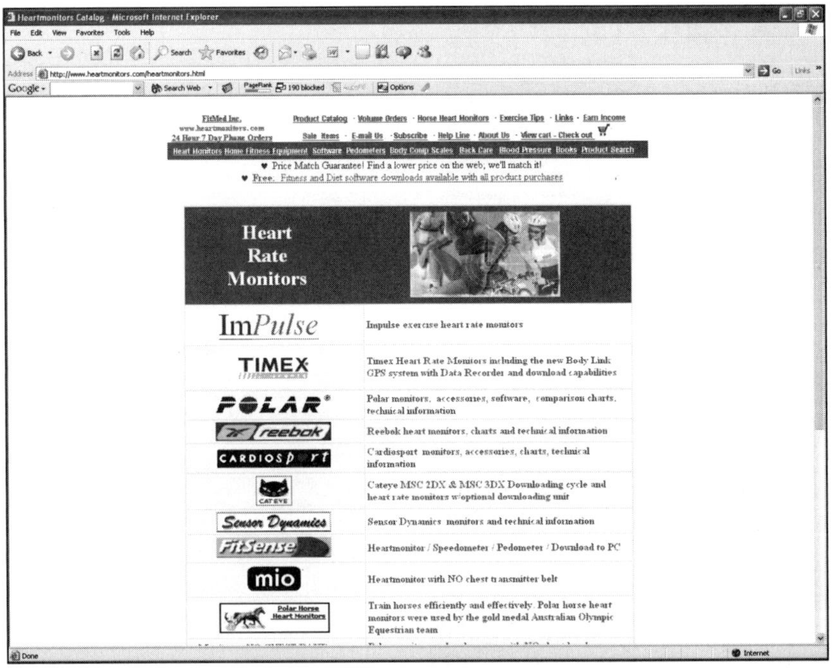

FIGURE 7.22 *Heart Monitors*

Heart Monitors includes software and other products, such as body composition scales, pedometers, and books, but not at anything near the selection level of their heart monitors.

BUYING DIRECT

Many fitness vendors will sell you products directly. Most of the companies profiled in Chapter 6, for example, provide a way for you to buy directly from them. Some of the time, this isn't a good idea. SportBrain, for example, sells its iStep pedometer for $99 on its Web site, but other vendors offer the same pedometer with the same Web-site features for $34.95. Other times, you can get the same or better pricing directly from the manufacturer. For example, NEW-LIFESTYLES, INC. (http://www.new-lifestyles.com) offers a full-service site promoting its pedometers, which are available from other vendors as well. While some vendors will not sell directly to you, NEW-LIFESTYLES' business is focused on doing just that.

NEW-LIFESTYLES offers a great deal of information about pedometers on its Web site, and produces a great product as well. The DIGI-WALKER and NL-2000 products are well regarded (see Figure 7.23).

When buying directly from a vendor, use one of the price-comparison sites mentioned earlier in this chapter to ensure that the vendor is offering you a competitive price.

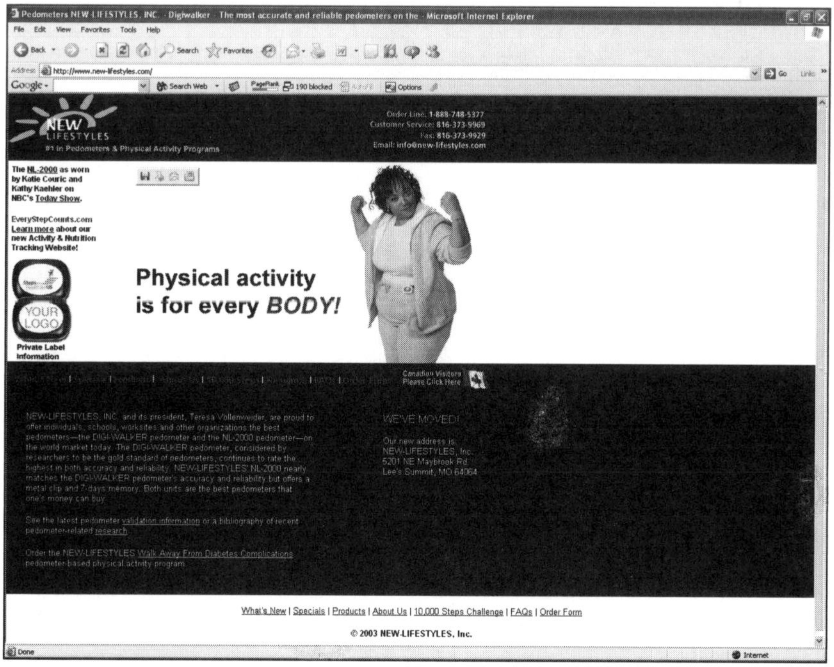

FIGURE 7.23 *NEW-LIFESTYLES features excellent information about pedometers and fitness, including the DIGI-WALKER and NL-2000 pedometers.*

Heartratemonitorsusa.com and Pedometersusa.com

http://www.heartratemonitorsusa.com

http://www.pedometersusa.com

Summary: You want a pedometer? This is a good place to find one. You want a heart monitor? This is also a good place. Cookware? Bad place.

Companion sites Heartratemonitorsusa.com and Pedometersusa.com offer competitive pricing and good information about a decent selection of pedometers and heart rate monitors, among other fitness devices (see Figures 7.24 and 7.25). Both sites also offer scales, body-fat measuring devices, stopwatches, books, and Timex speed and distance systems, which are watch devices that tell you how fast you went and how far. A third companion site is Targetzone.net (http://www.targetzone.net), which is basically the same site as Heartratemonitorsusa.com.

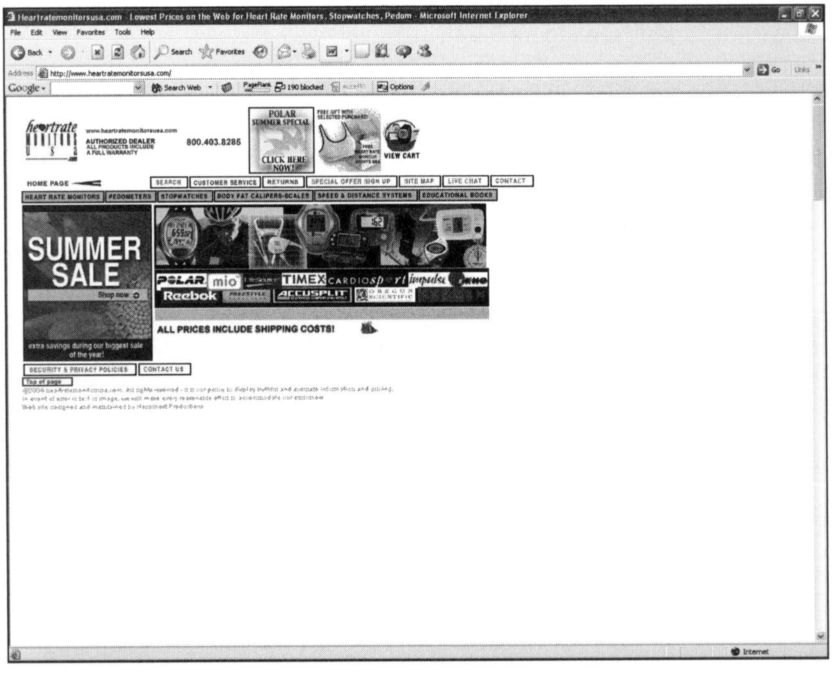

FIGURE 7.24 *Heartratemonitorssusa.com*

For support, each site offers live chats with customer service and sales representatives, a comparison chart to help users make intelligent purchase decisions, an 800 number for orders, 24-hour shipment of orders, and a price-match guarantee. Plus, the site is an authorized dealer for every device that they sell.

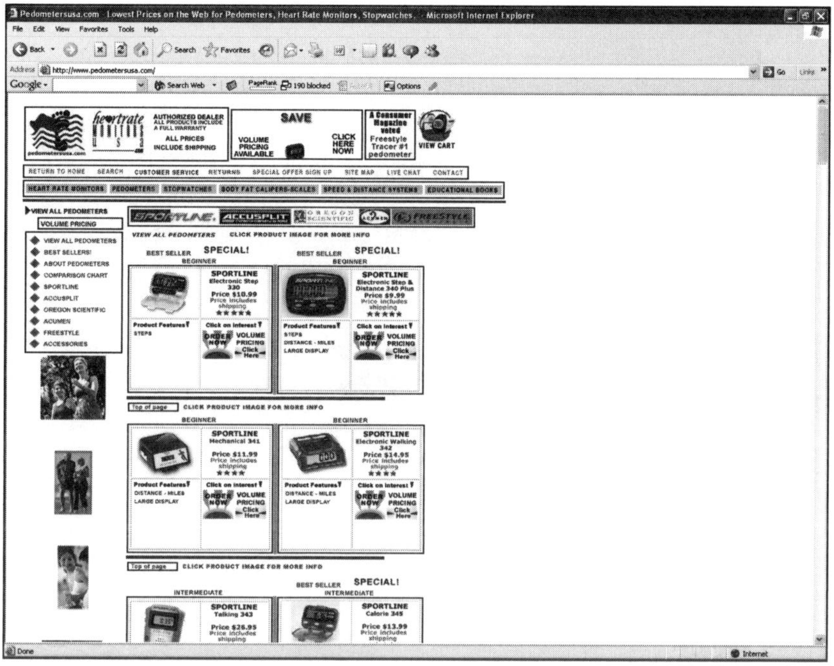

FIGURE 7.25 *Pedometersusa.com*

There isn't enough content on the site to explain each of the various devices. However, the selection criteria are easy to use. For heart monitors, for example, you can shop by manufacturer, your primary activity, and the level or type of heart monitor you want. The shopping process is easy, although we wish that they'd get rid of all of the flashing screens in the shopping process.

Sark Products

http://www.sarkproducts.com

Summary: Decent site that specializes in heart rate monitors.

Sark Products sells heart rate monitors, body-fat scales, calculators, and the Timex Bodylink System from its overly busy Web site, which has too many flashing devices and is hard to read (see Figure 7.26). If you can get past that, though, the company offers good prices and fast service. They promise to match anyone's price and to ship your order the same day they receive it (if it's before 6:30 PM EST).

The manufacturer's product information onsite is supplemented by the company's own commentary, making Sark Products a useful place to make decisions. Comparison charts also help guide you through the buying process.

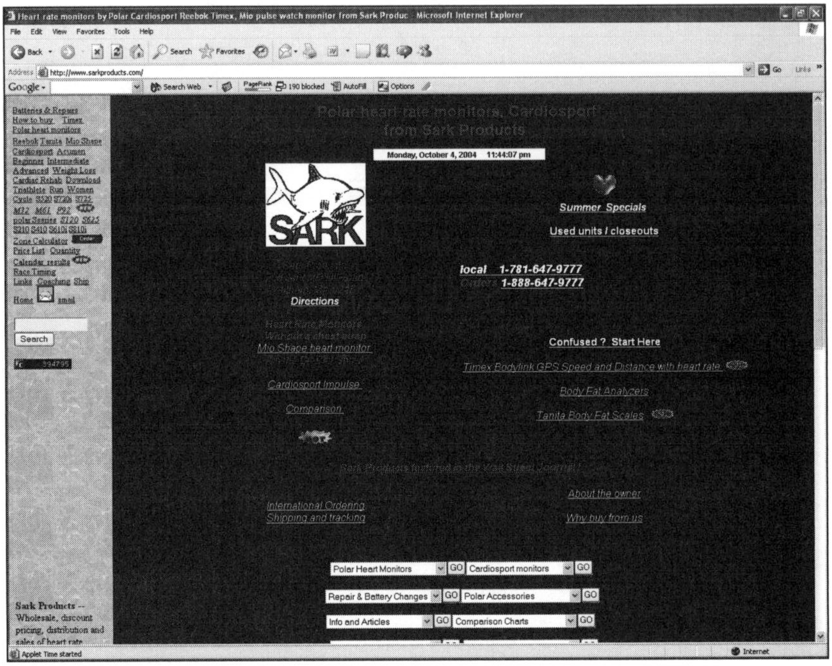

FIGURE 7.26 *Sark Products specializes in heart rate monitors.*

BIDDING YOUR WAY TO FITNESS

You don't have to pay retail for fitness products; in fact, you don't have to pay much at all if you hunt in the right places, such as at auction sites like eBay and Yahoo! Auctions.

End users offer products that they aren't using, and vendors sell products online. You just have to be careful to make the right purchase from the right person when bidding on auction items at eBay, Yahoo!, or other auction sites.

First, check out the seller. What's his or her rating, and what kind of feedback does he or she get? If the seller has too much negative feedback, don't buy there. Sometimes, prices *are* too good to be true.

Other times the prices seem to be good but they really aren't, thanks to shipping costs. Those can add unreasonably hefty amounts to your winning bid.

On a recent day at eBay, there were some great buys and some not-so-great ones. Someone was selling an old $99 SportBrain pedometer for $19.99, but failed to mention that you had to pay a membership fee to use it. That was not so good. Another was selling the Timex Bodylink System for about 40% off of the list price, a very good deal.

BIDDING YOUR WAY TO FITNESS *(CONTINUED)*

There are some eBay vendors who specialize in selling refurbished merchandise, which is fine as long as you know that it has been refurbished. There are others, such as Buy Essex, who offer tremendous values online, but make no bones about the fact that their merchandise is used. They tell you the condition and that items are sometimes missing. You then make the decision about whether to bid on it.

A few other words: When bidding, bid late—very late—like in the last minute or so. Don't bid early; just watch the bidding, be patient, make sure this is a product that you want to buy, and then swoop in at the last minute and buy it. This, of course, goes for much more than just fitness equipment (see Figure 7.27).

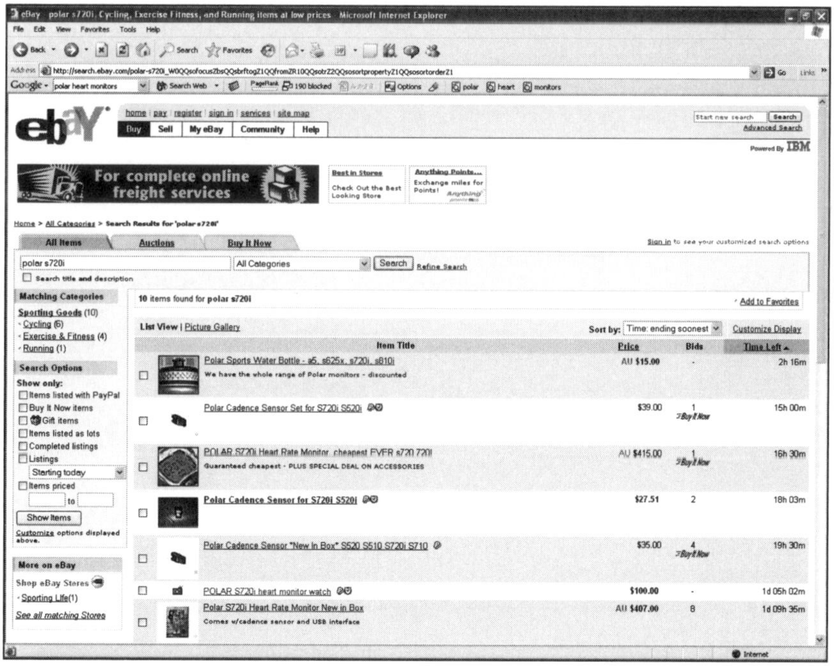

FIGURE 7.27 *Bidding on fitness products at eBay*

VKRshop.com

http://www.vkrshop.com

Summary: Not a lot of products, but they believe in what they sell.

VKRshop.com only offers a few products, but they are strong evangelists for pedometers (see Figure 7.28). They believe that if you walk 10,000 steps per day, you'll lose weight. (We think it's more like 15,000 steps, but they're on the right track.) They provide a spreadsheet to let you count your steps along the way. VKR checks out its equipment before they agree to sell it, so their pages include mini-reviews of each item. They offer their own models, plus offerings from DIGI-WALKER, SportBrain, and Sportline. VKR offers only a few heart rate monitors, a private brand model and a few others from Go and Impulse. Clearly, their main goal is to sell pedometers.

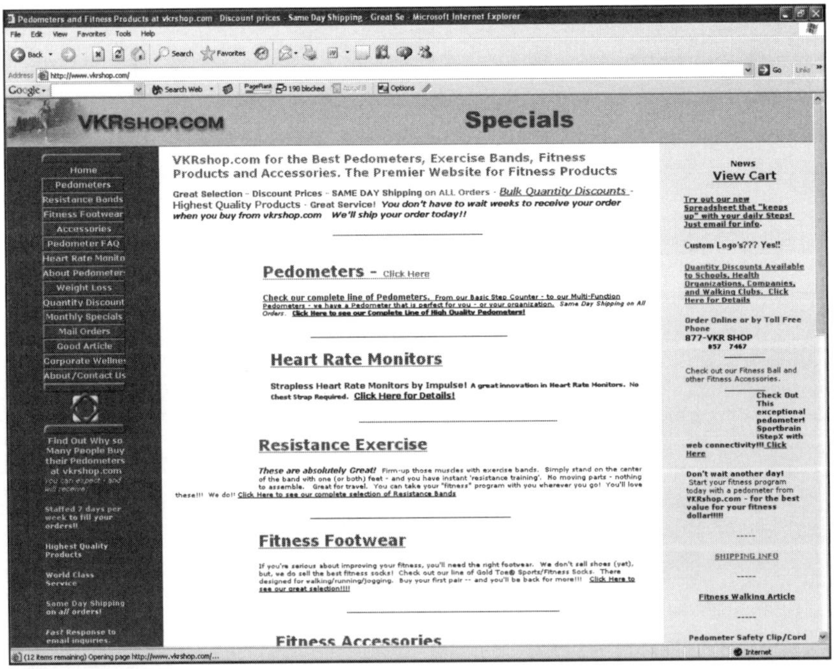

FIGURE 7.28 *VKRshop.com*

ALL'S FAIR IN LOVE AND SPORTING GOODS

There are many good sporting goods on the Internet. In fact, little separates the Web presences of the major sporting goods retailers. Dick's Sporting Goods, Modell's, Sportmart and The Sports Authority all feature great selections, almost identical pricing, and very similar inventory. This makes sense; most of these retailers don't compete with each other offline because each has carved out its own regional niche.

Each site has fitness equipment, gear, gadgets, shoes, camping equipment, and clothing (see Figure 7.29). They all carry the major heart rate monitors, pedometers, and other fitness gadgets. And they all carry game tables and other items to put in your rec room. The only differences between the sites are their weekly specials and clearance items, so you might have to visit each site to find the best pricing on a particular item.

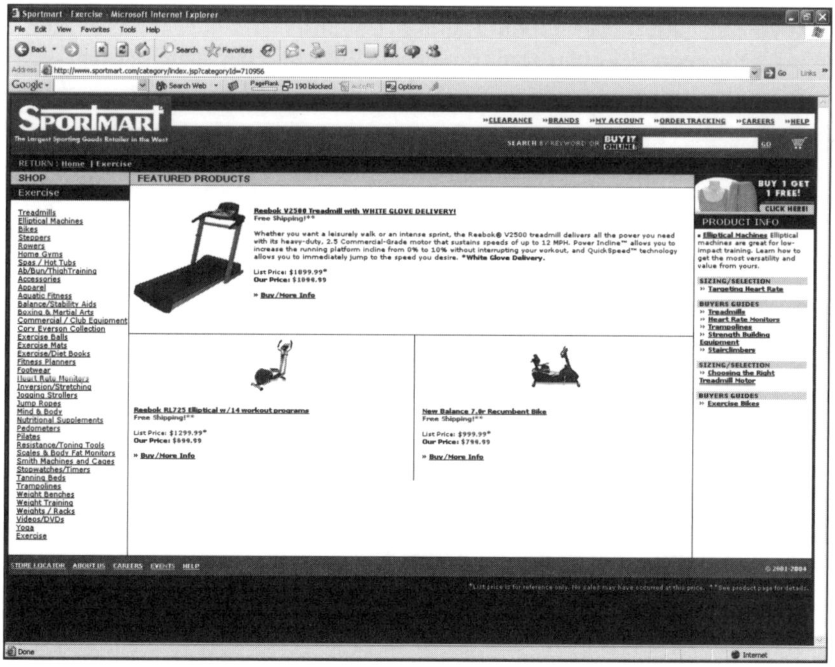

FIGURE 7.29 *Sportmart.com's Fitness section*

The Walker's Warehouse

http://www.walkerswarehouse.com

Summary: Lots of great walking-related products.

In the late '80s and early '90s, when Spike Lee was making those marvelous TV commercials for Nike, his character insisted to Michael Jordan that it "had to be the shoes." The Walker's Warehouse helps you get the right shoes for your fitness program and offers lots of other walking and exercise equipment to go along with the shoes (see Figure 7.30). They offer shoes and fitness socks from all major manufacturers, fitness clothing, a wide range of fitness gadgets, exercise equipment, and exercise media.

As far as the "warehouse" part of their title is concerned, The Walker's Warehouse has competitive pricing for its regularly priced items and very aggressive pricing in its clearance center. A recent visit to The Walker's Warehouse clearance center featured shoes that listed for $89 or more selling for $29 or less. You can get a 5% discount on all orders by paying $20 for a one-year membership and joining The Walker's Warehouse VIP Shopping Club, which also gets you priority shipping and a free walking kit.

The Walker's Warehouse includes a variety of resources for walkers, including pedometer and shoe comparison charts, articles about walking, tips and techniques for exercising effectively, a walking log, a footwear guide, an event finder, and links to other exercise sites (see Figure 7.31).

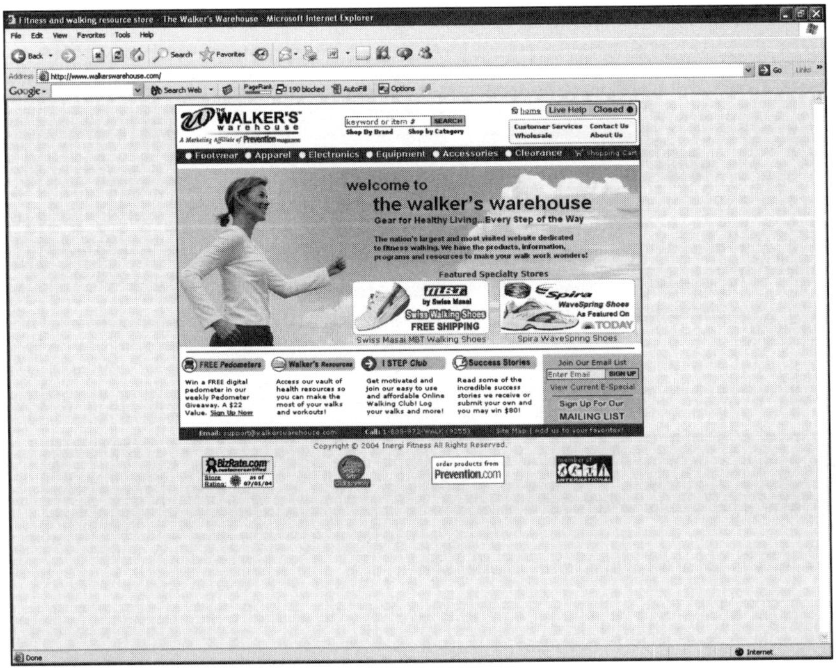

FIGURE 7.30 *The Walker's Warehouse*

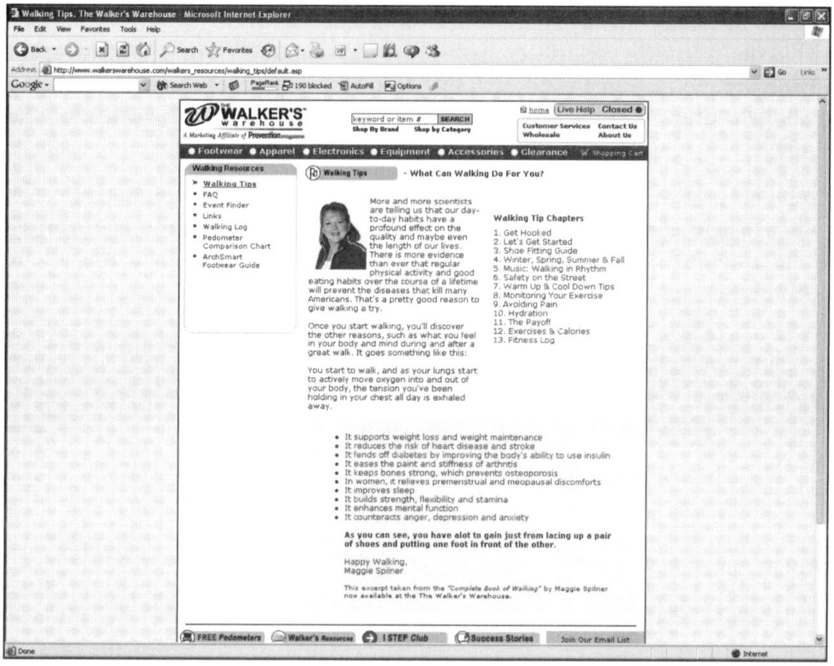

FIGURE 7.31 *The Walker's Warehouse offers many resources for walkers.*

The Walker's Warehouse also features the I Step Club, which is also offered by *Prevention* magazine. The Club, which costs $49.95 per year at the premium level, includes a variety of tips and logs to motivate you to walk more, plus a free pedometer from *Prevention* magazine.

Summary

Thanks to the Internet, you can do all your shopping online. Many sites offer the products you need to succeed. It's your choice whether to shop at a specialty store or a superstore.

Keeping fit and losing weight is not an easy process; it's a daily battle. And that's how you have to treat it—one day at a time. Do your best every day, and you'll lose weight and keep it off. Fall for a "lose weight quick" scheme, and you'll do okay while it lasts and fall off the wagon the first time you slip up. Gadgets can help you keep the weight off because they take away some of the drudgery of weight loss and substitute fun. I'm a big fan of fun. I think we should all have more of it.

I've found that wearing a pedometer, being vigilant about portion control, and eating right have let me keep off that weight. I'm always in search of the next fun gadget that will add motivation and make this process even more fun than it already is.

I've also been helped greatly by support networks on SportBrain (http://www.sportbrain.com), Bearykirby.com (http://bearykirby.com/sb), Steptracker.com, Weight Watchers, and other sites that provide the motivation I need each day to exercise more, eat less, or both. Joining SportBrain's 500,000 Steps Club was a great move because it made me walk more and keep the weight off.

Happy trails on your weight loss and fitness quest. If you find any sites of interest that you think I should add to a new edition of this book or my Web site, please e-mail me at jordango@gmail.com. And be sure to visit the Web site, at http://www.GetFitWithTechnology.com. I look forward to hearing from you.

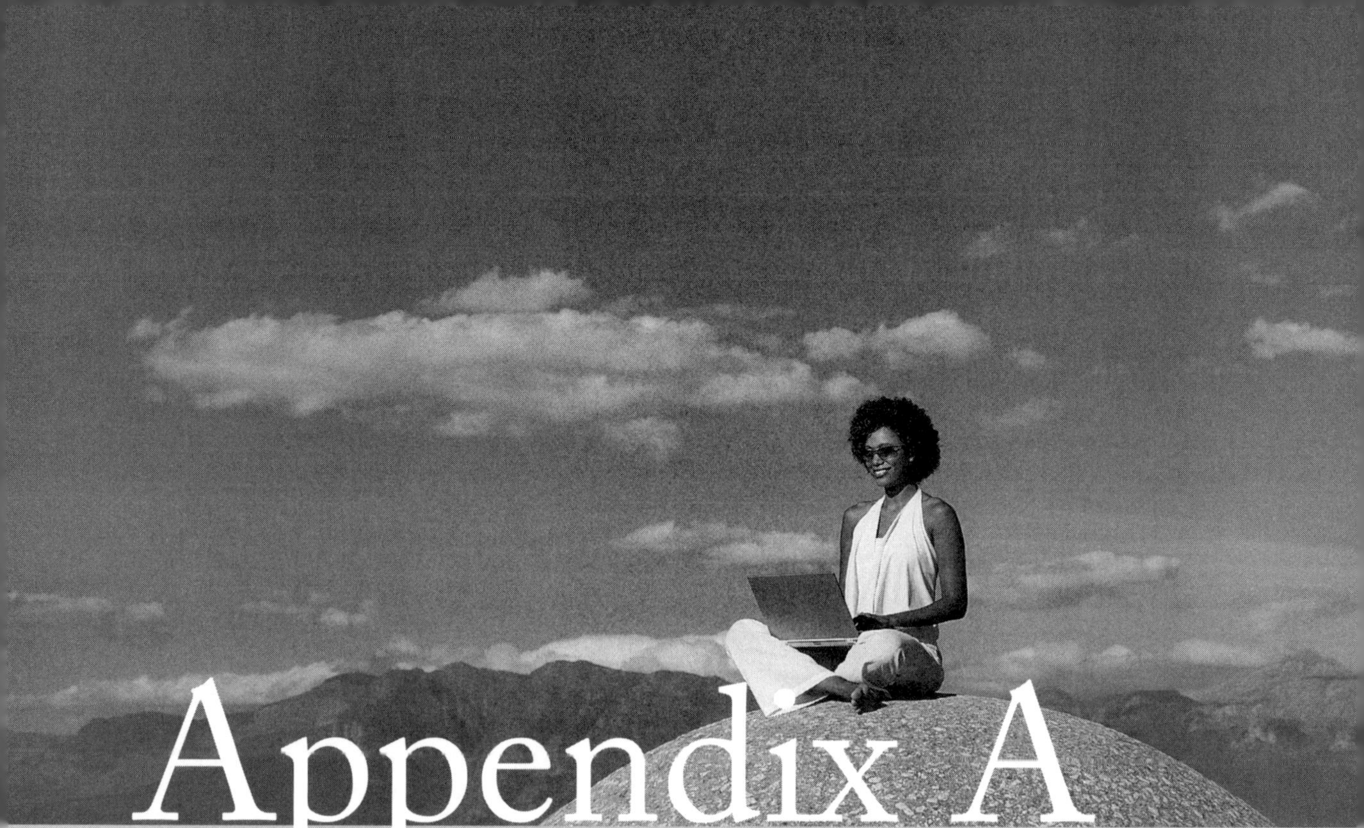

Appendix A

Sites for Specific Diseases and Conditions

As mentioned throughout the book, there are a number of Web sites that specifically offer support, content, encouragement, and advice for a wide variety of different diseases and conditions. This appendix will cover each major disease in alphabetical order.

A Few Sites That Cover It All

Many of the sites mentioned in the book cover all, or almost all, of the conditions covered in this appendix. Some of these sites are tailored toward men, women, or seniors, while others are more comprehensive. In addition to the sites mentioned here, the World Health Organization (http://www.who.int) has some excellent, if somewhat clinical, materials, and MedicineNet.com provides useful information as well. This section includes a few other sites that cover it all.

> **CAREFULLY RESEARCH THE WEB SITES YOU VISIT**
>
> Many, but not all, of the Web sites mentioned in this chapter are created by nonprofit organizations. That's because many for-profit organizations build Web sites with useful information that is targeted toward helping you become informed enough to choose their product. We were careful not to include most of those Web sites here. Some sites promote a product, but also provide very helpful information about a disease or condition, and we included those here. I welcome your feedback about this, so please feel free to e-mail me your comments and suggestions at jordango@gmail.com.

AARP

http://www.aarp.org

AARP employs the Healthwise Knowledgebase in its comprehensive Health Guide, which is intended for those over 50. It includes tips on healthy living, a guide to medications, a glossary of medical tests, a guide to Medicare, and more than 1,000 support groups for various topics. It also includes the MedlinePlus directory, which includes interactive tutorials and slideshows, listings of clinical trials, healthcare provider directories, and information on alternative medicine sources.

iVillage

http://www.ivillage.com

Thanks to the cooperation of the Women's Health Resource Center, iVillage includes comprehensive information about diseases and conditions, usually accompanied by a message board. These message boards are specifically intended for women. The Women's Health Resource Center also includes an A–Z health dictionary, an overview, diagnosis and treatment information, prevention, facts, questions to ask, and tips, as well as a test to see how much you know about a subject.

MayoClinic.com

http://www.mayoclinic.com

MayoClinic.com covers all major diseases and conditions in three different ways: A–Z order, in a Disease & Condition Center, which goes into much more detail in 14 different categories, and in Health Decision Guides, which provide exhaustive information about eight different diseases and conditions (see Figure A.1). In A–Z format, MayoClinic.com discusses causes, treatment, prevention, screening and diagnosis, self care, and treatment for these diseases and conditions, and also advises you about when to see a doctor.

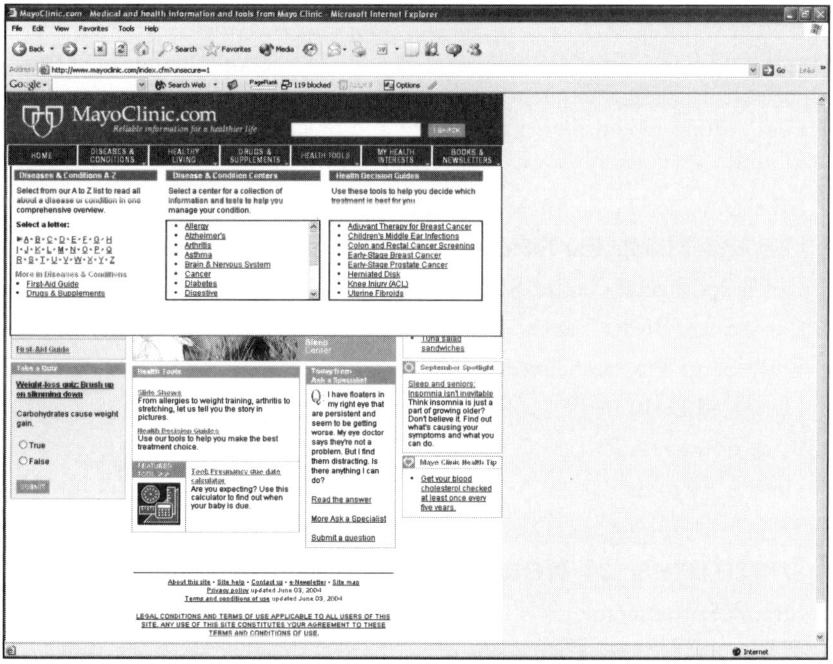

FIGURE A.1 *MayoClinic.com Diseases & Conditions page*

The Disease & Condition Centers go even further, with expert advice, slideshows, support groups, and more information. MayoClinic.com offers the following Disease & Condition Centers:

- Allergy
- Alzheimer's
- Arthritis
- Asthma
- Brain & Nervous System

- Cancer
- Diabetes
- Digestive
- Heart
- High Blood Pressure
- Infectious Disease
- Mental Health
- Pain Management
- Skin

Each Health Decision Guide includes treatment options, about 30 minutes of videos of a Mayo Clinic specialist discussing frequently asked questions, personal stories of people who've had the condition, things to consider, a dictionary, and links to related information. Eight Health Decision Guides are currently available on MayoClinic.com:

- Adjuvant Therapy for Breast Cancer
- Children's Middle Ear Infections
- Colon and Rectal Cancer Screening
- Early-Stage Breast Cancer
- Early-Stage Prostate Cancer
- Herniated Disk
- Knee Injury (ACL)
- Uterine Fibroids

National Institutes of Health

http://health.nih.gov

The National Institutes of Health (NIH) features health information for everyone, and then breaks it down for men, women, children, minorities, and seniors. Its Health Information pages feature an A–Z index of diseases and conditions, the latest research information, quizzes, articles, a category breakdown of diseases and conditions, a number of health databases, and links to additional federal government Web sites for more information (see Figure A.2).

The A–Z index provides links to other databases for further information. Click on gout, for example, and you'll get to a page that provides links to other information. There's a Q&A section that features a comprehensive article about gout that answers frequently asked questions. There's a link to the definition in the MedlinePlus database, which in turn links to 14 more gout-related articles. You can call the supplied phone number for further information, investigate the latest clinical trials, and decide whether to participate. There's also a link to the government agency most responsible for dealing with gout—in this case, the National Institute of Arthritis and Musculoskeletal and Skin Diseases.

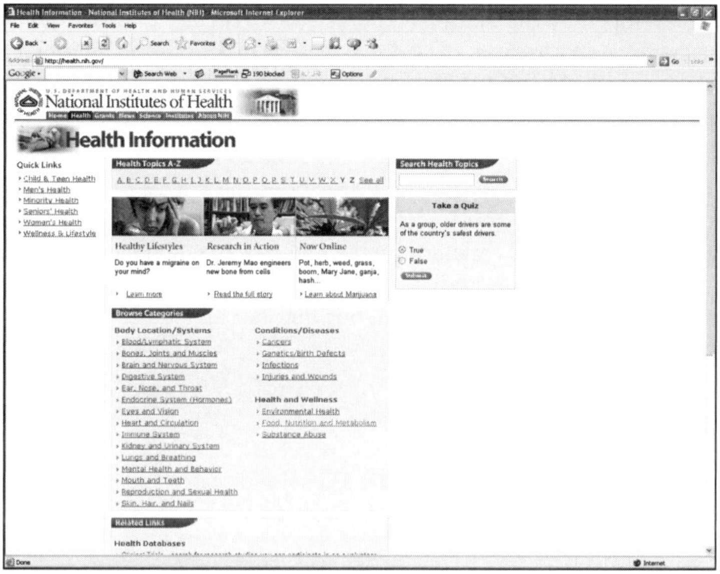

FIGURE A.2 *The NIH Health Information area is one of the most comprehensive on the Internet.*

The category search essentially breaks the A–Z index into sections based on three major categories—Body Location/Systems (Blood/Lymphatic, Brain and Nervous System, Eyes and Vision, and so on), Conditions/Diseases (Injuries and Wounds, Cancer, Infections, and so on), and Health and Wellness (Food, Nutrition and Metabolism; Substance Abuse; and so on). Clicking on Brain and Nervous System, for example, brings you to a page that provides links to all the conditions and diseases related to the brain and nervous system. Clicking on one of those brings you to a page similar to the gout example mentioned earlier.

As we mentioned, the NIH features links to a number of health databases, including:

- **Clinical Trials.** Provides links to clinical trials at NIH or around the country that are either currently underway or about to start. Users can often participate in these as volunteers, assuming they meet the eligibility criteria. This also provides links to results of clinical trials that have already occurred, at ClinicalTrials.gov (http://www.clinicaltrials.gov).
- **MedlinePlus.** Maintained by the NIH National Library of Medicine, MedlinePlus features comprehensive information about more than 650 health-related topics, plus a drug information resource, a medical encyclopedia and dictionary, news, directories to help you locate a doctor, interactive tutorials, and links to other resources on the Internet.
- **Healthfinder.** Developed by the U.S. Department of Health and Human Services, Healthfinder provides a health library, topics oriented for specific groups (men, women, children, seniors, minorities, age groups, and so on), healthcare directories, health news, and more than 50 quizzes and tests about health topics.

- **PubMed.** Developed by the National Library of Medicine, PubMed is the card catalog of medical information, providing more than 15 million citations for medical articles written since the 1950s.
- **International Bibliographic Information on Dietary Supplements (IBIDS) Database.** IBIDS contains more than 730,000 citations about dietary supplements. Highly technical, these articles generally are about the effects of these supplements on the human body. For example, searching for calcium netted 38,701 articles, including one that explored "calcium intake and risk of colon cancer in men and women." It said that in some studies, higher intake of calcium results in a reduced risk of colon cancer in men and women, but that not all studies confirm this.

WebMD.com

http://www.webmd.com

WebMD is a comprehensive site that covers nearly all major diseases and conditions. It includes A–Z guides, an interactive symptom checker, tips, quizzes, articles, message boards, live events, and much more.

The Diseases & Conditions Center includes an exhaustive directory of diseases and conditions, complete with tips, articles, medical data from the Cleveland Clinic, a directory of clinical trials about the condition, quizzes and tools, and a section called We Knew You'd Want to Know, which covers tips and techniques for dealing with the condition.

The Medical Library features an interactive symptom checker, an A–Z library of medical terms, a directory that describes nearly all medical tests, a drug and herb guide, and a listing of all clinical trials. There's also expert advice, more than 200 message boards, and live events. The message boards include options from users as well as expert advice.

Specialized Sites

We'll cover the major conditions and diseases and highlight the most useful sites on a content and community basis, as well as providing a brief synopsis of each.

DON'T FORGET ABOUT NEWSGROUPS

Topic-specific newsgroups are great sources of information about diseases and conditions, as well as lots of other things. Literally hundreds of thousands of newsgroups abound on the Internet. To find one, do a Google search for your interest using misc.health.name as the format—for example, misc.health.diabetes, which is a great newsgroup providing support for people with diabetes. Newsgroups are essentially the same as message boards on Web sites.

AIDS

AIDS.ORG

http://www.AIDS.org

The aim of AIDS.ORG is to educate people about AIDS, raise awareness about AIDS, and build a community to support people with AIDS. The site includes FAQs, streaming videos of doctors discussing AIDS, fact sheets, news, and links to other sites (see Figure A.3).

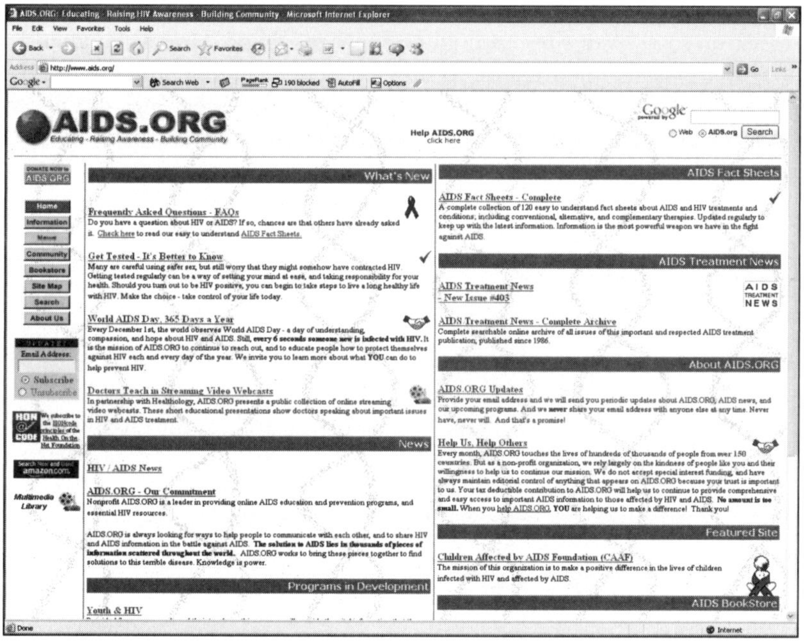

FIGURE A.3 *AIDS.ORG*

AIDS Online

http://www.AIDSonline.com

The official journal of the International AIDS Society, AIDS Online is published 18 times per year. All articles older than 12 months are available for free on this Web site.

Elizabeth Glaser Pediatric AIDS Foundation

http://www.pedaids.org

This site provides educational information about pediatric AIDS, particularly highlighting events and fundraisers.

ALS

See the "Lou Gehrig's Disease" section.

Alcoholism

Alcoholics Anonymous

http://www.aa.org

This site provides both offline and online resources for alcoholism, including group locations and how to set up local Web sites and online support groups. Several hundred local support groups throughout North America have set up Web sites, including http://www.aasandiego.org, http://www.aanashville.org, and http://www.aaboston.org. Local sites include links to other sites, information about meetings, a hotline to call, and guides that explain how the organization works.

Alzheimer's Disease

Alzheimer's Association

http://www.alz.org

This is the Web site of the national Alzheimer's Association (see Figure A.4). It provides news and information about Alzheimer's disease, including the latest research information, additional resources, articles and publications, contact information, and links to local chapters throughout the U.S.

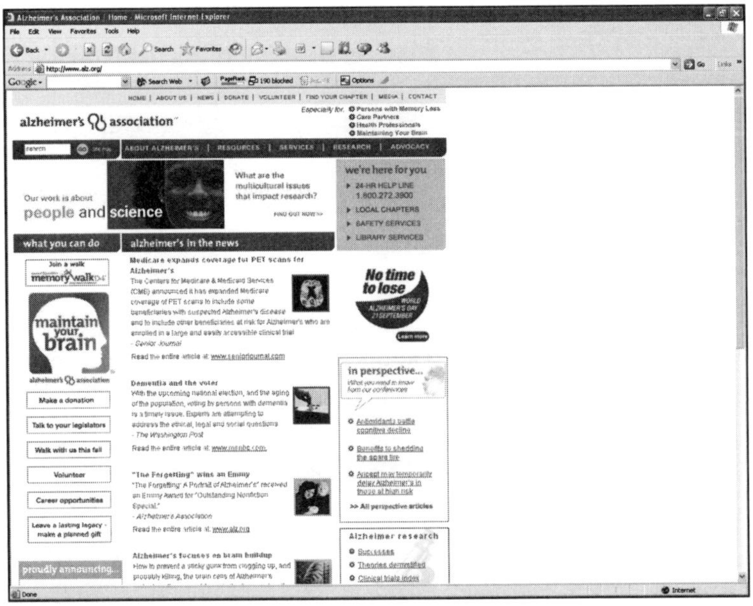

FIGURE A.4 *The Alzheimer's Association provides the latest information about Alzheimer's disease.*

Alzheimer's Disease Education & Referral Center (ADEAR)

http://www.alzheimers.org

This government site provides the latest information about Alzheimer's disease.

Alzheimer's Society

http://www.alzheimers.org.uk

This is the leading U.K. care and research charity for Alzheimer's and related diseases. It provides information, the latest news and articles, caregiver directories, fundraisers, and more.

Arthritis

Arthritis Foundation

http://www.arthritis.org

The Arthritis Foundation is a nonprofit association dedicated to providing information about arthritis. The site includes articles, condition and treatment centers, resources, brochures, tips, and more. It also includes a store that sells arthritis materials (including *Arthritis Today* magazine), as well as active message boards.

Arthritis.com

http://www.arthritis.com

Drug-maker Pfizer offers a user-friendly site that features news; resources and guides about arthritis; medical information from Johns Hopkins; an arthritis symptom checklist; treatment options; a free newsletter; and a graphical causes, symptoms, and animations feature.

Asthma

Asthma and Allergy Foundation of America

http://www.aafa.org

The Asthma and Allergy Foundation of America, founded in 1953 and dedicated to helping those who suffer from asthma and related allergies, offers an informative Web site that includes a comprehensive overview of asthma, information about who gets it and how, articles featuring the latest asthma-related news, case histories, links to support groups and regional chapters, and information about clinical trials. It also includes expert information from allergists, a bulletin board, and an area for teens with asthma.

Attention Deficit/Hyperactivity Disorder

Children and Adults with Attention-Deficit/Hyperactivity Disorder

http://www.chadd.org

This site covers the disorder for both children and adults. It includes FAQs, fact sheets, symptoms, message boards, links to other sites, local chapters, the latest research, and a store that sells educational resources.

Back Injuries

SpineUniverse

http://www.spineuniverse.com

Although this site isn't much to look at, it's information-packed. It covers all back- and spine-related injuries, with treatment options, videos, wellness advice, tips on pain management, and more. It includes articles from the Cleveland Clinic, the American Association of Neurological Surgeons, the Scoliosis Research Society, the International Spinal Injection Society, the National Association of Orthopaedic Nurses, and the National Pain Foundation. To get specific information about a condition, users select the appropriate condition center (see Figure A.5), which takes them to an area that offers definition and diagnosis of the condition, and then provides non-surgical as well as surgical solutions for dealing with that condition.

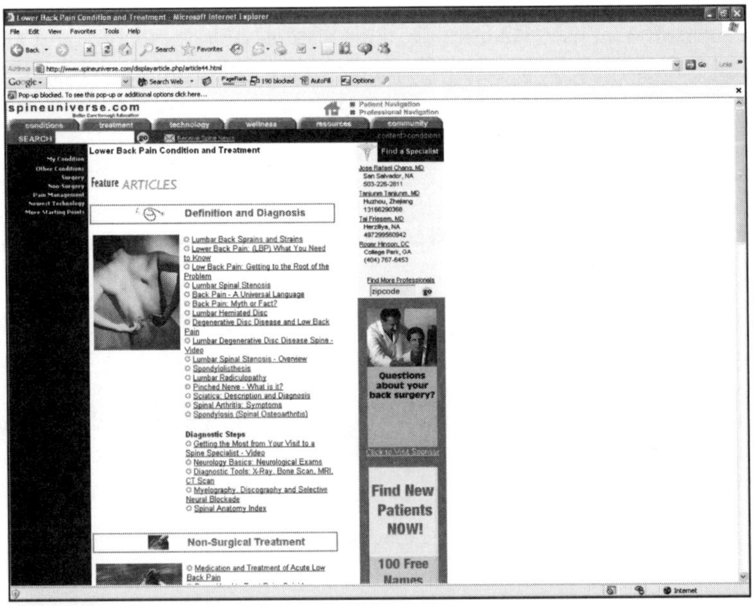

FIGURE A.5 *SpineUniverse offers a number of condition centers that provide helpful advice and information about many conditions, including this one that explores lower back pain.*

Spine-Health.com

http://www.spine-health.com

This site provides comprehensive information about spinal injuries and back pain. It includes message boards, articles, a doctor finder, a store, clinical trial results, polls, surveys, and much more.

Bipolar Disorder

Bipolar.com

http://www.bipolar.com

Developed by GlaxoSmithKline, this site provides the latest information about bipolar disease, as well as links to more information. It helps users recognize the condition and teaches them how to live with it and how to help others deal with it. It also provides links to support information about bipolar disorder. The Web site covers medication, but it is not a site that continually tries to sell GlaxoSmithKline's offerings.

Blindness

Foundation Fighting Blindness

http://www.blindness.org

The Foundation Fighting Blindness takes the informative approach to blindness, fighting blindness through awareness and raising money for research. It also provides information about the major retinal diseases that cause blindness, including macular degeneration, retinitis pigmentosa, Stargardt disease, and Usher syndrome.

Prevent Blindness America

http://www.preventblindness.org

Building awareness, Prevent Blindness America focuses on safety and prevention. For example, one article points out that 90% of eye injuries each year could be prevented by simply wearing safety goggles. It also offers seminars about macular degeneration and teaches prevention by strongly suggesting that everyone get their eyes examined on a regular basis. The site also includes an online catalog featuring educational material aimed at spreading the word about blindness.

Breast Cancer

BreastCancer.org

http://www.breastcancer.org

BreastCancer.org is a nonprofit site dedicated to helping women and their loved ones deal with breast cancer. It includes more than 2,000 pages of information, including articles, prevention information, symptoms and diagnosis, treatment, research news, expert advice, recovery and renewal information, and community support. It includes very active message boards and provides support in many different ways. It includes information for women at all stages of the disease, from those just diagnosed, to those going through treatment, to those dealing with chemotherapy, to those going forward after treatment is over. The site was founded in 1999 by Dr. Marisa Weiss, an oncologist who believed that doctors don't have enough time to spend with their patients, so she created a site to help women learn about breast cancer themselves. The site claims 300,000 unique visitors per month.

The Susan G. Komen Breast Cancer Foundation

http://www.komen.org

Before Susan Komen died of breast cancer in the early 1980s at the age of 36, she asked her sister, Nancy, to do everything possible to put an end to the disease. So, shortly after Susan's death, Nancy founded the association in Susan's memory. Nancy Brinker shares this extremely touching story on the Web site which, like the foundation, is dedicated to helping women with breast cancer and helping to eradicate the disease (see Figure A.6). There are hundreds of offline affiliate organizations dedicated to helping cure breast cancer. The organization sponsors many events to raise money to find a cure, and it publicizes those online. There's also lots of excellent information for patients, survivors, and others who want to learn about breast cancer. In addition, there are message boards and information about the corporate sponsors who help fund breast cancer research.

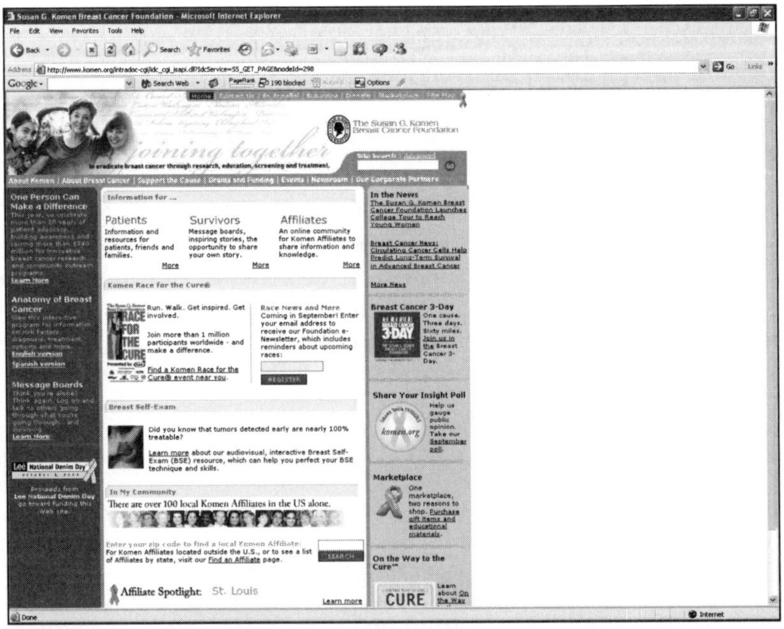

FIGURE A.6 *The Susan G. Komen Breast Cancer Foundation was founded in 1982 in memory of Susan G. Komen.*

Cancer (General)

The National Cancer Institute

http://www.nci.nih.gov

The National Cancer Institute is the NIH's principal agency for cancer research. As such, their Web site is a phenomenal resource for cancer information (see Figure A.7). It provides information about all major types of cancers, the latest research, a dictionary of related terms, and guides to all forms of cancer. There's also information about cancer prevention and treatment, screening and testing, and coping with cancer. Because the NCI leads the way in cancer research, there's a lot of information about research, results, and clinical trials. There are also cancer statistics and the latest news about cancer.

The American Cancer Society

http://www.cancer.org

The American Cancer Society's Web site features a great deal of information about cancer, including information about all types of cancer, treatment options, clinical trials, coping, and surviving. It also includes a community feature with message boards, survivor stories, volunteer opportunities, and the ability to take donations online.

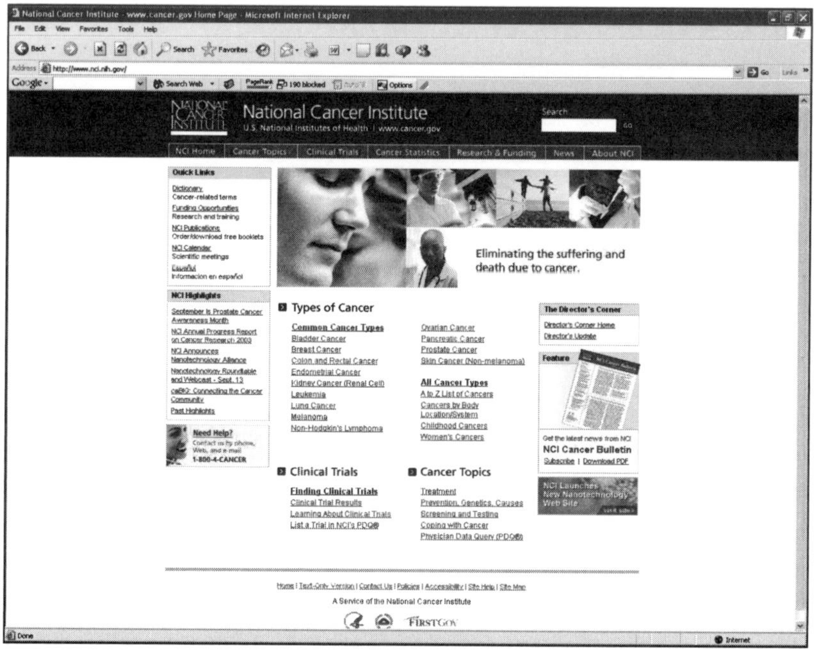

FIGURE A.7 *The National Cancer Institute boasts a wealth of data about all types of cancer.*

Carpal Tunnel Syndrome

CTS Place

http://www.ctsplace.com

A site free of bells and whistles, but sporting plenty of information about carpal tunnel syndrome, CTS Place provides an overview of the condition, articles and books about it, links to many related sites, a bookstore, health and safety information, suggested preventative measures, support groups and other resources, and a message board featuring questions and answers on the most popular topics.

Cerebral Palsy

United Cerebral Palsy

http://www.ucp.org

This site features facts about cerebral palsy, plus FAQs, products and services, treatment options, and more. It also includes a great deal of information about the Americans with Disabilities Act (ADA).

Cervical Cancer

National Cervical Cancer Coalition

http://www.nccc-online.org

This site includes information about cervical cancer, prevention and treatment options, news, events, links to local chapters, expert advice, and support groups.

Chlamydia

See the "Sexually Transmitted Diseases" section.

Chronic Fatigue Syndrome

CFIDS Association of America

http://www.cfids.org

The Chronic Fatigue and Immune Dysfunction Syndrome Association of America (CFIDS Association of America) hosts this informative Web site about chronic fatigue syndrome. It includes articles about the syndrome, tips for dealing with it, help diagnosing the condition, a store that sells related materials, resources for more information, and community help, including a support group.

Colitis

Crohn's & Colitis Foundation of America

http://www.ccfa.org

CCFA is a nonprofit organization dedicated to helping those with Crohn's disease and colitis. This site includes information about the diseases, research, clinical trials, news, local events, and information for physicians and other medical professionals.

Crohn's Disease

See the "Colitis" section.

Cystic Fibrosis

Cystic Fibrosis Foundation

http://www.cff.org

This site provides information about cystic fibrosis, including the latest research, local events, clinical trials, publications, Webcasts, surveys, and much more.

CysticFibrosis.com

http://www.cysticfibrosis.com

This site provides information about cystic fibrosis, answers to FAQs, treatment options, message boards, advice, and much more.

Deafness

The Alexander Graham Bell Foundation for the Deaf and Hard of Hearing

http://www.agbell.org

The Alexander Graham Bell Foundation for the Deaf and Hard of Hearing is dedicated to helping people who have suffered hearing loss. Founded in 1890 by Dr. Alexander Graham Bell, the inventor of the telephone and a teacher of the deaf, the Association is the largest information and support center for pediatric hearing loss and oral/deaf education. The Association promotes the latest technologies to help the deaf and hard of hearing, and it serves as an advocate for individuals who are deaf or hard of hearing. Their Web site features resources, articles, links to other sites, message boards, a store, and links to the latest events (see Figure A.8).

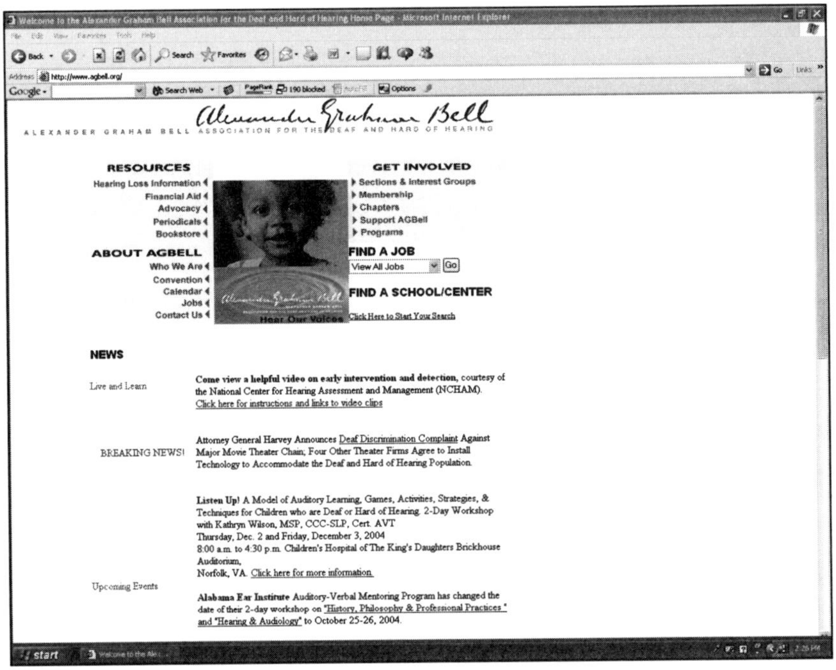

FIGURE A.8 *The Alexander Graham Bell Foundation for the Deaf and Hard of Hearing*

Dental Health

The American Dental Association

http://www.ada.org

This is a great site for finding a dentist, and it also includes news about dental health for adults and children, an A–Z dental topic list, answers to frequently asked questions, and animations and games to help children feel more comfortable with going to the dentist. There are also career resources for anyone interested in going into dentistry as a profession.

Depression

The National Alliance for Research on Schizophrenia and Depression (NARSAD)

http://www.narsad.org

NARSAD is a nonprofit organization whose goal is to raise funds for researching the causes, cures, treatments, and prevention of psychiatric brain disorders, such as schizophrenia and depression. The site features research, the latest news, an A–Z topic list, and more about depression.

Focus on Depression

http://www.focusondepression.com

This standalone site was recently folded into MedicineNet.com, a comprehensive Web site similar to WebMD and MayoClinic.com. It offers a library of information about depression, including the signs, causes, and diagnoses, plus comprehensive information about drugs and research. It also includes a message board about depression.

Diabetes

American Diabetes Association

http://www.diabetes.org

The American Diabetes Association is a nonprofit health organization that provides diabetes research, information, and advocacy. The Web site provides information about diabetes, treatments, and the latest news, plus research, prevention, a dictionary, a store, and information about local events. A large part of the Web site is devoted to diabetes-friendly recipes, weight loss, and exercise. There are also a number of active message boards on the site.

Diabetes Forums

http://www.diabetesforums.com

This site features a number of diabetes-specific message boards.

Juvenile Diabetes Research Foundation

http://www.jdf.org

The Juvenile Diabetes Research Foundation is a nonprofit organization dedicated to finding a cure for diabetes. The organization, which has Mary Tyler Moore as its spokesperson, claims that 85 cents of every dollar received is used for research to find a cure for Type 1 diabetes. The site provides research information, plus tips on living with diabetes, and more.

Drug Abuse

National Institute on Drug Abuse (NIDA)

http://www.drugabuse.gov

This is another great NIH site that features news about drug abuse; information for parents, teachers, students, researchers, and health professionals; plus a teen site (http://teens.drugabuse.gov), the latest research data, and links to other sites. The NIDA is all about research, so there is lots of information about the latest research as well as the latest clinical trials.

Streetdrugs.org

http://www.streetdrugs.org

This information-packed site is for students, educators, and parents. It includes a top 10 list of most abused drugs, frequently asked questions, information on how to get help, signs of drug abuse for parents, and lots of advice for dealing with drugs for kids. For example, the site admonishes people not to leave beverages unattended, to only take beverages from someone they trust, and not to drink from a punchbowl. This will help them avoid being drugged at a party or bar.

Death and Dying

GriefNet.org

http://www.griefnet.org

http://www.kidsaid.com

These sites provide help and support for those dealing with death and dying. GriefNet.org includes 47 message boards, and KIDSAID allows children to ask questions and receive support. Both sites provide healing, remembrance, support, and education.

Dementia

See the "Alzheimer's Disease" section.

Epilepsy

Epilepsy Project

http://www.epilepsy.com

This comprehensive site provides information about epilepsy. It features comprehensive information about epilepsy, plus news; clinical trials; drug interactions; diagnosis; treatment; information for men, women, children, teens, families, and seniors; and message boards. The site is a service of The Epilepsy Project, a nonprofit research organization.

Foot Injuries

American Podiatric Medical Association

http://www.apma.org

This site provides information about foot health, dealing with injuries, FAQs, dos and don'ts, and facts about foot health with arthritis and with diabetes. It also includes an online version of the *Journal of the American Podiatric Medical Association*.

Gonorrhea

See the "Sexually Transmitted Diseases" section.

Hair Loss

American Hair Loss Council

http://www.ahlc.org

This informative Web site covers both male and female hair loss with causes, treatments, options, and a directory of specialists. There are also message boards and forums.

Head Injuries

Brain Injury Resource Center

http://www.headinjury.com

This nonprofit organization was founded and is operated by head injury activists. The site provides links to doctors, answers to FAQs, support, a checklist for selecting the right doctor, links to rehab centers, information about assistive devices, and more.

Headaches

National Headaches Foundation

http://www.headaches.org/consumer

This nonprofit organization is dedicated to helping headache sufferers and the professionals who treat them. The site includes educational materials, events, drug information, clinical trials, and a newsletter available for subscription. There is a sister site for professionals at http://www.headaches.org/professional.

American Council for Headache Education

http://www.achenet.org

This site from a nonprofit headache relief organization features general headache information and specific data about kids' headaches and women's migraines, prevention, message boards with expert advice, a physician finder, a free newsletter, and more (see Figure A.9).

Hearing Disorders

See the "Deafness" section.

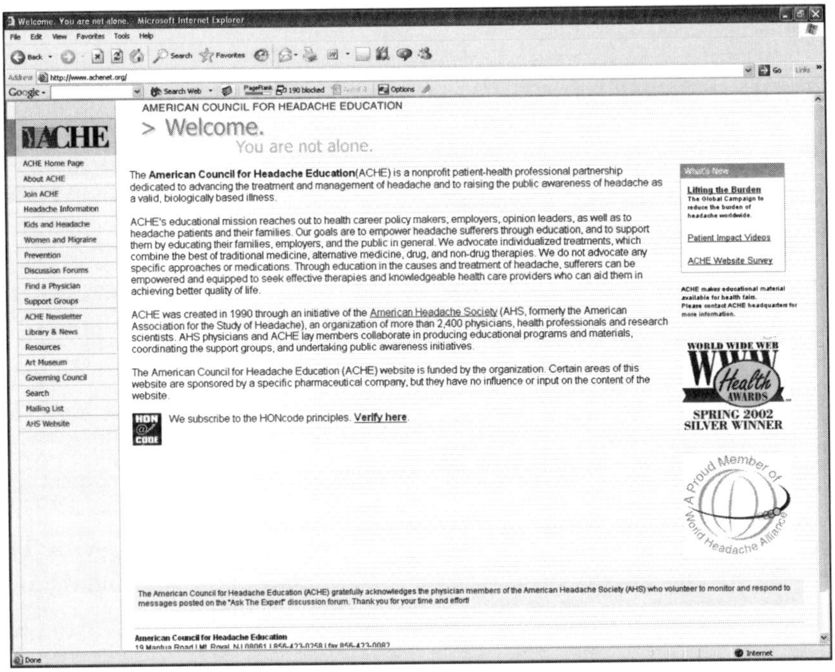

FIGURE A.9 *The American Council for Headache Education helps headache sufferers and their families.*

Heart Disease

American Heart Association

http://www.americanheart.org

This informative site features the warning signs of heart disease, prevention, CPR, how to live healthily, an encyclopedia, research information, local chapters, and a variety of publications. It also includes articles listing the warning signs of heart attacks, strokes, and cardiac arrest.

HeartCenterOnline

http://www.heartcenteronline.com

This is an information-rich site for cardiologists and heart patients (see Figure A.10). It provides comprehensive information about heart disease, high cholesterol, heart failure, irregular heartbeat, diabetes, and diet and nutrition. The Web site offers a healthy-living program to help people lose weight and lower their cholesterol through meal plans, diet and exercise, and stress relief.

The site also includes news about heart disease, quizzes, an A–Z heart-related dictionary, animations of various heart-related problems, FAQs, message boards, a panel of experts, and information about dealing with doctors, finding a doctor, and finding associated hospitals.

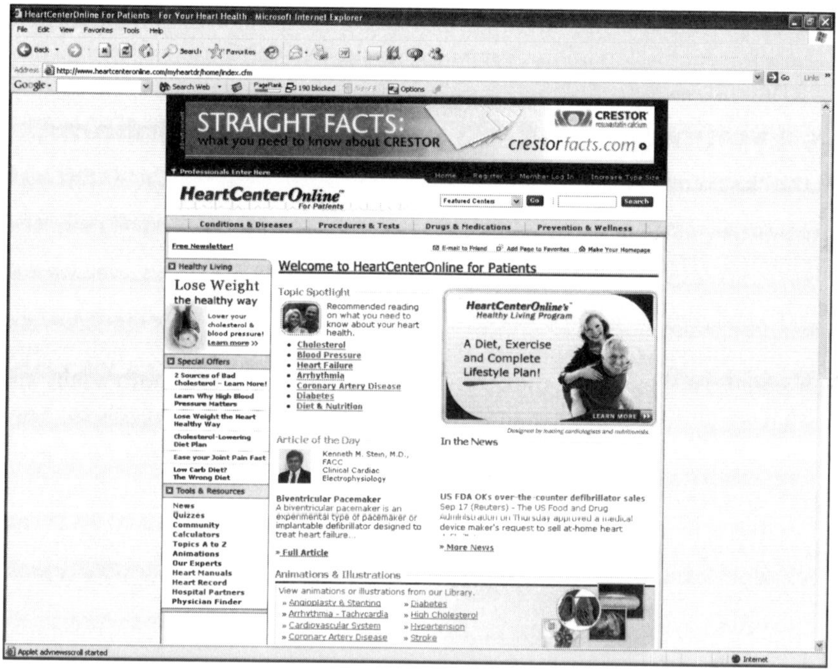

FIGURE A.10 *HeartCenterOnline features comprehensive information for cardiologists and their patients.*

Hepatitis

Hepatitis-Central.com

http://www.hepatitis-central.com

This Web site features more than 2000 pages of information about hepatitis, including descriptions of all known variations of the disease (hepatitis A, B, C, D, E, and G). It also includes survivor stories, message boards, news, doctors, links, and information about related diseases, such as cirrhosis and liver cancer.

High Blood Pressure

See the "Heart Disease" section.

Herpes

Also see the "Sexually Transmitted Diseases" section.

Herpes.com

http://www.herpes.com

This resource features an overview of herpes, provides symptom information, and answers frequently asked questions about the condition. A store on the site also sells herpes-related medications.

Hodgkin's Lymphoma and Non-Hodgkin's Lymphoma

Also see the "Leukemia" section.

Lymphoma Information Network

http://www.lymphomainfo.net

This site covers all types of lymphoma, as well as treatment, diagnosis, and resources. It contains areas specific to Hodgkin's and Non-Hodgkin's lymphoma for both adults and children. It also includes a glossary of terms, links to other sites, and books available for sale.

Huntington's Disease

Huntington's Disease Society of America

http://www.hdsa.org

This site provides information about Huntington's and help for those who need treatment and support. It includes a physician finder, links to other sites, and information about the latest research and clinical trials. It also includes links to local chapters, events, and other information.

Hyperactivity

See the "Attention Deficit/Hyperactivity Disorder" section.

Hypoglycemia

Hypoglycemia Support Foundation

http://www.hypoglycemia.org

This site includes a comprehensive glossary of terms, a description of the condition, a recommended diet, quizzes, case studies, support groups, links to other sites, and a store that sells products related to hypoglycemia.

Impotence

Impotence.org

http://www.impotence.org

Sponsored by the Sexual Function Advisory Council of the American Foundation for Urologic Disease, this Web site includes information about impotence, diagnosis, treatments, FAQs, links and resources, a physician finder, and live chats.

Infertility

International Council on Infertility Information Dissemination, Inc.

http://www.inciid.org

This site provides information about infertility, including prevention and treatment, a directory of specialists, message boards, news, fact sheets, articles, and an encyclopedia of terms.

RESOLVE

http://www.resolve.org

This information-packed site provides support and encouragement for couples trying to conceive, parenting advice, areas for men only and areas for women only, treatment options, adoption resources, and support for those who decide to live without children. It also includes message boards, local chapter information, and a physician finder.

Kidney Diseases

National Kidney Foundation

http://www.kidney.org

This site includes an A–Z health guide about kidney disease, brochures in PDF format, message boards, information for parents of children with kidney problems, clinical trials, and a cookbook for people on dialysis. There's also an area for health professionals.

DaVita

http://www.davita.com

The largest provider of dialysis services in the U.S. also provides a Web site with lots of information about kidney disease, message boards, animations, news, a dialysis-center finder, and information for health professionals.

Knee Injuries

KNEEguru

http://www.kneeguru.co.uk

This site features information about knee injuries, including a medical dictionary, types of knee injuries and how to treat them, current issues and news, and a bulletin board to get support from others who have suffered the same types of injuries. It also includes a worldwide directory of knee clinics and surgeons.

Leukemia

The Leukemia & Lymphoma Society

http://www.leukemia.org

This site provides educational information about leukemia, lymphoma, myeloma, and other blood cancers. It includes information about events, inspiring stories, local chapters, plus comprehensive disease information, and support and treatment options for patients with decision tools to help them select the option that works best for them. It also includes links to clinical trials, message boards, and an area for scientists and medical professionals.

Liver Disease

American Liver Foundation

http://www.liverfoundation.org

This site includes articles, links, and information about liver disease, including treatment, prevention, message boards, clinical trials, transplants, local chapters, news and events, and the latest research.

Lou Gehrig's Disease (ALS)

Also see the "Muscular Dystrophy" section.

ALS Association

http://www.alsa.org

This site includes information about local chapters, the latest research, clinical trials, case studies, and more. It also includes a description of ALS, symptoms, diagnosis, genetic information, facts, and new hope and challenges. There is a separate area of the site for healthcare professionals.

Lung Cancer

Lung Cancer Online

http://www.lungcanceronline.org

This is a support area for people with lung cancer and their families. It includes a physician finder, support groups, information about lung cancer, treatment options, symptoms, side effects and complications, tests and procedures, links to other sites, survivor stories, and a comprehensive medical library of information. It also includes a guide for lung cancer survivors.

Lyme Disease

Lyme Disease Network

http://www.lymenet.org

This is an information center about Lyme disease, including its causes, symptoms, treatment options, news, and related materials. The site includes links to support groups around the world, books, FAQs, and a newsletter.

Malaria

Malaria Foundation International

http://www.malaria.org

This site provides information about malaria, global initiatives, scientific resources, literature, and travel advisories.

Melanoma

The SHADE Foundation of America

http://www.shadefoundation.org

Founded by Shonda Schilling, a skin cancer and melanoma survivor and the wife of baseball star Curt Schilling, the SHADE Foundation focuses on prevention of skin cancer. The organization focuses on teaching children about the dangers of skin cancer. The site includes educational information, message boards, school programs, and events.

Melanoma Patients' Information Page

http://www.mpip.org

This information-packed site includes pictures, news, treatment options, bulletin boards, a research library, clinical trials, and drug news.

Meningitis

Meningitis Foundation of America

http://www.musa.org

This site includes symptoms, treatment options, prevention, recovery, FAQs, message boards, articles, and more. It also includes statistics, links to international sites, surveys, and mailing lists.

Mental Health

See the "Depression" section.

Multiple Sclerosis

National Multiple Sclerosis Society

http://www.nmss.org

This site includes information about MS, treatments, research, news, clinical trials, local chapter information, message boards, and a site for professionals.

All About Multiple Sclerosis

http://www.mult-sclerosis.org

This informative site was created by a patient with multiple sclerosis (Paul Jones). It includes an encyclopedia of terms, and explanation of what MS is, Jones' personal experience with the disease, symptoms, treatments, possible causes, research information, links to other sites, and a list of famous people who have MS.

Muscular Dystrophy

Muscular Dystrophy Association

http://www.mdausa.org

The MDA Telethon has been hosted by Jerry Lewis for decades, making this association one of the best known in the world. The Web page includes lots of information about MD, including the latest research information, publications, a directory of clinics, message boards, articles, and more (see Figure A.11). The association also provides information and research support for other muscular diseases, including Lou Gehrig's disease.

Myeloma

See the "Leukemia" section.

Osteoporosis

National Osteoporosis Foundation

http://www.nof.org

This site provides information about osteoporosis, including prevention, tips for men and women, FAQs, facts, and information about bone density. It also includes a physician finder, support groups, and expert advice. There is also a separate site for medical professionals.

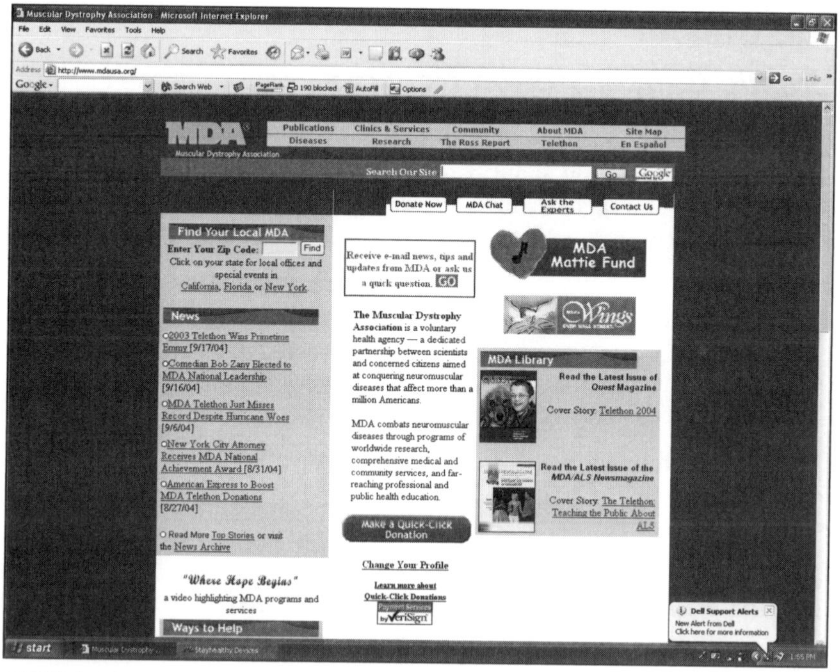

FIGURE A.11 *The Muscular Dystrophy Association home page*

Ovarian Cancer

Ovarian Cancer National Alliance

http://www.ovariancancer.org

This site provides information about ovarian cancer, approaches to treatment, clinical trials, and support for dealing with the disease. The site is divided into information for those who are newly diagnosed, survivors, and people with a general interest in the disease.

The Lynne Cohen Foundation for Ovarian Cancer Research

http://www.lynnecohenfoundation.org

Dedicated to the memory of Lynne Cohen, who died of ovarian cancer at the age of 54 in 1998, the site provides information about ovarian cancer, plus prevention, warning signs, and clinics. It also includes message boards, clinical trials, and the latest research news.

Pancreatic Cancer

Pancreatic Cancer Action Network

http://www.pancan.org

This site includes information about pancreatic cancer, treatments, symptoms, support, and links to resources. It also includes links to related information, research, and information for healthcare professionals.

Parkinson's Disease

Parkinson's Disease Foundation

http://www.pdf.org

This site includes information about Parkinson's disease, the latest news, expert advice, message boards, drug news, FAQs, and much more. It also includes publications and videos about the disease available for purchase.

American Parkinson's Disease Association

http://www.apdaparkinson.org

This is the Web site of a research organization dedicated to finding a cure for Parkinson's disease. It includes information about Parkinson's disease, the latest news, local chapter information, and publications and videos about the disease available for purchase.

Polio

Global Polio Eradication

http://www.polioeradication.org

Once one of the most feared diseases on Earth, polio has been limited severely over the last several decades, after Dr. Jonas Salk developed a vaccine for it in the 1950s. Now, in the largest public health initiative the world has ever known, according to the World Health Organization, the global eradication of the disease continues. Since 1988, the WHO has worked to eradicate polio from the face of the Earth, and it has made tremendous progress. The site includes information about polio, advisories about locations in the world where the disease is still active, and a listing of how many cases there are in the world and where at any one time (690 in 2004 as of mid-September, with 80% of those in Nigeria). Many countries, including the U.S., are certified to be polio free.

Prostate Cancer

PSA Rising

http://www.psa-rising.org

This site is dedicated to supporting survivors of prostate cancer and informing others about the disease (see Figure A.12). The site includes diet recommendations, symptoms, detection, treatment options, message boards, news, expert advice, and the latest research about the condition, as well as the most effective drugs for treating it.

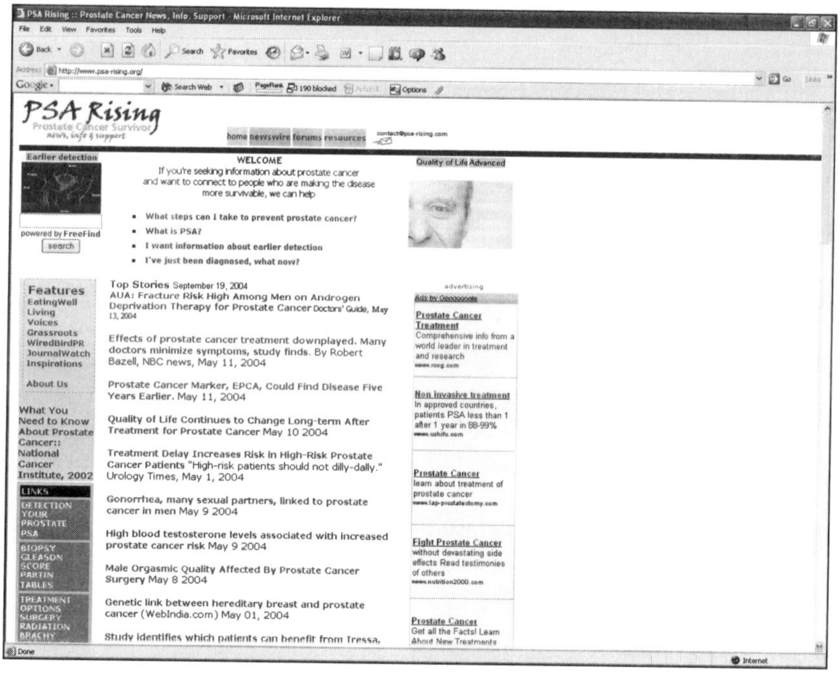

FIGURE A.12 *PSA Rising is dedicated to supporting those with prostate cancer and those who have survived it.*

Prostate Cancer Research Institute

http://www.prostate-cancer.org

This site is dedicated to informing and educating people about prostate cancer, providing options and information for those who have contracted it, and finding a cure. The site includes educational material, event listings, research papers, and a newsletter.

Reye's Syndrome

National Reye's Syndrome Foundation

http://www.reyessyndrome.org

This site includes information about Reye's syndrome, listings of events, treatment, research, videos available for rental, and the role that aspirin might play in developing Reye's syndrome.

Rotator Cuff Injury

See the "Sports Injuries" section.

SARS

Severe Acute Respiratory Syndrome

http://www.who.int/csr/sars/en

A service of the World Health Organization, this site features the latest scientific research about SARS and news about its containment in various places in the world.

Sexually Transmitted Diseases

American Social Health Association

http://www.ashastd.org

This Web site includes comprehensive information about sexually transmitted diseases, including AIDS, chlamydia, herpes, gonorrhea, and syphilis. It includes a glossary of terms, statistics, FAQs, chat rooms, publications, and much more.

Sickle Cell Anemia

American Sickle Cell Anemia Association

http://www.ascaa.org

This site includes educational materials, screening information, events, message boards, videos, and links to other sites.

Spina Bifida

Spina Bifida Association of America

http://www.sbaa.org

This site includes news, educational materials, screening information, events, message boards, FAQs, the latest research information, and links to other sites. It also includes information specifically for health professionals.

Spine Injuries

See the "Back Injuries" section.

Sports Injuries

SportsInjuryClinic.net

http://www.sportsinjuryclinic.net

This site features an A–Z directory of sports injuries, books, message centers, and physician referral, as well as links to injuries by type and by sport with a virtual diagnosis feature. The site also includes an area for physicians.

Stroke

American Stroke Association

http://www.strokeassociation.org

A division of the American Heart Association, this site is aimed at helping reduce the risk of strokes through research, prevention, and awareness (see Figure A.13). The site includes warning signs of strokes, an encyclopedia of stroke and heart terms, prevention and awareness information, risk factors, recovery and support, the latest news, and publications and resources. An area of the site for professionals includes education, resources, and initiatives aimed at helping medical professionals treat strokes more effectively.

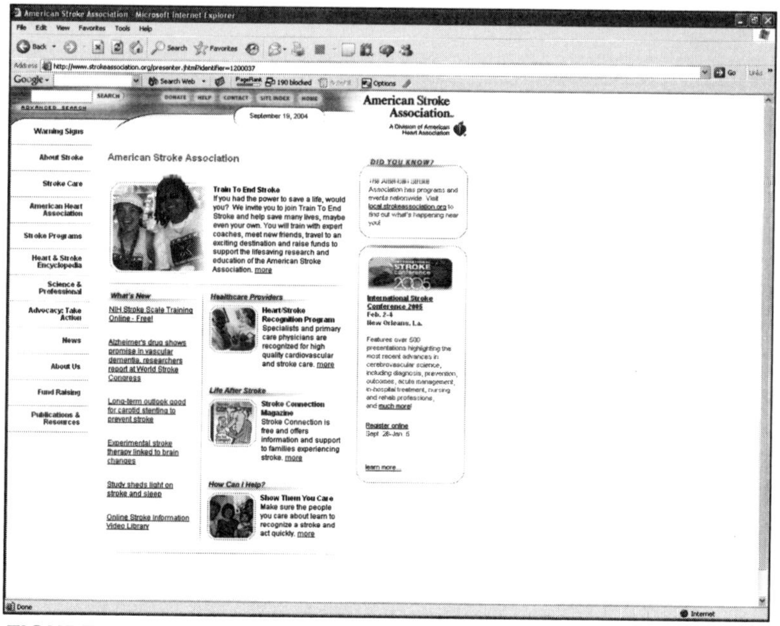

FIGURE A.13 *The American Stroke Association is a division of the American Heart Association.*

Sudden Infant Death Syndrome (SIDS)

American SIDS Institute

http://www.sids.org

This site provides resources for sudden infant death syndrome, explaining the causes and means that parents can use to prevent their child from dying from SIDS. (The most helpful thing is to have an infant sleep on his or her back. According to the Institute, stomach sleep is up to 12.9 times more dangerous than back sleep for an infant.) The Institute has research information, as well as information for prevention and awareness of SIDS. In fact, thanks to awareness, the SIDS rate in the U.S. has dropped every year since 1991, from 1.30 deaths per 1,000 live births in 1991 to 0.56 in 2001.

Syphilis

See the "Sexually Transmitted Diseases" section.

Thyroid Diseases

American Thyroid Association

http://www.thyroid.org

This site includes detailed information about the various thyroid conditions, with FAQs, Web brochures, expert advice, links to support organizations, and a physician finder. A section of the Web site is devoted to health and medical professionals.

Tourette Syndrome

Tourette Syndrome Association, Inc.

http://www.tsa-usa.org

This site includes information about Tourette syndrome, including articles for parents of children with Tourette syndrome (as well as for educators), a children's section, videos, treatment options, research, news and events, and newsletters (including specialized newsletters for children and young adults); see Figure A.14.

Tuberculosis

Tuberculosis.net

http://www.tuberculosis.net

Tuberculosis.net is an A–Z guide to tuberculosis, including FAQs and message boards. The site also includes teaching materials and information for healthcare providers.

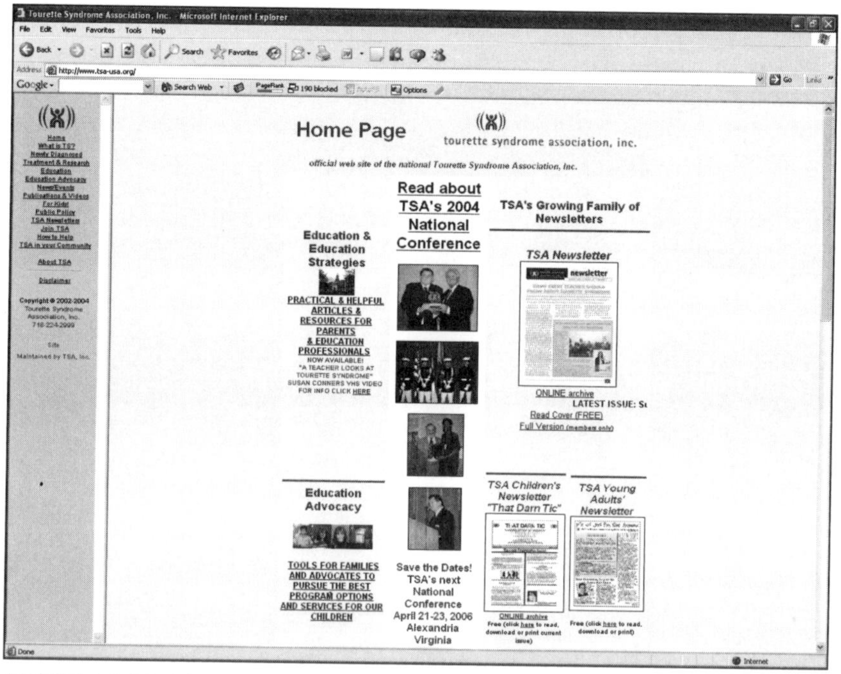

FIGURE A.14 *The Tourette Syndrome Association includes helpful advice for sufferers of the condition, their parents, and teachers.*

Uterine Cancer

See the "Cervical Cancer" and "Ovarian Cancer" sections.

West Nile Virus

West Nile Fever

http://www.westnilefever.com

West Nile Virus is a fatal disease that has spread (by mosquitoes) across the country over the last few years. This site includes information about West Nile, both for adults and children, as well as symptoms, treatment, prevention, dealing with mosquitoes, the latest news, and case reports.

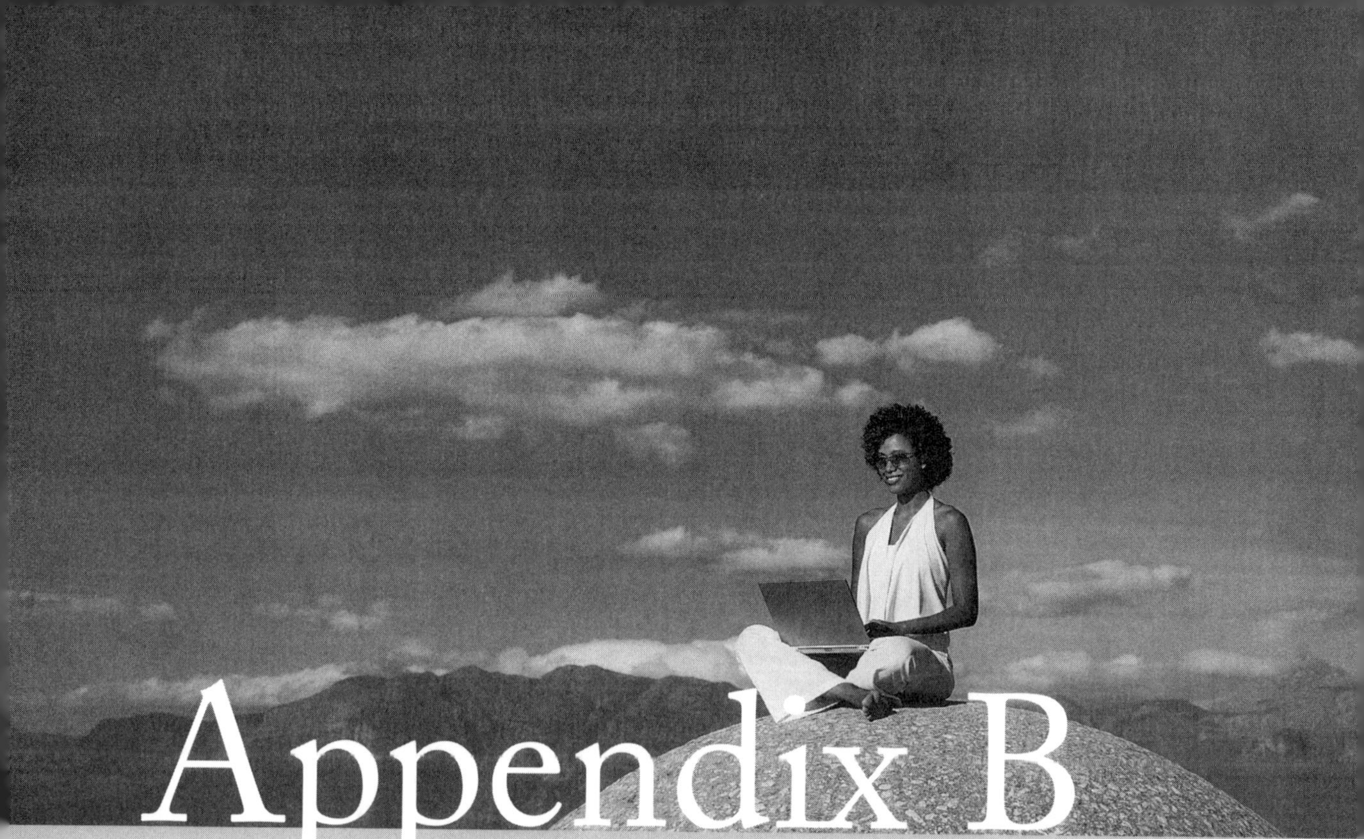

Appendix B

More Food and Exercise Diaries

As we mentioned in Chapter 2, there are an awful lot of food and exercise diary products out there. We profiled some of the best in that chapter, and we provide a more comprehensive listing here, in alphabetical order. It's not totally comprehensive; there are other software products available. However, if we questioned the viability of the company or if the program lacked any reasonable descriptions, we didn't include it here. By the way, many of the software programs mentioned here use a food database that is published by the USDA called the Nutrient Database for Standard Reference (SR-17). It includes more than 6,000 foods and nutrients and is freely available. You can search the USDA's database yourself at http://www.nal.usda.gov/fnic/foodcomp/search.

CalorieKing.com

$19.95/year Web site. Database software and diet diary (Windows, Mac, Palm, and Pocket PC) $19.95 each. (Windows or Mac version free with annual membership.)

http://www.calorieking.com

See Chapter 2 for a full description.

Crosstrainer

$49.95 Windows. $64.95 with Palm add-on.

http://www.crosstrainer.ca

Unlike most programs, which are diet software first and fitness second, Crosstrainer is just the opposite (see Figure B.1). It includes nutrition software with a 10,000-food database, but it also includes a complete fitness tracking program with modules for athlete tracking, nutrition tracking, strength training, and aerobics. It lets you track your basal metabolic rate, body measurements, heart rate zones, strength capacity, and aerobic levels. A Palm companion product is also available. A fairly active user community also is available on their Web site.

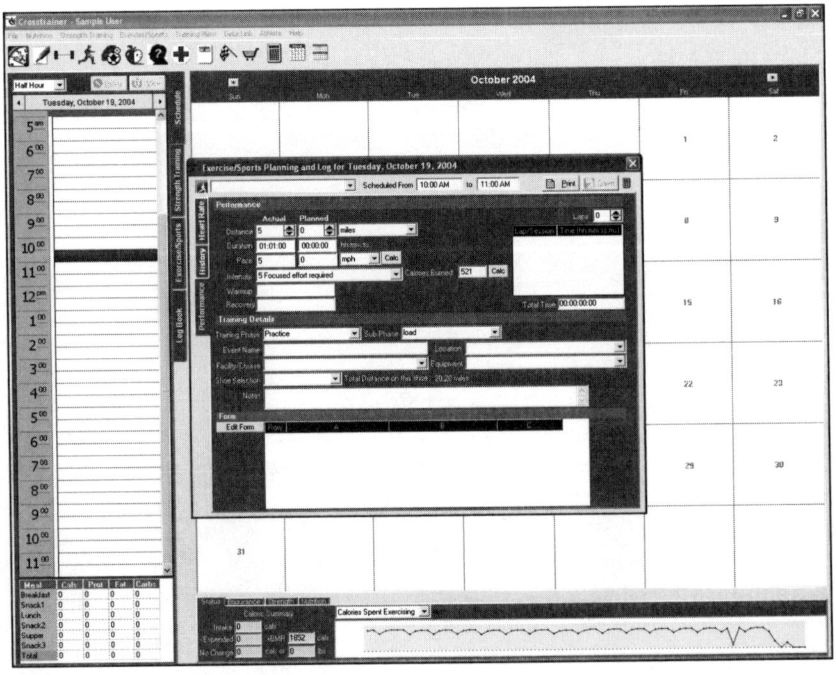

FIGURE B.1 *Crosstrainer is one of the few products that's a fitness program first and a diet program second.*

Cybernetic Dietician

$15.95 Windows and Mac.

http://www.satoripublishing.com/CyberDiet

This inexpensive product features a database of 2,500 foods and analysis software to help you analyze your diet. It provides data on the basic nutrients in your diet (carbs, fats, proteins, cholesterol, calcium, and sodium), and it works on both Mac and Windows computers.

Diet Cruncher

$75 Windows and Mac.

http://www.waydownsouthsoftware.com

This is fairly pricey for a software product whose main claim to fame is that it's from New Zealand (hence the name of the software company). It works with a variety of food databases, including the USDA, New Zealand's FOODfiles and the UK's McCance and Widdowson database. The USDA food database is free; the others are available for purchase at an additional charge. This is not a trivial charge—the New Zealand database is more than $400! Other than the ability to work with other databases, there isn't much different about this product. It includes a variety of reports, although the terminology may throw off some people (energy instead of calories, for example).

Diet & Exercise Assistant

$19.95 Pocket PC and Palm OS. $9.95 Windows.

http://www.keyoe.com

See Chapter 2 for a full description.

DietMaster 2000

$24.95 download; $29.95 CD-ROM. Windows only.

http://www.lifestylestech.com

The professional versions of this product sell for thousands of dollars. The personal version includes a 13,000-food database, a food and exercise diary, plus weight loss meal plan templates to help you get started. Additional meal plans, such as for low-carb, vegetarian, and bodybuilder programs, are available for $19.95 for each seven days worth of meal plans. Obviously, if you want a long-term plan, this could get expensive. Because this software is often used by companies offering weight-training programs, DietMaster includes protein requirements as well. A trial version is not available. You have to either download it or purchase a CD version.

DietOrganizer

$29.95 download. Windows, Palm, and Pocket PC.

http://www.dietorganizer.com

DietOrganizer offers a 6,000-food database and a simple user interface. It's a friendly, easy-to-use package that provides a variety of reports as well as an exercise diary and a food diary (see Figure B.2). It's a fairly large download because it requires a free, run-time version of the .NET Framework to run, but once you download it, it runs smoothly. A free trial version is available.

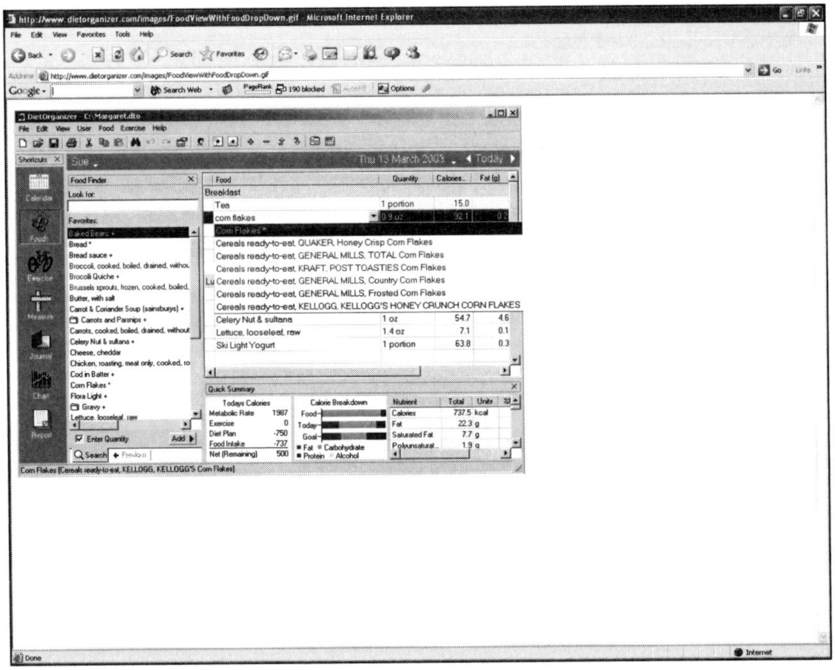

FIGURE B.2 *DietOrganizer runs on Windows PCs, plus Palm and Pocket PC devices.*

DietPower

$49.99 download; $54.99 CD-ROM. Windows only.

http://www.dietpower.com

See Chapter 2 for a full description.

Diet Pro

$64.95 download. Windows only.

http://www.dietpro.net

Diet Pro comes with 700 recipes, which isn't surprising, considering that Radium Technologies, the makers of the software, offer a sister product called Living Cookbook. As a result, its recipe management features set it apart from other software products. In addition to recipe management, Diet Pro provides weight management tools that let you track your weight, food intake, body-fat percentage, heart rate, blood pressure, and other factors. It includes the requisite reports and graphs as well.

Diet Sleuth with Health Tracker

$39.99 download. Windows and Mac.

http://www.blackcatsystems.com/software/diet.html

This is diet software with reporting module. It works on both Windows XP and Mac OS X, and it includes a database of more than 5,000 foods and a Recipe Editor that lets you add foods to recipes as well as the database.

Diet Tracker

$20 download. Windows only.

http://ourworld.compuserve.com/homepages/MCunningham/diettrak.htm

This inexpensive basic shareware product features diet tracking for up to five users. It includes a database of 1,000 foods and reports that show calorie intake and weight changes.

DINE Healthy

$129 for version 4.2 for Windows or 3.0 for Mac (runs in OS X in Classic mode).

http://www.dinehealthy.com

DINE Healthy is a pricey product because it's intended for professionals and for use in learning environments. But although it can be used for learning, there is no reason why end users can't use it as well. However, $129 is a steep price to pay for a nutrition software product. It includes a customizable 10,000-food database that analyzes 77 nutrients. It also includes an exercise database with 500 built-in exercises. The unique feature of the program is that it includes a DINE Score, which tells the user how healthy his or her eating habits are. A Mac version is available, but it was designed for Mac OS 9. It runs on OS X-based Macs in Classic mode.

Do-It!

$39.95 download. Windows only.

http://www.doithome.com

Do-It! offers an 8,600-food database that tracks 55 different nutrients (see Figure B.3). The vendor calls it a set of "Power Tools for Dieters" because it provides body-fat calculations, food diaries, goal setting, and recipe tracking that makes a Nutrition Facts label for each recipe. It also includes a food and exercise database.

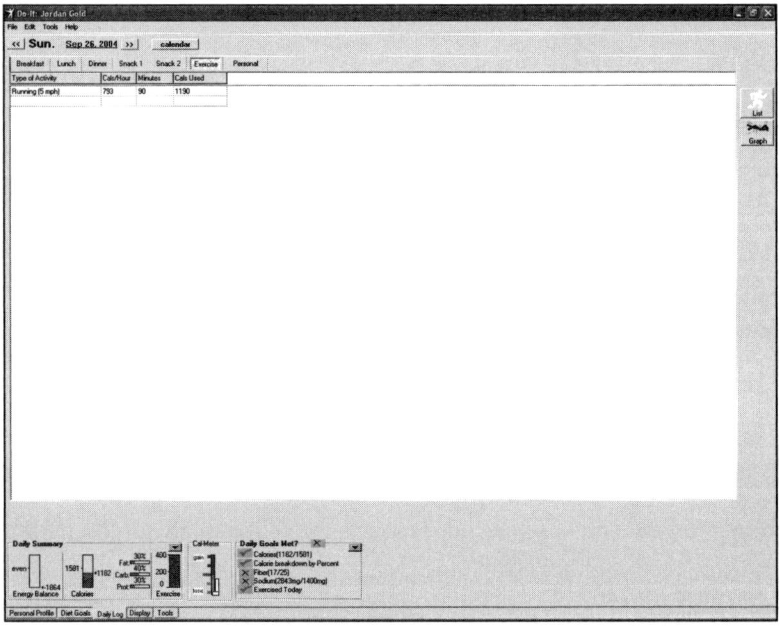

FIGURE B.3 *Do-It! offers an 8,600-food database that tracks 55 different nutrients.*

Eat Well-Be Well

$79 download. Windows only.

http://www.eatwell-bewell.com

The main purpose of this software is to help users decide the best diet program for them. It includes a food database with 6,200 foods, up to 99 meal plans, and an exercise manager. It also includes a series of self tests and tools that help you understand weight loss, including your personal illness risk, a scorecard that tells you how many of your daily meals are healthy (it can measure this for as long as a year), tests that measure your nutrition knowledge, and a calculator that tells you how many calories you've burned at a certain activity.

eDiets

$2.99 per week to $7.97 per week, depending on how many options you choose.

http://www.ediets.com

See Chapter 2 for a full description.

FitDay

Web version is free. $19.95 download for PC version; $24.95 for CD-ROM. Windows only.

http://www.fitday.com

See Chapter 2 for a full description.

Food Smart

$49.95 Windows only.

http://www.food-smart.com

Food Smart is the lowest end of a family of products that includes a number of professional editions for dieticians and fitness professionals. It includes a food diary and database and supports up to 12 users. Measurements can be displayed in either metric or non-metric form and can be modified to work with special diets, such as diabetes. It also breaks down foods into two categories—caloric values (protein, fat, and carbs) and types of fat (monounsaturated, polyunsaturated, and saturated—unfortunately no trans-fats yet).

FrenchDiet

$30 download. Windows and Mac.

http://www.diondine.com

FrenchDiet includes a 6,000-food database, but highlights a 1,400+ food subset of the most eaten foods. Users can add their own foods as well. It also includes subcategories, recipes, and favorites, and provides a comparison of your eating habits to both the USDA Food Guide Pyramid and a typical Mediterranean diet. This software is also available in a French-language version, called Diondine. It's the same software in either language.

Kathleen's Diet Planner

$79 Canadian download. Windows only.

http://www.betbyte.com/kdiet.htm

With a database of more than 30,000 foods from both the USDA and the Canadian Nutrient File, this is one of the largest on the market (see Figure B.4). It also tracks the glycemic index for foods and lets you decide what else you'd like to track, including things such as cigarettes smoked, body temperature, even headaches. This is a Canadian product, so the price is in Canadian dollars. However, the program includes a handy currency converter so you can see the price in US dollars at a glance. It doesn't have the friendliest interface in the world, but it is a pretty powerful product in any case.

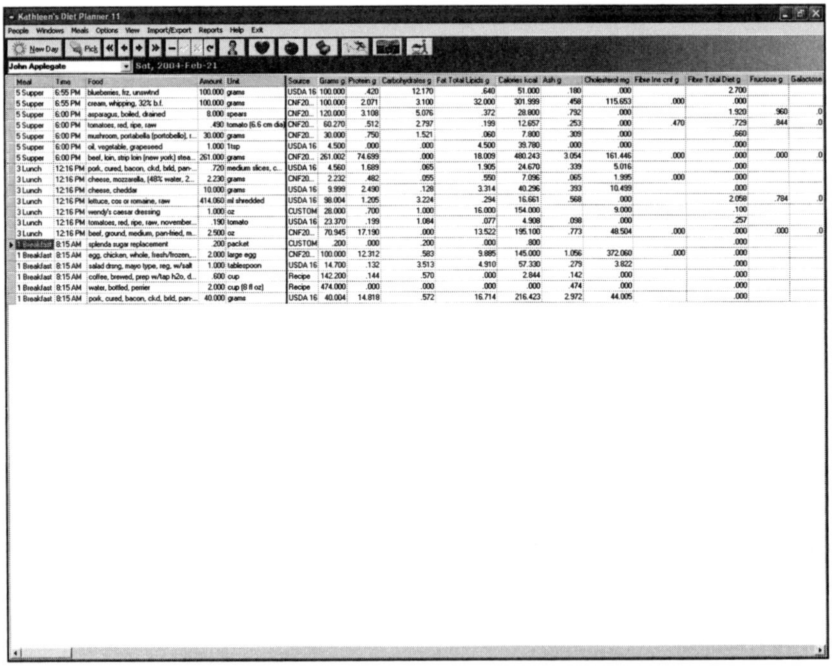

FIGURE B.4 *Kathleen's Diet Planner tracks a lot of vitamins and minerals in its 30,000+ food database.*

Life Form

$39 download; $49 on CD. Windows only.

http://www.fitnesoft.com

Developed by Pete Peterson, the founder of WordPerfect, Life Form is a health management program that monitors food intake, exercise, and even basic health information, including your doctors, prescription drugs, insurance policies, blood-test results, and other information (see Figure B.5). The food database includes 13,000 foods, and it tracks all basic nutrients. Although Life Form is a powerful product, it's a bit outdated. It was originally written for Windows 3.1, and it works on XP. However, it wasn't designed for XP, so don't expect the latest technology or the best performance. However, do expect a unique product.

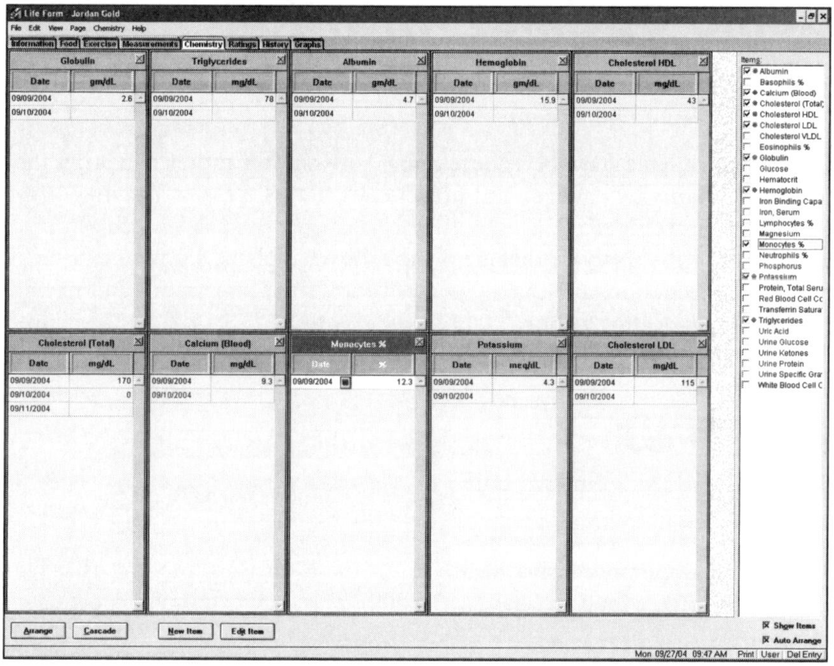

FIGURE B.5 *Life Form goes well beyond the normal food and exercise software, featuring blood chemistry, exercise, and emotional levels.*

Mealformation

$49.95 download. Windows or Mac.

http://www.mealformation.com

Mealformation is a basic software product with a food database, a recipe database, a shopping-list generator, and a meal planner. It includes a goal-setting capabilities feature, called the Profile Calculator, which tells you how much you should be eating; a Food Database that manages recipes, meal plans, and other items; and a Menu Manager, which is the Food Diary.

NutriBase

$29.95 to $69.95 download; $39.95 to $89.95 CD. Windows and Palm OS.

http://www.dietsoftware.com

See Chapter 2 for a full description.

NutriGenie Optimal Nutrition

$49.95. Windows only.

http://www.nutrigenie.com

The folks at NutriGenie have been developing software for more than a decade. Their software is used primarily by colleges and universities, and there is a dizzying array of products available, which probably explains why they haven't made much of a splash on the PC side. Unique features of the software include on-the-fly meal plans, a glycemic index for all foods, and a weight-projection feature that estimates your weight one month and/or one week in the future based on your eating habits.

NutriStrategy

$39 CD-ROM. Windows only.

http://www.nutristrategy.com

NutriStrategy is a comprehensive health and fitness software product that features a food diary, fitness tracking, a food database of 10,000 items, and extensive reporting capabilities.

Paraben's Diet Tracker

$19.95 download. Windows only.

http://www.paraben.com/html/diet.html

This inexpensive program tracks activity for up to four users. It includes a 6,000-food database, and it tracks weight, fat, protein, carbs, sodium, calories, and two other nutrients that the user picks. It doesn't have a lot of nutrient tracking, but again, this is an inexpensive program.

Pocket Diet Tracker and Pocket Diet Assistant

$24.95 (Diet Tracker) and $14.95 (Diet Assistant) download. Pocket PC only.

http://www.pocketdiettracker.com

These PDA-based products have many of the features of larger PC products, but without much of the power. However, some users will find that the convenience of a PDA-based product overcomes any inconveniences caused by a lack of power. The food database includes only 900 foods. You can download another database with 4,600 more, but that might take up much of your Pocket PC's storage space. There's no fitness module, but you can download MySport-Training, a fitness program available for $24.95 at http://www.mysporttraining.com and have it work seamlessly with either Pocket Diet Tracker or Pocket Diet Assistant. Pocket Diet Assistant, by the way, is a slimmed-down version of Pocket Diet Tracker.

ProTrack 2005

$24.95 download; $39.95 CD-ROM. Windows only.

http://www.dakotafit.com

This fitness-tracking program also has a meal-planning component. It includes a workout log, nutrition log, personal measurements and exercise maximums log, and the Daily Journal. The program includes workout templates and 82 predesigned strength-training plans (see Figure B.6).

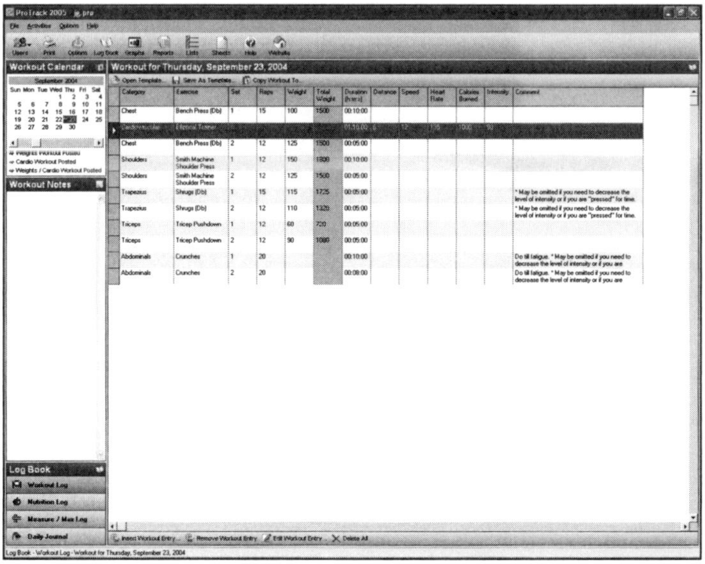

FIGURE B.6 *ProTrack 2005 includes a workout log that features workout templates and 82 preplanned strength-training plans.*

Recipe Calc

Shareware—free download, $24.95 after 20 days. Windows only.

http://www.recipecalc.com

This program's claim to fame is that it takes the foods you've eaten and gives you reports in "Nutrition Facts" format, so that your reports look just like the food labels you see on foods (see Figure B.7). It includes a database of approximately 3,000 foods.

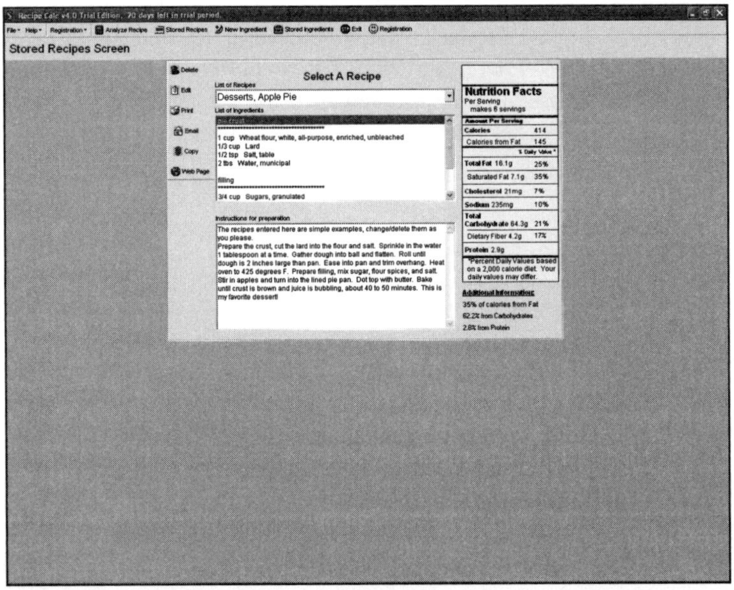

FIGURE B.7 *Recipe Calc uses a Nutrition Facts label as the basis for its reports.*

SparkPeople.com

$9.95 per year.

http://www.sparkpeople.com

See Chapter 2 for a full description.

Weight-By-Date

$21.95 download (Basic version); $39.95 download, $49.95 CD-ROM (Pro version); $19.95 download, $24.95 CD-ROM (Mobile versions). Windows, plus Pocket PC and Palm OS (Mobile versions).

http://www.weightbydate.com

Trying to hit a weight by a certain date? That's the premise of this software product, which includes a calendar-based entry system, color-coded weekly and monthly totals, and optional motivating music (see Figure B.8). The Pro version adds a food database with more than 7,500 foods, an exercise database, and a meal and exercise planner, plus a carb counter, a calorie counter, and other features. The Palm version works as a companion product to the main software product, while the Pocket PC version works as a standalone version. Both share much of the functionality of the Pro version.

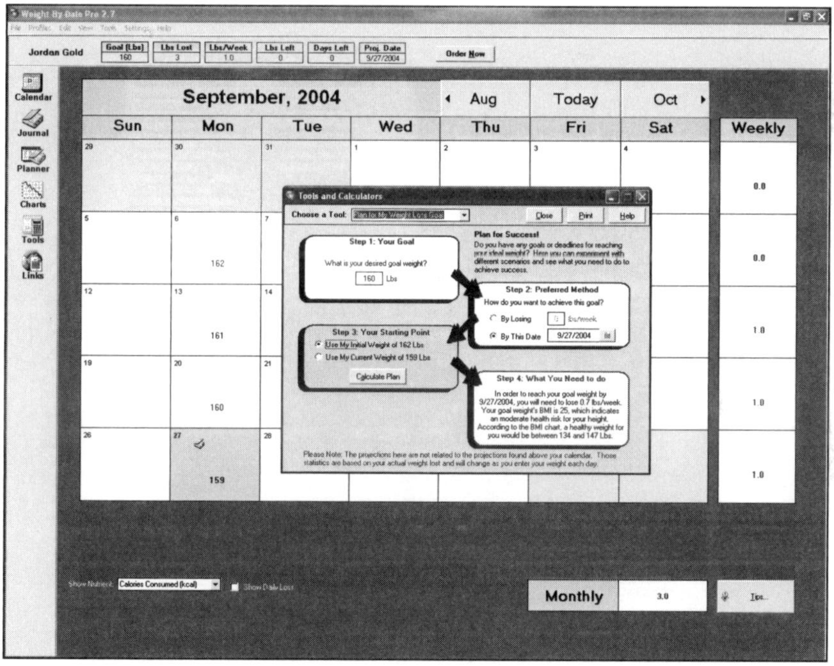

FIGURE B.8 *Weight-By-Date uses a calendar-based reporting structure.*

Weight Watchers Online/eTools

eTools (for Weight Watchers meetings members): $29.95 for prepaid three-month subscription or $12.95 per month. Weight Watchers Online (for people who don't attend meetings): $65 for prepaid three-month subscription and $16.95 per additional month, or $46.95 for the first month and $16.95 for each additional month.

http://www.weightwatchers.com

See Chapter 2 for a full description.

Index

G

H

M

N

T

Y

Z